13

AF764155

MANAGING MEDICAL TECHNOLOGICAL INNOVATIONS

Exploring Multiple Perspectives

World Scientific Series in R&D Management

Print ISSN: 2591-7498
Online ISSN: 2591-7501

Series Editor: Tugrul U Daim *(Portland State University, USA)*

Published

Vol. 5 *Managing Medical Technological Innovations: Exploring Multiple Perspectives*
edited by Tugrul U Daim and Alexander Brem

Vol. 4 *Managing Mobile Technologies: An Analysis from Multiple Perspectives*
edited by Tugrul U Daim and Alexander Brem

Vol. 3 *Cooperative Innovation: Science and Technology Policy*
by Frederick Betz

Vol. 2 *Technology Roadmapping*
edited by Tugrul U Daim, Terry Oliver and Rob Phaal

Vol. 1 *Managing Technological Innovation: Tools and Methods*
edited by Tugrul U Daim

World Scientific Series in R&D Management – Vol.5

MANAGING MEDICAL TECHNOLOGICAL INNOVATIONS

Exploring Multiple Perspectives

Editors

Tugrul U Daim

Portland State University, USA
Higher School of Economics, Russia
Chaoyang University of Technology, Taiwan

Alexander Brem

Friedrich-Alexander-Universität Erlangen-Nürnberg, Germany

World Scientific

NEW JERSEY • LONDON • SINGAPORE • BEIJING • SHANGHAI • HONG KONG • TAIPEI • CHENNAI • TOKYO

About the Editors

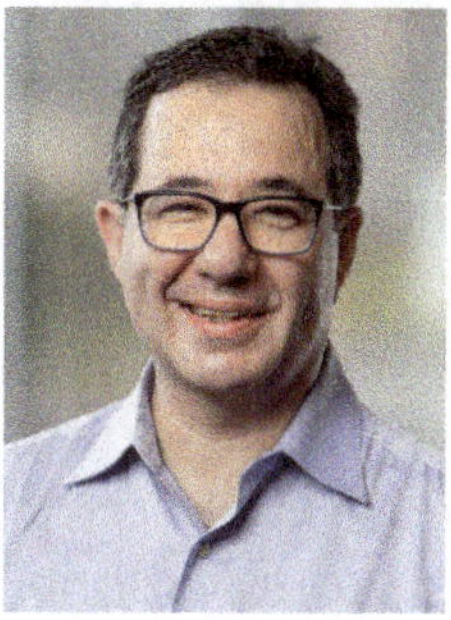

Tugrul U Daim is a Professor and the Director of the Technology Management Doctoral Program in the Maseeh College of Engineering and Computer Science at Portland State University, USA (PSU). He is also the Director of the Research Group on Infrastructure and Technology Management. He is a Faculty Fellow at the Institute for Sustainable Solutions. The US Department of Energy, National Science Foundation, National Cooperative Highway Research Program, and many other regional, national, and international organizations have funded his research. He has published over 200 refereed papers in journals and conference proceedings. He has edited more than 20 special issues in journals and more than 20 books and conference proceedings. He was the adviser for 17 Ph.D. graduates who are now in leading positions in government, industry, and academia.

He is the Editor-in-Chief of *IEEE Transactions on Engineering Management*. He has been in various editorial roles in many journals including the *International Journal of Innovation and Technology Management*, *Technological Forecasting and Social Change*, *Technology in Society*, *Foresight*, *Journal of Knowledge Economy*, and *International Journal of Innovation and Entrepreneurship*. Prior to joining PSU, Dr Daim worked at Intel Corporation for over a decade in varying management roles. At Intel he managed product and technology development. During his tenure at PSU, he has acted as a Strategic Consultant to the Chief Technology Innovation Officer of Bonneville Power Administration, a part of the US Department of Energy. He has helped develop regional and national technology roadmaps in the energy sector. He is a member of the R&D Advisory Board for TUPRAS, the largest industrial firm in Turkey. He has also consulted for many other international, national, and regional organizations including Elsevier, Biotronik, NEEA, Energy Trust of Oregon, EPRI, ETRI, Koc Holding, Arcelik, Tofas, Ford Otosan, Kirlangic, Siemens, Marks and Spencer, and Castrol.

He is also a visiting professor with the Northern Institute of Technology at the Technical University of Hamburg, Harburg, and Nottingham Trent University. He has given keynotes and distinguished speaker lectures at conferences, companies, universities, and research centers around the world, including IAMOT; EUROMOT; Samsung; Helmut Schmidt University, Germany; Kuhne Logistics University, Germany; Seoul National University, South Korea; Bogazici University, Turkey; Koc University, Turkey; University of Gaziantep, Turkey; Izmir Institute of Technology, Turkey; University of Pretoria, South Africa; Tampere University of Technology, Finland; Science and Technology Policy Institute (STEPI), South Korea; EPIC at UNC Charlotte, USA; Cambridge University, UK; National Taiwan University, Taiwan; Higher School of Economics in Moscow, Russia; Chinese Academy of Engineering, China; and Office of Naval Research, USA.

He was given the Research Publication Award by the International Association of Management of Technology (IAMOT) and Fellow Award by the Portland International Center for Management of Engineering and Technology (PICMET), both in 2014. He has been a Leading Research Fellow at the National Research University Higher School of Economics in Moscow, Russia since 2018. He was awarded the Honorary Chair Professor title by Chaoyang University of Technology, Taiwan in 2019.

Dr. Daim was the President of Omega Rho, International Honor Society in Operations Research and Management Science, between the years of 2014 and 2016. He received his B.S. in Mechanical Engineering from Bogazici University, Turkey, M.S. in Mechanical Engineering from Lehigh University, USA, M.S. in Engineering Management from Portland and Ph.D. in Systems Science: Engineering Management from Portland State University USA.

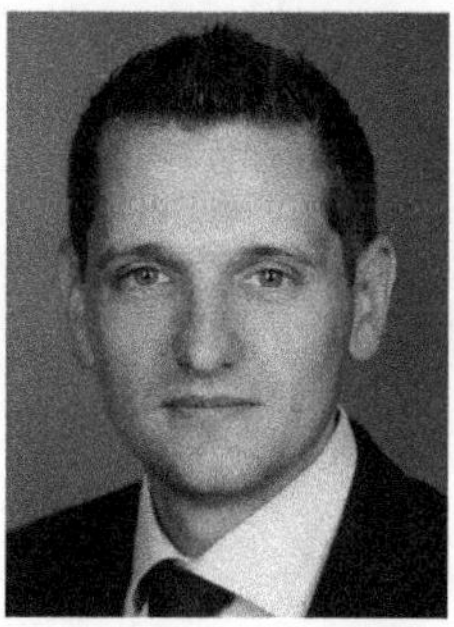

Alexander Brem holds the Chair of Technology Management at the Friedrich-Alexander-Universität Erlangen-Nürnberg (FAU), Germany, which is located at the Nuremberg Campus of Technology (NCT). He is a CCSR International Research Associate at DeMontfort University (UK) and a Visiting Professor at the EADA Business School in Barcelona (Spain) and HHL Graduate School of Management (Germany). Moreover, he serves as an Academic Committee Member of the Center of Technological Innovation, Tsinghua University, Beijing (China). In addition, he was appointed as Honorary Professor at the University of Southern Denmark (SDU) in May 2017. Further information can be found here: https://www.tm.rw.fau.eu.

Contents

Introduction

Managing Medical Technological Innovations*

Managing Medical Technological Innovations — Why a Book on This Topic?

First of all, we think that research these days has a problem. Most of the current results are only published in academic journals; for most journals, you need a subscription. Hence, this knowledge does not reach companies anymore, since these articles are too specialized and they are difficult and expensive to access. Hence, we thought it might be worth a try to put together key literature on medical technology management.

Hence, with this book, we want to present an in-depth portrayal of medical technical innovations and the whole organizational construct from the development via organizational and management tasks up until the technology adoption for our valued readers. Through this complete approach and high-quality research as the base across all studies, we hope to offer insights and analysis to this interesting sector, characterized by new technology developments.

With the constantly growing spread of new technologies across all fields in the current scenario, the medical sector has attracted more attention in the adaption of technology. The growing improvements and progress in human healthcare also lead to the implementation of new and innovative technologies, from wearables to smart IT systems.

*The book is partially funded by the Basic Research Program of the National Research University Higher School of Economics (HSE) and by the Russian Academic Excellence Project "5-100".

But these transitions in the medical sector can also lead to new challenges, especially for those companies that develop, produce, and distribute. They need to rethink their foci in management tasks and strategies to be equipped for future markets from an organizational point of view. Considering these "medical technological innovations", this book presents the complete concept from five different perspectives in the different parts: first, technology perspective as the basis for medical innovations in Part 1; in Part 2, the organizational perspective, which is a key factor in business strategy; then, innovation management perspective with its special issues under medical concern in Part 3; Part 4 discusses the new product development perspective; and finally, the technology adoption perspective in Part 5 to address the implementation of new technologies.

The first chapter in Part 1, Technology Perspectives, gives an overview on wearable technologies by analyzing publications on Scopus, a scientific database. A bibliometric analysis reflects the current research's status and direction, whereas technology trends are identified through a cluster analysis. Milad Dehghani concludes with insights on the identification of new trends and provides a few potential directions for future research. In Chapter 2, Japanese biotechnology start-ups are reviewed taking into account technology creation and development. Based on a case study including the review of policies and several interviews, comparisons are drawn to Europe and the United States. Shiaw Jia Eyo describes the strong positive impact of the new 1990 policies of the Japanese government but finds that many of the companies only operate at the start-up or even seed stage. The author explains the key issue as the lack of a sustainable funding system. Chapter 3 by James C. Benneyan and Claire Bond discusses possible applications of industrial engineering and systems engineering in the healthcare sector. With reusable medical equipment (RME) being a huge cost burden, illustrated by the use of practical examples, the management, understanding, and improvement of RME are focused on. Different perspectives are discussed, including inventory management, facility layout, quality, reliability, and more.

Part 2, named Organizational Perspectives, starts with Chapter 4 by Jörg Mahlich, who discusses the development in R&D management within pharmaceutical companies from Japan. The internationalization of their R&D, where heavy investments were made in foreign R&D centers during the 1980s and 1990s, is analyzed. As this led to only very limited knowledge transfer, the businesses are now shifting their strategies toward a better integration of their units abroad. In Chapter 4, a patent analysis, based on USPTO data from 1984 to 2005, is made with a focus on co-opetition strategies of stent manufacturers. Starting with the initial stages for both, growing competition and critical issues for companies to integrate patent information with their business strategies, Kuei-Kuei Lai, Fang-Pei Su, Calvin S. Weng, Mei-Lan Lin, and Chiau-Ling Chen find co-opetition as a way to keep sustainable competitive advantage in Chapter 5. The authors proved their conclusions by inspecting the changes on perspective and business scope, describing the relationship between business strategies and technology, and discussing the technological position and strength. Chapter 6 in this perspective presents empirical data to analyze strategic partnerships in the biotechnology sector regarding success factors. Therefore, the research collaborations of 23 companies are analyzed and three structural as well as three dynamic factors are examined. Describing a high number of more than 50% failures of the research partnerships in this sector, Uwe Kehrel, Kai Klischan, and Nathalie Sick derive implications for better company strategies, while finding a significant influence of several success factors.

For the Innovation Management Perspectives in Part 3, Hua-Hsin Wan and Xiaohong Quan start Chapter 7 with a case study on Acclarent, a medical device manufacturer and subsidiary of Johnson & Johnson.[1] The effective management of

[1]https://www.acclarent.com/home.

knowledge flow and an innovation process integrating third-party payer's policies as well as FDA[2] regulations are discussed as a key for Acclarent's success. In the conclusion, a framework for open innovation in the medical device industry is proposed. Chapter 8 studies the catch-up efforts of pharmaceutical firms in China facing technology complexity in the past few decades. Hao Hu and Liming Zhang describe this complexity as a major challenge for affected businesses. Reasons are an increase in capability requirements, the necessity for more networking, the possible effect of a complicated institutional design, as well as a lengthened catch-up process itself. To counteract these effects, an evolutionary strategy with self-investment into system capability as well as network competence is needed. The results of the study provide references for such efforts across other industries and branches. Chapter 9, from the innovation perspective, introduces a legitimacy-based view of innovations in biotechnology using a sequential construct of cognitive legitimacy, regulative legitimacy, and normative legitimacy. Mark J. Ahn, Anne S. York, So Young Sohn, and Payam Benyamini find great promises in disruptive technology platforms on the one hand and discuss the legitimacy hurdles faced by these technologies on the other hand, thereby suggesting that nascent firms must learn new responsibilities. The conclusions provide insights on how breakthrough technologies can achieve legitimacy and mobilize resources and talent and attain commercial success.

In Part 4, New Product Development Perspectives, Chapter 10 opens by exploring and explaining the relation between ambiguity management and contextual ambidexterity in innovation with both quality case data and a model. Eric Christian Brun describes several factors that help in generating ambiguity to achieve exploration: perspective-taking, requisite variety, interpretive skills, and a factor helping to reduce ambiguity to achieve exploitation — analytical skills. It is stated that low ambiguity tolerance levels emphasize exploitation, whereas

[2]Food and Drug Administration of the United States.

high ambiguity tolerance levels emphasize exploration. The results of the study can help innovation projects through achieving contextual ambidexterity. Chapter 11 by Eric Christian Brun, Alf Steinar Sætre, and Martin Gjelsvik identifies ambiguity as an undesirable element in new product development and explores how companies can sustain or even increase ambiguity during new product development. The study is based on qualitative case data of four different developmental projects in the medical device industry and provides a model to better understand the processes. The authors derive four ways to improve new product development projects by temporarily sustaining ambiguity, e.g., saving cost and time. Chapter 12 continues with in-depth studies of four new product development projects in the medical device industry. Alf Steinar Sætre and Eric Christian Brun provide a model for effectively managing ambiguity at the fuzzy front end of innovation projects and also characterize innovation processes by exploitative and explorative activities. Ambiguity oscillates in the short run, whereas it decreases in the long run. The study's outcomes lead to a management model of ambiguity: Innovation teams with a higher tolerance level for ambiguity are better able to exploit it.

The final part, Technology Adoption Perspectives, is introduced by Nathasit Gerdsri and Chonyacha Suebsin in Chapter 13 with four interview-based case studies from different hospitals expounding key issues impacting the adoption of IT in healthcare organizations. The chapter finds decisions to adopt new technologies based on project-related costs and restrictions due to human-related issues through complication of implementation processes on an individual level. Based on the technology acceptance model, a mental framework of IT adoption in healthcare is presented. Chapter 14 examines a construct measuring the Escalation Prevention Potential (EPP), describing the escalation of commitment in innovation projects, with a survey among 1062 clinicians in Dutch hospitals. Ferry Koster and Mattijs Lambooij explain the three components of EPP: goals, process, and ability. These components add up to a single measure. A large share of EPP is found and explained with four organizational characteristics: employee involvement, leadership reflexivity, organizational routines, and support staff quality. The book's final chapter, Chapter 15, by Christian Barrot, Jan Kuhlmann, and Andrea Popa, investigates the influence of personal communication networks in innovation adoption based on an empirical study of the US market for innovative medical devices with a survey in a network of anesthetists of 151 hospitals. The authors can confirm the influence of personal communication on individual adoption decisions through hazard regressions. They conclude with a framework showing that the identification of seeding strategies would be optimal for a fast market penetration.

Hopefully, you will also conclude as we did: This kind of research is important, and more needs to be done.

Part 1

Technology Perspectives

Chapter 1

A Bibliometric Review of Wearable Technologies

Milad Dehghani

Department of Computer, Control, and Management Engineering, Sapienza University of Rome, Italy

milad.dehghani@uniroma1.it

Abstract

This study analyzes publications in the field of wearable technologies (WTs) recorded in the Scopus database during the period 2000–2016. Using bibliometric analysis, we probe into the current status and direction of research on WTs. In addition, we use cluster analysis to reveal keywords with highest frequency and identify technology trends over time amongst research activities. The study provides researchers and practitioners with insights that help to identify trends in WTs research. The study also highlights potential research directions, and is therefore expected to benefit researchers in the area of WTs.

Keywords: Wearable technology, bibliometric analysis, cluster analysis.

1. Introduction

Innovations in the field of wearable technologies (WTs) have led to new notions of human–computer interaction in the context of pervasive computing (Conti, 2012), enhancing the sense of connectedness and possibility of ubiquitous communication (Wasik, 2013). "Smart wearable technologies" or "wearable devices" are phrases that describe seamlessly embedded portable computer and advanced electronics that allow interaction between users and a smart environment (i.e., smart home appliances) at any time and from anywhere (Dehghani and Dangelico, 2017). As WT becomes ubiquitous in everyday life, they become a platform for connected mobile devices to leverage, due to the nature of their use on or near the human body (Kooroshnia *et al.*, 2015). The ultimate goal of WT is not only to establish the best network with multiple and different interconnected devices, but also to embed portable computers and advanced electronics seamlessly into people's daily lives (Fang and Chang, 2016). The field of WT is constantly changing. In addition to new hardware, software and social technologies, innovative planning and development are also at the center of this trend (Bryson, 2009). Over the past few years, much research has focused on the ways in which people have or have not sought to incorporate smart technology initiatives (Soh *et al.*, 2015).

WT attracts diverse users from the fields of education, entertainment, gaming, sport, music, and military. In the past few years, there has been an explosion in the range of smart wearable products in the market. According to a WT database (Vandrico),[1] 421 different devices exist across a range of sectors, including medical, entertainment, fitness, industrial, gaming, and lifestyle. Wearables are expected to grow in range into smart clothing, smart coaching, reading technology, hearables, wearable toys, lifesaving and even pet monitoring, and GPS mapping (Wright and Keith, 2014; GSMA, 2015). Some of the examples of already popular wearable devices include: Fitbit, Nike+, Apple Watch, Google Glass and Google Cardboard, Oculus Rift, Samsung Gear, and Microsoft Band. The WT market is anticipated to dramatically change

[1]http://vandrico.com/wearables [Accessed 12 April 2017].

the way we live and do business. A recent report on wearable products indicates that the market is expected to grow annually from 2013 to 2018 at the rate of 17.7%, with a market revenue exceeding 8 billion dollars by 2018 that global wearable vendors would account for roughly 214 million shipments by 2020. According to wearable technologies database (Vandrico, 2019), 431 devices have been identified as WTs across a range of industries, including the medical, entertainment, fitness, industrial, gaming, and lifestyle sectors. Wearable devices are anticipated to speed up in penetration rates to account for 46% of the total market by 2018. Furthermore, the healthcare sector will continue to be the dominant sector in the WT market (Wright and Keith, 2014). Today, the technical uncertainty for WT is high and the changes of the production development are frequent. In addition, following the evolution and growth of the field and the development of different products for this new technology, a great number of studies have recently appeared that show insights into the research activity of various researchers in academic institutions. With advanced menu driven application tools for monitoring research performance, and with journal indicators and the mapping and ranking of universities, bibliometric methods have now gained an arsenal of very reliable and informative instruments in research measurement practice (Van Raan and Anthony, 2014).

However, despite a great amount of research having been carried out in the domain of WT, no research has been conducted into WT in terms of trends and technology analysis. Therefore, this is the first study that aims to make an original contribution to the literature and to fill the gap in this relevant area, by using bibliometric and cluster analysis on WT. Hence, it is fundamentally significant for researchers interested in this new technology to understand the *status quo* of studies being undertaken worldwide and to have an overall perspective of it. Here we report on a bibliometric analysis of papers based on research about WT that have been published over a period of 15 years. Our aim is to examine two issues. First, we aim to identify the topics that were addressed, and facilitate a sophisticated understanding of the points and options to be considered in order to stimulate collaboration in the development of this new technology. Second, we intend to shed light into the various potential domains in a manner that is meaningful to future researchers, and to understand WT and its products as a whole, as well as the distribution of WT research in terms of knowledge maps, professional networks, key players and potential collaborations for future development of this field. In addition, a bibliometric and cluster analysis can offer significant potential for the better understanding of scientific activity trends as well as analyses of the current topics of research interest into WT. The two parts of the analysis, each based on a different methodological approach, are aimed to be complementary to each other. The remainder of this paper is structured as follows. The paper starts with a description of the theoretical background (Section 2), and then presents the methodology adopted (Section 3). This is followed by the presentation of results from bibliometric and cluster analysis (Section 4), and finally, our conclusions (Section 5).

2. Theoretical Background

2.1. *Overview of smart wearable technologies*

WT (also referred to as wearables, wearable devices) have become one of the fastest growing segments in the domain of the Internet of Things (IOT) (Cheng and Mitomo, 2017). Nowadays, smart devices are introducing new trends in terms of the functionalities they exhibit, from products with static functionalities to products that exhibit dynamic functionalities (Dehghani and Kim, 2019). In the literature, several definitions of WT have been presented (Table 1).

According to the definitions in the table, there is a shift for WT over the past decade, from "self-contained computer" to any accessory and embedded portable device that can be worn

Table 1. Definitions for WT.

Author(s)	Year	Definition
Barfield and Caudell	2001	Self-powered, fully functional and self-contained computer that provides access to information, and interaction with human body at anytime and anywhere.
Viseu	2003	A shift from digital simulation (separation and replication) to digital augmentation (responsiveness and connectivity).
Tehrani and Michael	2014	Accessories or clothing that incorporate advanced electronic techniques and incorporate computers, which can be worn on the body.
Nyan and Tay	2014	Wearable devices that merge wireless connectivity for the aim of seamlessly accessing, interacting with and exchanging contextually relevant information.
Wright and Keith	2014	Computers and electronics that are integrated into textile or clothing and other accessories that can be worn comfortably on the body.
Bower and Sturman	2015	The target of WT is exchanging and interacting with relevant information through seamless access via wireless connectivity.
Yang *et al.*	2016	Wearable technology can be attached as either an accessory or embedded in clothes, which can be used in various applications equipped with sensors, processors, internet connections and operating systems.

on any part of body. Therefore, we define WT as embedded portable computers and advanced electronics that integrate seamlessly into people's daily lives in order to have them interact with a smart environment anytime and anywhere.

Much of the optimism for the future of this industry is based on the notion that WT will become ubiquitous in the near future due to increased reliability, reduced cost, enhanced connectivity, improved usability and long battery life (Bartlett, 2014). The built-in infrastructure of some of these smart devices, such as the Apple Watch and Google Glass, present early signs of the potential of such products to meet the WT market needs and consumers' individual personality (Bartlett, 2014; Dehghani, 2016). Research by Bower and Sturman (2015) identified several barriers from the consumer's point of view to the usage of WT for education purposes: potential distraction, overreliance on WT, cost, technical problems, lack of support and technology before pedagogy. On the other hand, due to the nature of wearable devices, factors such as product design, aesthetic appeal and acceptability will become increasingly significant determinants (Cho, 2009). Several companies have successfully commercialized sports applications of smart clothing, particularly in the market segments for healthcare, sports & outdoor clothing, and work wear (Chuah *et al.*, 2016). Many proprietary market intelligence reports predict a huge potential growth in the smart clothing market in the future (Seyrkammer, 2015). Recent studies show the greatest potential for WT is concentrated on sport and healthcare (Sultan, 2015; Lee and Lee, 2016). Moreover, different studies see an emerging trend in WT for products with high-tech functionality that are designed to look more like fashion accessories (e.g., watches, eyeglasses, and jewelry) than enhanced sensors (Jost *et al.*, 2013; Wu *et al.*, 2015). Research by Chuah and her colleagues (2016) also proved that fashion and technology (aka Fashionology) are both important in the strategy of communicating with potential consumers in order to involve them in the purchase intention. Finally, the report on "Wearable Technology 2014–2024: Technologies, Markets, Forecasts (Harrop *et al.*, 2014)" predicts that the dominant sector in the WT market will be at the intersection between the medical and fitness sectors due to the high number of famous brand companies — such as

Adidas and Nike — developing products in this field together with technology companies like Apple. In addition, the report concludes that the smart wearables market is now starting to grow rapidly, according to leading indicators such as patent filings over the years, increased functionality of devices, and the cost reduction of key enabling technologies.

Despite the diffusion of this new technology, WT is still at the beginning stage, and some analysts are already predicting that smart WTs will become the next mass consumer adoption after smartphones (GSMA, 2015; Kelly, 2014). Although there is considerable literature investigating the development and use of WT across multidisciplinary fields (Son *et al.*, 2014), there is less research into the technological trends and the research background of WT. One of the reasons for this could be that scholars are not familiar with the different potential future domains in WT.

3. Methodology and Data Collection

3.1. *Bibliometrics for emerging technologies*

The quantitative analysis, frequency distribution and statistics of publications are a significant component of science policy in many countries (Adenle *et al.*, 2013). The analysis of written publications based on mathematical and statistical methods is referred to as bibliometrics. The initial concept of bibliometrics was noticed by James McKeen Cattell in the early 1900s (Godin, 2006). The main aim of bibliometrics is the performance evaluation of science and technology both on an international and a national level within a given field or body of literature study. The bibliometric analysis of scientific papers has long been recognized by research scholars as indicative of the theoretical foundations of the study (Yan, 2015; Adenle *et al.*, 2013). Basically, researchers distinguish publication patterns by using bibliometric data as part of their statistical analyses (McBurney *et al.*, 2002). A variety of disciplines such as the life sciences, telecommunication, social sciences, and health sciences have used this methodology (Gómez-Barroso *et al.*, 2016; Daim *et al.*, 2006). Since 2000, the literature regarding bibliometrics has expanded into text mining, where full texts and document abstracts are examined (Guo *et al.*, 2012). Bibliometrics is the measurement of information data and literature by using statistics and mathematics to organize, analyze and explore large amounts of historical data in order to assist researchers to recognize "hidden patterns" by classifying information according to authors, keywords, organizations, phrases, countries, and citations to help with the decision-making process as well as forecast emerging technologies (Kostoff, 2001). The method helps to organize and explore large amounts of data in order to reveal hidden patterns, which in turn helps the decision making process (Li *et al.*, 2015a, 2015b). In addition, the scientific community has begun to focus on this information in an attempt to distinguish the functions and process of identifying research patterns for the benefit of society. For example, a study by Yeo *et al.* (2015) was able to identify research papers that measure the uncertainty in a product's technological innovation by using bibliometric analysis.

Several analysis tools have been applied in the field of bibliometrics, such as text analysis, simple document counting, co-word analysis, citation analysis, cluster analysis, and cooperation analysis (Gerdsri *et al.*, 2017; D'Auria *et al.*, 2017; Fetscherin *et al.*, 2010; Xin *et al.*, 2010). There are typically two steps in the process of bibliometric analysis, *performance analysis,* and *science mapping* (Yataganbaba and Kurtbaş, 2016). The first step of performance analysis (network extraction, data retrieval, preprocessing, and normalization) determines bibliometric parameters according to authors, type of document, source of publication, year, institutions, citations and country. The second step (mapping and visualization) determines the relationship between fields, disciplines, individual papers or authors, and provides an understanding of the relationships between citations in a scientific research field, which is called co-citation

(Yataganbaba and Kurtba, 2016; Small, 1999). The ISI Web of Science, Scopus and Google Scholar are common sources of bibliometric data. To map and explore patterns in the structure, there are software tools that can be used for the processing and mapping of scientific data, such as UCINET, Cite Space, VOSviewer, and Science of Science (Cobo *et al.*, 2011; van Eck and Waltman, 2009). Each of these tools has certain benefits and limitations that may affect a study. For example, with Sci2, it is not possible to convert from one format to another, and there are limitations when running certain algorithms to detect duplicate records or nodes (Gomez *et al.*, 2014).

3.2. *Cluster analysis*

Clustering has been utilized in many fields and by diverse approaches (Gerdsri *et al.*, 2013; Li *et al.*, 2015a, 2015b). Document clustering is an approach for text-based data (Hung, 2012; Boyack *et al.*, 2011). It is used in many applications including natural language processing, web information retrieval, bioinformatics, telecommunication, and technology analysis (Yeo *et al.*, 2015; Kwon and Cho, 2015; Takano *et al.*, 2017). Technological trends and associations can be discovered by analyzing these *document* clusters (Han and Jin, 2015). Cluster analysis was employed for the research in this paper in order to identify words with similar characteristics, as well as to highlight research activity trends in WT. To this end, the VOSviewer software (van Eck and Waltman, 2009) was used to construct and visualize journal and keyword networks since it has already been tested and proven in other technological research (Mohammadi, 2012; Leydesdorff *et al.*, 2013). Co-occurrence networks provide a graphical visualization of the relationship between keywords in articles. These networks are useful for studying the kind of knowledge that is contained in subfields or different research topics. Titles, abstracts and keywords of the articles are the best place to find trends in a domain (Hsu *et al.*, 2006). Thus, VOSviewer uses processing techniques to yield a list of all noun phrases from the title and abstract. In addition, a list of word clusters can be generated using VOSviewer. This allows words that may be considered highly related to one another to be grouped, and distinguishes them with the same color set in the visual representation of mapped terms.

3.3. *Data collection*

The Scopus database was systematically searched to collect all of the published documents relating to WT. This database can be used without the necessity of separating the different sections of published documents in order to analyze the assessment of the research field (Burnham, 2006). The data retrieval strategies utilize topic, abstract and keyword data. In other words, this means that the words located in titles, abstracts and keywords are collected for analysis. The year range covers 2000–2016. The search covers up to December 2016. To search for publications, different combinations of keywords were used to identify papers that were most likely to be related to WT. To select the keywords, scientific publications and the websites of top companies in the smart wearable industry were carefully reviewed in order to distinguish the most popular products and keywords in WT.

The selection of search strings is usually performed by using textbooks that include subject glossaries and indexes. To the best of our knowledge, no textbook regarding WT exists. Therefore, by using the terms and definitions in publications, top registered patents in the WT domain (from Thomson innovation database) and a wearable database (vandrico), 19 words were chosen to be tagged in order to search on Scopus. This data collection resulted in a total of 8,242 published documents being retrieved from the Scopus database. We controlled the title and abstract of each published document for whether relevant topics are included accordingly, and we used bibliometric methods to analyze the publication output based on institution, author, journal, country, and categorized terms of WT research. Table 2 shows the number of publications registered per year for each keyword combination.

Table 2 summarizes the total number of publications contained in the Scopus database based on our chosen keywords for WT. In general, it can be seen that the number of keywords has been rising rapidly in recent years, and especially in 2016. To ensure the validity of the collected data, the titles of publications were read in order to verify that the selected papers do refer to our chosen keywords. This led to the deletion of 963 duplicates, and 7,279 publications were included in our final sample set.

4. Results

4.1. *Descriptive analysis (bibliometric analysis)*

Figure 1 illustrates the increase in the academic research output in WT that has taken place between 2000 and 2016. In the period 2000–2013, the output was conservative. In contrast, the period between 2013 and 2015 shows a sharp rise in the number of WT publications. 2016 was the most productive year for WT with ~3,170 publications.

As depicted in Figure 2, the majority of WT publications are conference papers (4,391), followed by journal articles (2,293) and book chapters (197). It can be concluded from the analysis of document types that researchers prefer to publish their study results in conferences, possibly because of the lack of specialized journals in the WT field. In addition, this is a new topic and results are therefore first published in conferences.

The geographic distribution of publications based on author affiliations for WT is reported in Figure 3. The United States of America is the most dominant country in terms of the number of publications, contributing to 19% of the papers. This is based on our analysis of global trends in academic activities when viewed from the perspective of whole countries. China is in the second position in terms of its share of the world's scientific

Table 2. The rapidly increasing number of publications each year that relate to WT keyword combinations.

Keywords	**<2007**	**2007**	**2008**	**2009**	**2010**	**2011**	**2012**	**2013**	**2014**	**2015**	**2016**	**Total**
Wearable technology/ies	220	42	26	38	39	44	43	64	415	2035	2326	**5292**
Smart textile/s	182	56	61	50	74	66	74	94	115	158	222	**1152**
Smart clothing/cloth/clothes	106	28	13	37	15	35	21	30	36	44	61	**426**
Smart glasses	14	1	2	1	2	5	8	20	58	109	133	**353**
Smart watch/watches	8	5	2	2	2	0	4	19	90	202	333	**667**
Smart shoes	3	0	5	7	10	8	13	17	13	22	40	**138**
Smart T-shirt/jacket	2	0	1	5	9	15	9	16	9	11	12	**89**
Smart helmet	2	2	0	1	0	1	0	4	6	11	15	**42**
Smart bracelet	0	0	0	0	0	0	0	2	7	11	16	**36**
Smart wristband	2	0	1	0	1	0	0	0	3	5	2	**14**
Smart ring	1	0	0	1	2	1	1	3	0	6	3	**18**
Smart eye wear	0	0	0	0	0	0	0	0	2	3	6	**11**
Smart jewellery	0	0	0	0	0	0	0	0	1	2	1	**4**
All products	**540**	**134**	**111**	**142**	**154**	**175**	**173**	**269**	**755**	**2619**	**3170**	**8242**

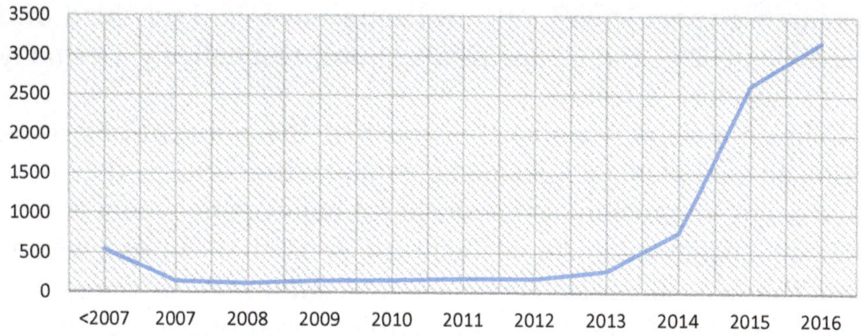

Figure 1. Distribution of academic output over the years.

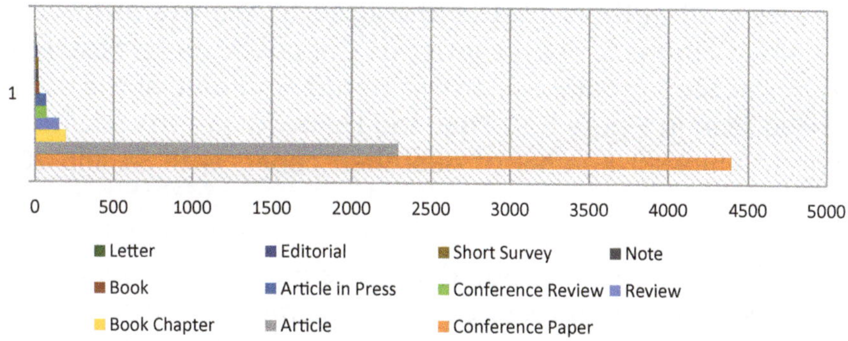

Figure 2. Distribution of publications according to document type.

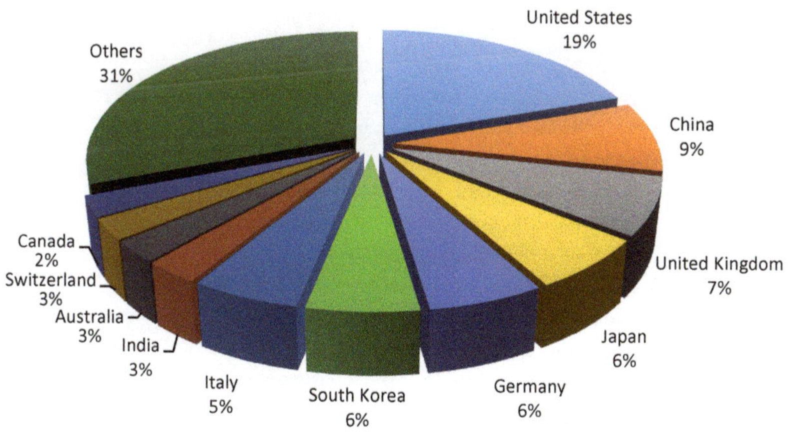

Figure 3. Geographic distribution of publications for WT.

research papers in WT. UK and Japan are ranked third and fourth with 7% and 6% of publications, respectively. Germany and South Korea follow.

Figure 4 demonstrates that most of the publications come from universities. As can be seen from the figure, the most prominent institution in the world for conducting research into WTs is Georgia Institute of Technology, with 113 publications over the last 10 years. The Chinese Academy of Sciences and Eidgenossische Technische Hochschule Zurich published 99 and 89 papers, respectively, which placed them in second and third place.

The lead authors that contributed to the literature are shown in Figure 5. The majority of the publications acquired from the Scopus database are written by multiple authors. As can be seen in Figure 5, Tröster and Lukowicz are the scientists with the highest number of published papers with 38 and 28, respectively.

Figure 6 shows the research activities that were published in journal or conference proceedings. The journal that published the most articles was *Lecture Notes in Computer Science* (325), followed by *Proceedings of Conference on Human Factors in Computing Systems* (124), and *ACM International Conference Proceeding Series* (121).

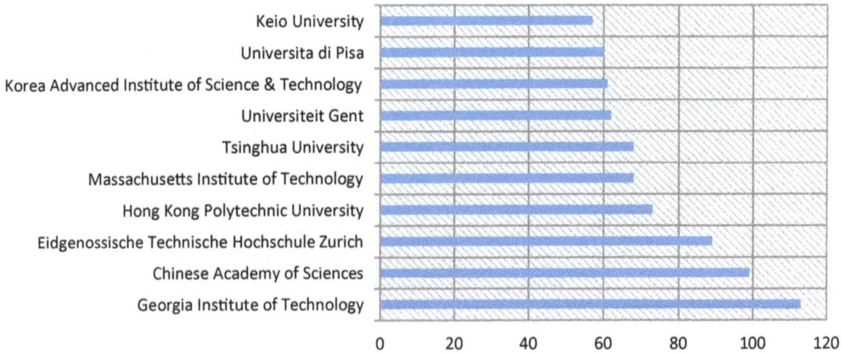

Figure 4. Distribution of publications of the top 10 institutions.

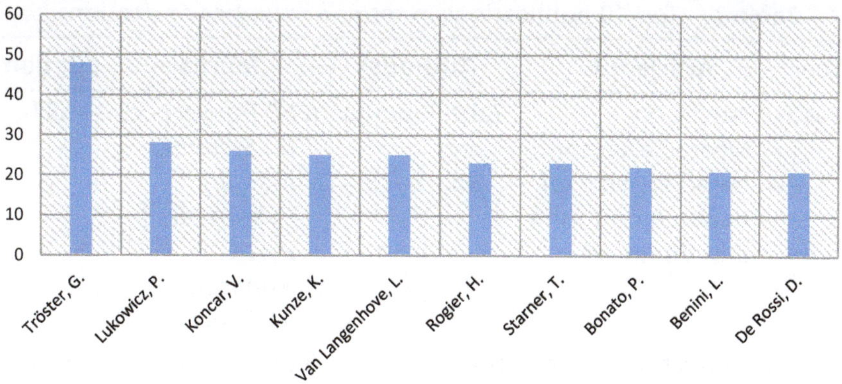

Figure 5. The top 10 most productive authors according to the number of publications.

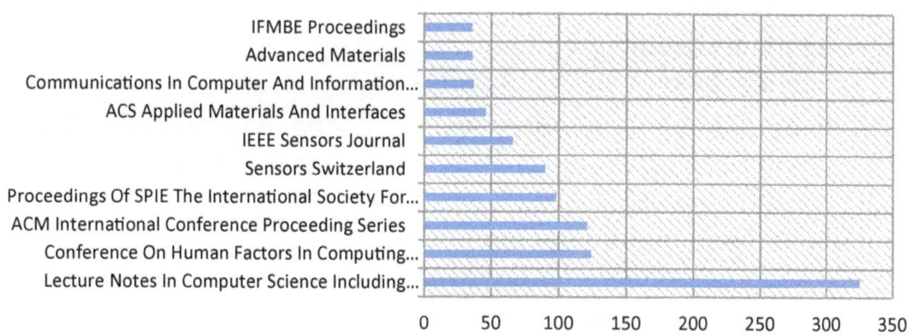

Figure 6. The top 10 leading conference proceedings and journals.

Table 3 shows the most cited articles. Most of these articles are either examining healthcare as a whole, or are specialized in its application. The top cited articles are quite young in terms of the year in which they were published. For example, the most cited article describes work on wearable sensors to direct the requirements of applications for health monitoring and prognosis, and was published in the year 2010.

4.2. *Results from the cluster analysis*

The overall terms acquired from 6,585 publications are displayed in Figure 7. An interesting next step is the combination of the

Table 3. Top 10 publications in terms of number of citations.

Year	Article title	Author(s)	Journal	Citation
2010	A survey on wearable sensor-based systems for health monitoring and prognosis	Pantelopoulos and Bourbakis	*IEEE Transactions on Systems, Man and Cybernetics Part C: Applications and Reviews*	537
2004	Introduction to the special section on m-Health: Beyond seamless mobility and global wireless healthcare connectivity	Istepanian *et al.*	*IEEE Transactions on Information Technology in Biomedicine*	358
2008	Phase change materials for smart textiles — An overview	Mondal	*Applied Thermal Engineering*	342
2011	Shape-memory polymers and their composites: Stimulus methods and applications	Leng *et al.*	*Progress in Materials Science*	337
2003	Enhancing the quality of life through WT	Park and Jayaraman	*IEEE Engineering in Medicine and Biology Magazine*	263
2012	A review of wearable sensors and systems with application in rehabilitation	Patel *et al.*	*Journal of Neuro Engineering and Rehabilitation*	220

(*Continued*)

Table 3. (*Continued*)

Year	Article title	Author(s)	Journal	Citation
2004	Gait assessment in Parkinson's disease: Toward an ambulatory system for long-term monitoring	Salarian *et al.*	*IEEE Transactions on Biomedical Engineering*	202
2012	Facile fabrication of light, flexible and multifunctional graphene fibers	Dong *et al.*	*Advanced Materials*	177
2005	Flexible technologies and smart clothing for citizen medicine, home healthcare, and disease prevention	Axisa *et al.*	*IEEE Transactions on Information Technology in Biomedicine*	176
2003	Large-area smart glass and integrated photovoltaics	Lampert	*Solar Energy Materials and Solar Cells*	167

two bibliometric methods and citation analysis. To this end, the relative citation impact of each term is indicated with a color. For a term to be included in the analysis, it needs to occur in a minimum of 10 publications. 62,481 terms were extracted from the titles and abstracts, and 17,633 terms met the threshold and were mapped. For each of the 17,633 terms, a relevance score was estimated, and on the basis of this score, the most relevant terms were selected. The number of citations of each publication is divided by the average number of citations of all publications that were published in same year, in order to correct for the age of a publication. This yields a publication's

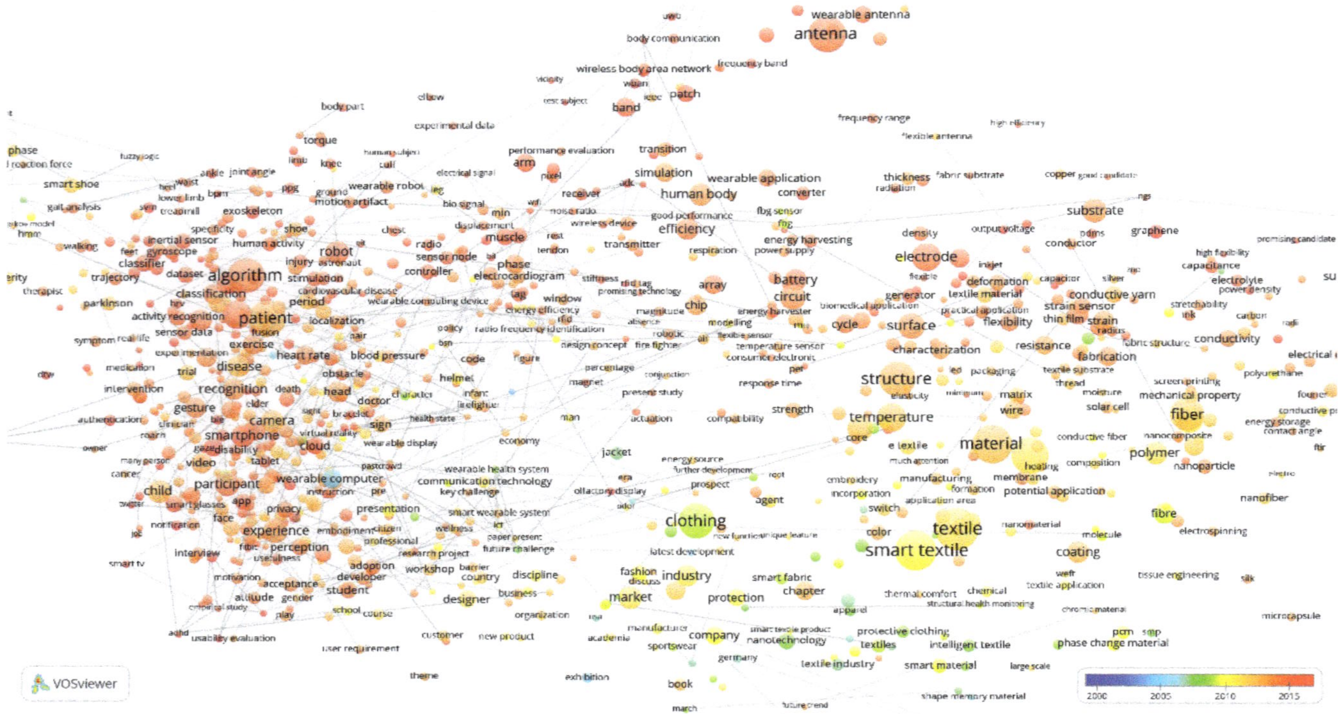

Figure 7. Overlay map based on WT publications from the period 2000 to 2016. The color of a term indicates the average year of the publications in which the term occurs (closer to red is more recent).

normalized citation score. Finally, a total of 1,077 terms were selected and mapped. Each of the 1,077 topics is marked in an algorithmic way. This process is performed by extracting the most relevant terms from the titles and abstracts of the publications belonging to a topic. As is clear from the overlay visualization in Figure 8, the larger words represent those with the highest frequency. These words attract the highest degree of attention and accordingly demonstrate the research hotspots in the field. The larger the number of publications in which two terms co-occur, the stronger the relationship between these terms in the two-dimensional space (visualized as the closeness of the terms), while terms that do not have a strong relationship are consequently located further away from each other.

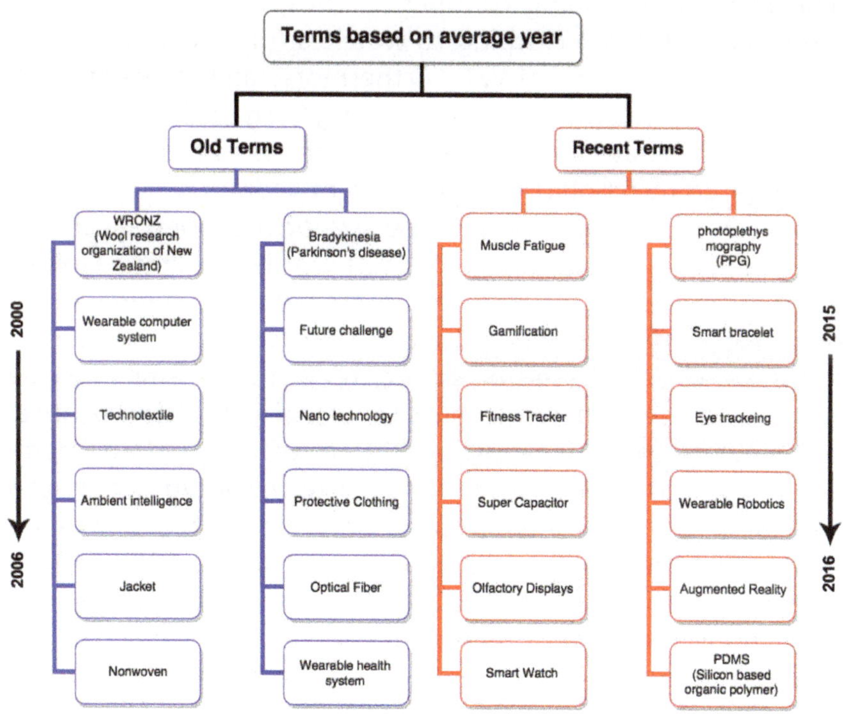

Figure 8. Chart elaboration of old and recent terms based on the average year and number of occurrences.

The different colors on the banner represent different periods of time from 2000 to 2016, and the gradation from cool colors on the left to warm colors on the right signifies that time is moving from the past toward the present. In the visualization, each term is colored according to the average year of the publications in which the term occurs. The closer the color of a term is to blue, the older the publications are in which the term occurs. On the contrary, the closer the color of a term is to red, the more recent the publications are in which the term occurs.

The publications trend can be better seen in the word analysis visualization shown in Figure 8. This shows that textile and clothing are older terms that were considered interesting. On the contrary, smart bracelet and smart watch are recognized by scholars as being the most interesting more recent terms upon which research is being conducted. Thus, it can be seen that there is a shift from clothing to watches for research into the product development of WT. Furthermore, new concepts such as "wearable robotics", "eye tracking", "gamification" and "olfactory displays" are the newest categories that are being investigated by scholars over the current year.

As can be seen in Figure 9, the size of the labels illustrates the frequency of occurrence of each word. The link between different labels means that co-occurrence exists between the keywords, and the colors show word clusters. For each cluster, terms are chosen based on two criteria. First terms must be unique, and second terms must be of sufficient significance, which means that they must occur in a sufficiently large number of publications. In other words, a term should not be too general, in order for it to properly determine a topic. Thus we leave out terms that relate to many different topics. More detailed information regarding the term selection process can be found in the study by Waltman and Van Eck (2012). The co-occurrence analysis grouped the 1,077 terms into five clusters of significant size. The shorter the distance between two terms, the closer their relationship, and thus the higher the number of co-occurrences in groups of keywords for each cluster. The red

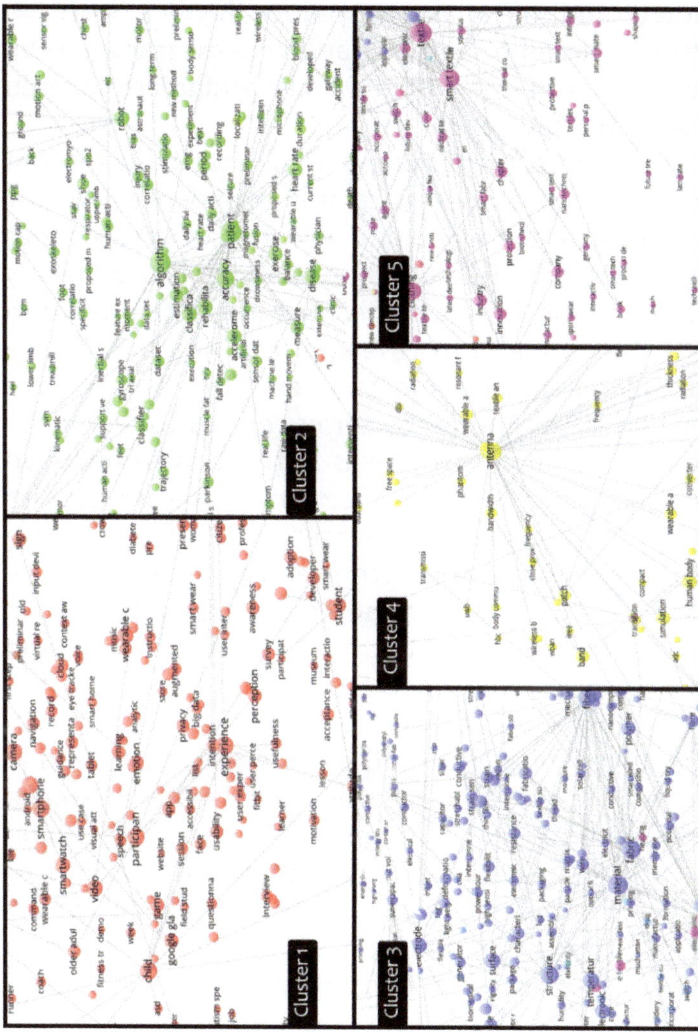

Figure 9. Map view of WT clusters. Terms are shown by label and marked with circles. The higher the occurrence of the terms, the larger are their labels and circles. The color of the circle is used to distinguish between different clusters, which are based on the VOS technique e.g., Cluster 1 (red), Cluster 2 (green), Cluster 3 (blue), Cluster 4 (yellow), Cluster 5 (violet).

cluster in the visualization (Cluster 1), consists of terms/phrases frequently occurring in human interaction and WT products. The green cluster (Cluster 2), covers terms related to healthcare and its measurement. The blue cluster (Cluster 3), exclusively describes power and material. The yellow cluster (Cluster 4) consists of terms related to antenna and wireless transmission. Finally, terms related to smart textile and clothing are covered in the purple cluster (Cluster 5).

To further elaborate, cluster one is dominated by terms that refer to the interaction of users (e.g., user experience and user interfaces). Research into models and newer product categories (e.g., smart watch, google glasses and bracelet) are heavily represented by scholars in this cluster. The interesting point in this cluster is that it contains research into smart wearable products across three sectors: entertainment, fitness and education. Cluster two is dominated by terms related to algorithm and physical internal controls. Terms in this cluster focus on patients, disease diagnosis, and subjects in healthcare. Studies on "rehabilitation", "Parkinson's disease" and "disability disorders" are examples of hot topics, recognized by researchers. The high-value research that has been carried out among scholars in this cluster can be noted as relating to "wearable robots" and "exoskeletons". However, it seems that these terms are still in their infancy of use by scholars. Cluster three is focused on terms relating to new materials and adding relative advantage to smart wearable products. In regards to new materials, terms relating to "composite" and "nanofibers" are words with high frequency. On the other hand, research on advantages of supercapacitors for wearable devices that can retain energy for longer periods, is a point of interest in this cluster. The research in cluster four focuses on simulation of the human body and wireless smart antennas. This cluster has the lowest number of term occurrences in comparison to the other clusters. Terms relating to smart textiles and clothing are exclusively represented in cluster five. An interesting point in this cluster is related to emerging terms such as "fashion" and "technology".

Moreover, protection clothing was highlighted as a hot topic among scholars in this cluster. Another interesting point that emerges is that scholars tend to be focused on "smart mate" and its relationship with wearable products. Table 4 outlines the list of the top 10 words in terms of number occurrences for each cluster.

5. Conclusions

This study employs bibliometric analysis to evaluate the quantity and quality of research into WT and its applications, and addresses the identified literature gap. Furthermore, several future directions are also identified from the evaluation, and the association of these directions with smart WT will help consolidate the growing literature in this field.

By employing the bibliometric technique, this study identified emerging and fading themes of academic research in the field of WT. The lists of most productive journals, institutions and authors can serve as a useful guidance for those who are interested in this particular discipline as they look for professional advice in forming their future policy and making better decisions. The results highlight the increase in the importance of WT in today's research environment over the past couple of years. They also highlight the noticeable contributions made by researchers from different disciplines and disciplines that are still forthcoming in their pursuit of WT. In our cluster analysis, we observed that five categories dominate the cluster networks and that internally-oriented WT activities enhance technical innovations from different sides. The cluster analysis results also show that new terms and clusters are emerging over time. One of the significant technology trends identified from clustering is the gradual transfer of products from smart textiles and wearable computers to augmented reality products such as smart eye contacts and glasses. Furthermore, scholars have mostly focused on healthcare over the studied timeframe, such as on rehabilitation and disabled patients. In addition, scholars

Table 4. Word clusters to display sets of terms according to their degree of relatedness and the number of co-occurrences as generated by VOSviewer.

Cluster 1 (frequencies)	Cluster 2 (frequencies)	Cluster 3 (frequencies)	Cluster 4 (frequencies)	Cluster 5 (frequencies)
Experience (226)	Patient (619)	Material (720)	Antenna (637)	Clothing (919)
Child (201)	Algorithm (588)	Fabric (637)	Circuit diagram (243)	Textile (766)
Head (147)	Robot (193)	Fibre (498)	Human body (196)	Coating (195)
Smart watch (123)	Rehabilitation (180)	Temperature (336)	Efficiency (179)	Technological innovation (139)
Physical activities (115)	Disease (177)	Electronic (352)	Simulation (138)	Protection (114)
Designer (101)	Accelerometer sensor (176)	Battery (176)	Arm (110)	Fashion (90)
Google glass (101)	Hear rate (143)	Supercapacitor (162)	Thickness (100)	Nanotechnology (81)
Game (99)	Smart shoes (126)	Resistance (130)	Bandwidth (76)	Heating (66)
Augmented reality (96)	Diagnosis (98)	Composite (128)	Wireless (72)	Smart mate (61)
Learning (73)	Parkinson (67)	Flexibility (114)	Transmission (63)	Sport wear (58)

have been adding features that provide relative advantage to products such as water resistance, new high-tech materials (e.g., nanofiber), the possibility of interaction with a smart environment and also embedded devices for routine daily life such as smart mate.

The theoretical contribution of this research is three-fold. First, research on WT is still scarce, so this study adds to the limited body of literature. Therefore, this paper has enhanced the understanding of the evolution and definition of WT as a whole and of its technological trends. Second, scholars need to be concerned with which terms are the most frequent within the five specific clusters of innovation identified in our analysis, and redefine and rearticulate their supporting plans for the future research of WT accordingly. Third, from a clustering perspective, we found diverse areas of interest in WT, such as computer human interaction, health measurement, power optimization, and motion recognition. Consequently, the development of WT requires extensive collaboration between different players from research laboratories and technological universities, and fostering such collaboration can be more efficient than the market regulators designing general policies for the development of the field. Thus, this collaboration would strongly contribute to the co-development of high value products and the enhancement of the future direction of WT research. Indeed, WT are still in their early stage, so investigating essential publication portfolios will be important as scholars and industry decide on future cooperation strategies based on their current directions and the directions revealed from the publication trends.

The current study has certain limitations, which should be addressed carefully in future bibliometric studies of this type. Our data retrieval strategy, which decided to include only English articles in the Scopus-indexed journals, produced a bias against research articles published in non-Scopus journals and non-English journals. We also acknowledge that co-occurrence analysis and visualization are subject to technological limitations. Furthermore, the research methods in this study are limited to bibliometric and cluster analysis. Future studies need to go beyond these methods and our chosen keywords, and also incorporate registered patents in order to explore similarities between publication and patent trends in WT with the aim of identifying technology overlaps and convergences. Furthermore, it is acknowledged that the frequency analysis and visualization maps produced by the VOSviewer software are subject to technological limitations.

Indeed, given the growing nature of the smart wearables industry in different contexts, it is possible that different products and terms that currently constitute this industry may slowly move and pursue altogether different trajectories over time. Therefore, a relevant question that may be necessary for scholars and decision-makers to ascertain in this domain is what will be the new forms of integration that connect various parts of the field as a whole, as it continues to grow. The wearables market will move across devices and integrate more fully with other connected products such as IOT platforms for home or the enterprise. Furthermore, WT follows trends in innovation that other technologies have shown in recent years. We can predict that such smart devices will become increasingly connected, able to sense our location and environments, able to discretely function, and engage us with greater involvement. The future will favor these types of transparent, comfortable, WT breakthroughs that enable fitness and health technology in new ways.

Disclosure Statement

No potential conflict of interest was reported by the author.

References

Adenle, A. A., Haslam, G. E. and Lee, L. (2013). Global assessment of research and development for algae biofuel production and its potential role for sustainable development in developing countries, *Energy Policy*, 61, 182–195.

Barfield, W. and Caudell, T. (2001). Basic concepts in wearable computers and augmented reality, *Fundamentals of Wearable Computers and Augmented Reality*, 3–26.

Bartlett-Bragg, A. (2014). Wearable technologies: Shaping the future of learning, *Training & Development*, 41(3), 13.

Bower, M. and Sturman, D. (2015). What are the educational affordances of wearable technologies? *Computers & Education*, 88, 343–353.

Boyack, K. W., Newman, D., Duhon, R. J., Klavans, R., Patek, M., Biberstine, J. R., Schijvenaars, B., Skupin, A., Ma, N. and Börner, K. (2011). Clustering more than two million biomedical publications: Comparing the accuracies of nine text-based similarity approaches, *PloS One*, 6(3), e18029.

Bryson, D. (2009). Smart clothes and wearable technology for the health and well-being market, in *Smart Clothes and Wearable Technology*, The Textile Institute and Woodhead Publishing, Oxford, Cambridge, New Delhi, pp. 335–345.

Burnham, J. F. (2006). Scopus database: A review, *Biomedical Digital Libraries*, 3(1), 1.

Cho, G. (ed.) (2009). *Smart Clothing: Technology and Applications*, CRC Press. Taylor & Francis Group.

Cheng, J. W. and Mitomo, H. (2017). The underlying factors of the perceived usefulness of using smart wearable devices for disaster applications, *Telematics and Informatics*, 34(2), 528–539.

Chuah, S. H-W., Rauschnabel, P. A., Krey, N., Nguyen, B., Ramayah, T. and Lade, S. (2016). Wearable technologies: The role of usefulness and visibility in smartwatch adoption, *Computers in Human Behavior*, 65, 276–284.

Cobo, M. J., López-Herrera, A. G., Herrera-Viedma, E. and Herrera, F. (2011). Science mapping software tools: Review, analysis, and cooperative study among tools, *Journal of the American Society for Information Science and Technology*, 62(7), 1382–1402.

Conti, M., Das, S. K., Bisdikian, C., Kumar, M., Ni, L. M., Passarella, A., Roussos, G., Tröster, G., Tsudik, G. and Zambonelli, F. (2012). Looking ahead in pervasive computing: Challenges and opportunities in the era of cyber–physical convergence, *Pervasive and Mobile Computing*, 8(1), 2–21.

Daim, T. U., Rueda, G., Martin, H., and Gerdsri, P. (2006). Forecasting emerging technologies: Use of bibliometrics and patent analysis, *Technological Forecasting and Social Change*, 73(8), 981–1012.

D'Auria, A. *et al*. (2017). Multiple context of innovation: Insights from literature, *International Journal of Innovation and Technology Management*, 14(2), 1740007.

Dehghani, M. (2016). An assessment towards adoption and diffusion of smart wearable technologies by consumers: The cases of smart watch and fitness wristband products, in *HT* (*Extended Proceedings*).

Dehghani, M. and Dangelico, R. M. (2017). Smart wearable technologies: Current status and market orientation through a patent analysis, in *2017 IEEE International Conference on IEEE, Industrial Technology (ICIT)*, pp. 1570–1575.

Dehghani, M., and Kim, K. J. (2019). The effects of design, size, and uniqueness of smartwatches: Perspectives from current versus potential users. *Behaviour & Information Technology*, 1–11.

Fang, Y-M. and Chang, C-C. (2016). Users' psychological perception and perceived readability of wearable devices for elderly people, *Behaviour & Information Technology*, 35(3), 225–232.

Fetscherin, M., Voss, H. and Gugler, P. (2010). 30 Years of foreign direct investment to China: An interdisciplinary literature review, *International Business Review*, 19(3), 235–246.

Gerdsri, N., Kongthon, A. and Puengrusme, S. (2017). Profiling the research landscape in emerging areas using bibliometrics and text mining: A case study of biomedical engineering (BME) in Thailand, *International Journal of Innovation and Technology Management*, 14(2), 1740011.

Gerdsri, N., Kongthon, A. and Vatananan, R. S. (2013). Mapping the knowledge evolution and professional network in the field of technology roadmapping: A bibliometric analysis, *Technology Analysis & Strategic Management*, 25(4), 403–422.

Godin, B. (2006). On the origins of bibliometrics, *Scientometrics*, 68(1), 109–133.

Gomez-Jauregui, V., Gomez-Jauregui, C., Manchado, C. and Otero, C. (2014). Information management and improvement of citation indices, *International Journal of Information Management*, 34(2), 257–271.

Gómez-Barroso, J. L., Feijóo, C., Quiles-Casas, M., and Bohlin, E. (2017). The evolution of the telecommunications policy agenda: Forty years of articles in Telecommunications Policy. *Telecommunications Policy*, 41(10), 853–877.

GSMA (2015). New report backs mass adoption of wearables. Available at: http://gsma.com/connectedliving/news/new-report-backs-mass-adoption-of-wearables/ [Accessed 12 December 2016].

Guo, Y., Ma, T., Porter, A. L. and Huang, L. (2012). Text mining of information resources to inform forecasting innovation pathways, *Technology Analysis & Strategic Management*, 24(8), 843–861.

Han, Y.-J. (2015). Analysis of essential patent portfolios via bibliometric mapping: An illustration of leading firms in the 4G era, *Technology Analysis & Strategic Management*, 27(7), 809–839.

Harrop, P., Das, R. and Chansin, G. (2014). Wearable technology 2014–2024, in *Report, IDTechEx*.

Hsu, F.-C., Trappey, A. J. C., Trappey, C. V., Hou, J.-L. and Liu, S.-J. (2006). Technology and knowledge document cluster analysis for enterprise R&D strategic planning, *International Journal of Technology Management*, 36(4), 336–353.

Hung, J. L. (2012). Trends of e-learning research from 2000 to 2008: Use of text mining and bibliometrics, *British Journal of Educational Technology*, 43(1), 5–16.

Jost, K., Stenger, D., Perez, C. R., McDonough, J. K., Lian, K, Gogotsi, Y. and Dion, G. (2013). Knitted and screen printed carbon-fiber supercapacitors for applications in wearable electronics, *Energy & Environmental Science* 6, 2698–2705.

Kelly, H. (2014). Smartphones are fading. Wearables are next. Available at: http://money.cnn.com/2014/03/19/technology/mobile/wearable-devices/ [Accessed 29 April 2016].

Kooroshnia, M., Thornquist, C. and Clausen, L. (2015). Performative interactions between body and dress: Thermochromic print in fashion, *International Journal of Fashion Design, Technology and Education*, 8(1), 47–53.

Kostoff, R. N., Toothman, D. R., Eberhart, H. J. and Humenik, J. A. (2001). Text mining using database tomography and bibliometrics: A review, *Technological Forecasting and Social Change*, 68(3), 223–253.

Kwon, Y. and Cho, S. (2015). Defining a cluster market: The case of the Korean Internet portal service market, *Telecommunications Policy*, 39(11), 921–932.

Lee, T.-G. and Lee, S-H. (2016). Dynamic bio-sensing process design in mobile wellness information system for smart healthcare, *Wireless Personal Communications*, 86(1), 201–215.

Leydesdorff, L., Rotolo, D. and de Nooy, W. (2013). Innovation as a nonlinear process, the scientometric perspective, and the specification of an 'innovation opportunities explorer, *Technology Analysis & Strategic Management*, 25(6), 641–653.

Li, J., Jovanovic, A., Klimek, P. and Guo, X. (2015b). Bibliometric analysis of fracking scientific literature, *Scientometrics*, 105(2), 1273–1284.

Li, X., Zhou, Y., Xue, L. and Huang, L. (2015a). Integrating bibliometrics and roadmapping methods: A case of dye-sensitized solar cell technology-based industry in China, *Technological Forecasting and Social Change*, 97, 205–222.

McBurney, M. K. and Novak, P. L. (2002). What is bibliometrics and why should you care? in *Proceedings of IEEE International Professional Communication Conference, 2002. IPCC 2002*, IEEE, pp. 108–114.

Morganti, E., Angelini, L., Adami, A., Lalanne, D., Lorenzelli, L. and Mugellini, E. (2012). A smart watch with embedded sensors to recognize objects, grasps and forearm gestures, *Procedia Engineering*, 41, 1169–1175.

Nyan, M. N., Tay, F. E. H. and Murugasu, E. (2008). A wearable system for pre-impact fall detection, *Journal of Biomechanics*, 41(16), 3475–3481.

Seyrkammer, S. (2015). *Wearable Computing Technology: Potenzielle Einsatzmöglichkeiten in der Industrie*, DiplomicaVerlag.

Small, H. (1999). Visualizing science by citation mapping, *Journal of the Association for Information Science and Technology*, 50(9), 799.

Soh, P. J., Vandenbosch, G. A. E., Mercuri, M. and Schreurs, D. M. M.-P. (2015). Wearable wireless health monitoring: Current developments, challenges, and future trends, IEEE *Microwave Magazine*, 16(4), 55–70.

Son, D., Lee, J., Qiao, S., Ghaffari, R., Kim, J., Lee, J. E., Song, C., Kim, S. J., Lee, D. J., Jun, S. W., Yang, S., Park, M., Shin, J., Do, K., Lee, M., Kang, K., Hwang, C. S., Lu, N., Hyeon, T. and Kim, D.-H. (2014). Multifunctional wearable devices for diagnosis and therapy of movement disorders, *Nature Nanotechnology*, 9(5), 397–404.

Sultan, N. (2015). Reflective thoughts on the potential and challenges of wearable technology for healthcare provision and medical education, *International Journal of Information Management*, 35(5), 521–526.

Takano, Y., Yuya, K. and Makoto, A. (2017). Trends and typology of emerging antenna propagation technologies: Citation network analysis, *International Journal of Innovation and Technology Management*, 14(1), 1740005.

Tehrani, K., and Michael, A. (2014). Wearable technology and wearable devices: Everything you need to know. *Wearable Devices Magazine*, 26.

van Eck, N. J. and Waltman, L. (2009). Software survey: VOSviewer, a computer program for bibliometric mapping, *Scientometrics*, 84(2), 523–538.

Van Raan and Anthony F. J. (2014). Advances in bibliometric analysis: Research performance assessment and science mapping, *Bibliometrics. Use and Abuse in the Review of Research Performance*, pp. 17–28. The Biochemist.

Vandrico. (2019). Available in: https://vandrico.com/wearables/ [Accessed 25 October 2018].

Viseu, A. (2003). Social dimensions of wearable computers: An overview, *Technoetic Arts*, 1(1), 77–82.

Waltman, L. and Nees J. E. (2012). A new methodology for constructing a publication-level classification system of science, *Journal of the Association for Information Science and Technology*, 63(12), 2378–2392.

Wasik, B. (2013). Why wearable tech will be as big as the smartphone. Wired. Available in: https://www.wired.com/2013/12/wearable-computers/.

Wright, R. and Keith, L. (2014). Wearable technology: If the tech fits, wear it, *Journal of Electronic Resources in Medical Libraries*, 11(4), 204–216.

Wu, L., Fan, A. A. and Mattila, A. S. (2015). Wearable technology in service delivery processes: The gender-moderated technology objectification effect, *International Journal of Hospitality Management*, 51, 1–7.

Xin, L., Jiwu, W., Lucheng, H., Jiang, L. and Jian, L. (2010). Empirical research on the technology opportunities analysis based on morphology analysis and conjoint analysis, *Foresight*, 12(2), 66–76.

Yan, S.-M. and Sun, J.-Q. (2015). Assessing China's salt lake resources R&D based on bibliometrics analysis, *Scientometrics*, 105(2), 1141–1155.

Yang, H., Yu, J., Zo, H. and Choi, M. (2016). User acceptance of wearable devices: An extended perspective of perceived value, *Telematics and Informatics*, 3(2), 256–269.

Yataganbaba, A., and Kurtbaş, İ. (2016). A scientific approach with bibliometric analysis related to brick and tile drying: A review. *Renewable and Sustainable Energy Reviews*, 59, 206–224.

Yeo, W., Kim, S., Park, H. and Kang, J. (2015). A bibliometric method for measuring the degree of technological innovation, *Technological Forecasting and Social Change*, 95, 152–162.

Chapter 2

A Review of Japan's Bioventures

Shiaw Jia Eyo

Department of Global and Interdisciplinary Studies,
Hosei University, Tokyo, Japan

sjeyo@hosei.ac.jp

Abstract

This chapter reviews the creation and the development of biotechnology start-ups in Japan known as "bioventures". In the early 1990s, the Japanese government began to introduce new policies to promote the development of bioventures. Within the span of a decade, the number of bioventures grew five times. However, majority of them continued to operate at the seed or start-up stage. This chapter seeks to explore the underdeveloped state of bioventures in Japan, based on the case study method which includes the use of interviews and reviews of several policies and regulations. This chapter also compares the development of the biotechnology industry in Japan with that in the US and Europe. This chapter concludes that the lack of a sustainable system of funding is the real issue hindering the development of bioventures in Japan.

Keywords: Biotechnology start-ups, Japan, funding, venture capital.

1. Introduction

Biotechnology has been one of the most flourishing sectors from the beginning of the 21st century. It has an increasingly important impact on a range of economic sectors and disciplines ranging from medical to agricultural to environmental, so much so that its pervasiveness allows it to be seen as an example of "general purpose technology", which has a significant impact on economic activities and a wide technological diffusion (Malerba, 2004; Gambardella and McGahan, 2010).

The role of new entrants or start-ups in biotechnology is pivotal. Biotechnology start-ups were the engine behind the creation of the modern biotechnology industry in the United States (US). According to Orsenigo (1989), their role was fundamental in two ways. First, they were responsible for most of the research in genetic engineering in the early years and heavily contributed to the directions of technical change; and second, they were a major source of knowledge for established corporations. According to Grabowski and Vernon (1994), in the early days of biotechnology, new biotechnology start-ups had greater capabilities and knowledge in biotechnology than large incumbent companies in pharmaceuticals. Lerner (1999) documented that biotechnology start-ups were the pioneer of the biotechnology revolution and they made unusual contributions to innovation, particularly during the early 1980s, as measured in patent applications in both products and processes. In another recent study, Kneller (2010) reported that drugs initially discovered in new biotechnology firms or universities accounted for approximately half of the 252 new drugs approved by the US Food and Drug Administration from 1998 to 2007.

The biotechnology industry emerged in the 1970s in the US because of two key scientific technology discoveries, namely recombinant DNA and monoclonal antibodies. Recombinant DNA (a method for manipulating the genetic characteristics of a cell so that it could be induced to produce a specific protein) was invented by Stanley Cohen from Stanford University and Herbert Boyer from the University of California, San Francisco in 1973. The creation of Genentech in 1976 by Herbert Boyer and venture capitalist Robert Swanson gave birth to the new biotechnology industry because it was the first company to achieve success in commercializing the scientific breakthroughs of biotechnology. Genentech developed the first biotechnology drug called *Humulin* in 1978. Humulin was cloned from human insulin using recombinant DNA techniques. Genentech's success in Humulin as well as its initial public offering (IPO) in 1980 created a model and a pattern for biotechnology start-ups in the US to explore and exploit innovations in biotechnology.

Twenty years later, a similar pattern of biotechnology boom was observed in Japan. With the bursting of the speculative "bubble economy" and the longest recession in Japan's post-war history that followed it, an array of reforms unfolded in Japan. These included among others an increase in the government R&D budgets for basic research; changes in legal and policy framework to encourage university–industry linkages; and intellectual property reforms and promotion of start-ups. The Japanese government also targeted biotechnology as one of its new frontier industries.

As a result, in the last decade, Japan has created a plethora of biotechnology start-ups known as bioventures. Despite its large number, biotechnology firms in Japan trailed far behind their counterparts in the US and Europe in terms of revenue, size, pipelines, and patents (OECD, 2009). Due to the lack of a sustainable system of funding, a vicious cycle has emerged among the bioventures. The lack of R&D funding from the government and angel investors pushed bioventures to seek venture capital funding at an early stage. However, with venture capital firms investing only in small amounts of funding, it did not take long for these bioventures to run out of capital. Going for an IPO became their last resort of funding, but even after they were listed, they continued to face funding problems. The lack of funding led to delays in milestones and sales projections which ultimately drove their share prices and market capitalization down. The chain of negative events discouraged new investments in bioventures and the whole vicious cycle became more entrenched.

Given the imperative role of new entrants in the biotechnology industry, this chapter seeks to address why biotechnology start-ups in Japan have not been successful and to find out what the real issue is that is hindering their development.

2. Research Methodology and Literature Review

This chapter uses the case study method to explore the recent development of the biotechnology industry in Japan. The case study method is chosen because it provides a detailed contextual analysis of a complex issue. Contextualization gives a greater understanding as to how an issue occurs and develops (Yin, 1984). In this research, the complex issue refers to the underdeveloped state of bioventures in Japan.

To analyze the current state of Japanese bioventures, representatives from eight bioventures were interviewed (see Appendix A). These bioventures were shortlisted because they fulfilled the following requirements of this research: (1) considered as a biotechnology start-up, (2) involved in drug discovery and development, (3) owned or partnered with academic institutions for the core technology, and (4) established for the purpose of commercializing the technology. The interviews were conducted for a period of one and half years from February 2009 to August 2010. The interviews lasted between 1.5 and 2 h. In total, 12 interviews were conducted, and 17 individuals including founders, CEOs, scientific advisors, managers, and venture capitalists were interviewed for this research.

The interviewed bioventures made up an illustrative sample of Japanese bioventures because both listed and unlisted bioventures were included. Furthermore, bioventures that were established in the late 1990s as well as those that were established in the recent years were included. At the same time, this chapter also recognizes that findings based on this small sample may not necessarily represent the general population of bioventures in Japan. The interviewed bioventures are more established compared to the rest of the bioventures out there. Therefore, one should be cautious when making a generalization about Japanese bioventures based on findings from these interviewed bioventures.

In addition to the use of interviews, this chapter also reviews several science and technology policies and institutional regulations. Since 1995, the Japanese government began to focus its investment in science and technology as a key prerequisite to the return of Japan's industrial competitiveness. Thus, this chapter focuses on policies and regulations implemented after 1995.

This chapter utilizes four different sources of data. The first group of data is interview data. The second group of data is published information from Japanese bioventures. The third group of data is reports and survey results from the government, industry associations, and international organizations. The last group of data is databases such as patent database and medical database. Collectively, these sources provide an understanding to explain the issues faced by bioventures and the overall development of the biotechnology industry in Japan.

Issues surrounding the development of the biotechnology industry in Japan have also been recognized by other scholars in the past. Prior to institutional changes in the late 1990s, Zucker and Darby (1994, 1996, 2001) found that Japan's innovation system for biotechnology deters the formation of new biotechnology firms because of the university structure, the financial market, and cultural differences with respect to entrepreneurialism. After Japan implemented a series of institutional changes, some scholars were positive that such changes would become more favorable for science-based industries such as biotechnology (Odagiri, 2004, 2006; Lynskey, 2004). Scholars pointed that institutional changes promoted the biotechnology industry by allowing greater university–industry collaboration

(Odagiri and Nakumura, 2002; Motohashi, 2005), higher bioentrepreneurship (Lynskey, 2004) and increased labor mobility in Japan (Lynskey, 2004; Braguinsky *et al*., 2010).

However, the positive effects of institutional changes on funding for biotechnology are less apparent. Odagiri and Nakumura (2002) found that procurement of capital is one of the major challenges faced by biotechnology start-ups during their establishment. Likewise, Kneller (2007) documented similar findings and attributed them to the "low-risk, low-return" strategy of venture capital investing in Japan. On the contrary, Lysnkey (2004, 2006) pointed out that because of amendments to Japanese corporate laws and stock exchange rules, there is now greater availability of venture capital for bioventures. This chapter extends the works of Kneller and Lynskey and argues *how* and *why* despite the various institutional changes, funding remains the real impediment for bioventures.

3. The Emergence of Bioventures

"Bioventure" (*baio bencha* in Japanese) is a term used in Japan to describe what is closest to be a biotechnology start-up or biotechnology venture irrespective of the sources of funding. The official agency responsible for conducting and compiling yearly data on bioventures is the Japan Bioindustry Association (JBA). JBA defines a bioventure as a company that fulfills the following main criteria:

(1) A company which does business with biotechnology as a means or objective.
(2) A company that has the required number of employees to be defined as a small and medium enterprise (SME) under the Basic Law on Small and Medium-sized Enterprises.
(3) A company established prior to 1986. The objective here is to distinguish *new biotechnology* from *old biotechnology*. The latter focuses on the use of genetic engineering such as recombinant DNA, hybridoma technology, cell fusion, and other novel bio-processing techniques.

It is reported that as late as 1990, there were hardly any signs of dedicated biotechnology start-ups in Japan, while some 250 dedicated biotechnology firms were listed on stock exchanges in the US, with another 1,100 unlisted, and Europe had nearly 500 biotechnology firms (Lynskey, 2006). However, in the span of a decade, a couple hundred biotechnology start-ups were created and the number more than quadrupled from 132 in 1996 to 587 in 2006 (JBA, 2009) (see Figure 1).

This unprecedented event changed the landscape of Japan's biotechnology industry, which was traditionally dominated by large, incumbent companies from various industries such as food, chemical, and pharmaceuticals (Collins, 2004). In 1999, a "national strategy" was unveiled to prepare Japan toward a biotechnology nation with a goal of achieving a market size of JPY25 trillion or approximately US$250 billion by 2010 with 1,000 new biotechnology-related companies (JBA, 2002). The new policy was important because for the first time, the Japanese government harbored hope to promote the biotechnology industry through the creation of start-ups. The creation and growth of bioventures were also heavily influenced by changes in Japan's innovation system, particularly in the

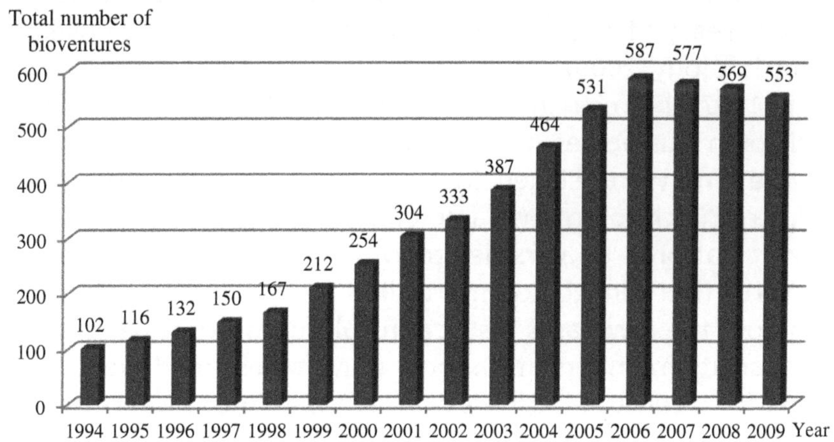

Figure 1. Cumulative number of bioventures (1994–2009).
Source: JBA (2010).

following areas: university–industry linkages, intellectual property, and funding for start-ups.

3.1. *University–Industry linkages*

Universities are the origin of many discoveries that become the basis for innovative new technologies developed by bioventures (Kneller, 2007). Prior to 1998, technology transfer in Japan was informal and disadvantageous for small companies. It lacked a standard mechanism to select the most appropriate development partner from among potentially interested companies and relied instead on existing personal relationships between individual academics and established companies (Kneller, 1999).

In May 1998, the Japanese government passed a law to promote the transfer of university technologies. The Technology Transfer Law, otherwise known as the Technology Licensing Offices (TLO) Law, allows the establishment of TLOs, independent of, but affiliated with particular universities. The Technology Transfer Law legitimizes and facilitates transparent, contractual transfers of university discoveries to industry. Professors can also voluntarily assign their individually owned inventions to TLOs. Since the law was enacted, the number of TLOs increased from 5 in 1998 to 48 by the end of 2007 (Nikkei Biotechnology, 2009).

In 1997, the restrictions preventing professors from starting their own businesses or becoming directors or employees of private firms were relaxed. In April 2000, the Law to Strengthen Industrial Technology was implemented. The law permits faculty at national universities to work for or establish private ventures that aim to commercialize their research efforts. In addition, the law eases restrictions placed on outside work so that faculty members at national universities could work after hours for a venture business or even take up to 3 years of sabbatical leave to work for the venture. The law encourages the development of academic spin-offs by faculty members.

Academic spin-offs increased from 62 in year 1999 to 179 in the year 2003. Biotechnology start-ups accounted for a fifth of these spin-offs (Kondo, 2009).

In April 2004, the National University Incorporation Law was implemented. The law changed the status of all national universities to independent administrative institutions, which gave universities greater autonomy in budget, accounting, salary system, and property rules from central government. With this law, inventions made by faculty members of Japanese national universities changed ownership from the nation to the respective universities. This cleared the previously ambiguous issue of ownership of university research results. Hence, universities can now grant bioventures exclusivity on intellectual property rights (IPRs) and derive revenues from licensing agreements.

3.2. *Intellectual property reform*

IPRs such as patents and copyrights have strategic importance in biotechnology because they serve as a means of appropriating returns to R&D investment. Prior to 1999, IPR for inventions developed at national universities in Japan belonged either to the individual inventor or to the nation. Most IPRs, however, were returned to the individual inventors, who most commonly transferred the title of their inventions to private companies for little or no fees, without filing for patents. In return for the IPR, companies provided university faculty with grants and endowments in the form of donations. Such a system was a disadvantage to small companies because they could not compete with the large companies in terms of the number of laboratories to which they could give donations or offer attractive jobs to the students of the faculties.

In October 1999, the Law of Special Measure to Revive Industry was passed that was modeled after the 1980 Bayh–Dole Act legislation in the US. The law allows the private sector to hold ownership of IPRs generated under government-funded research. This law was not immediately applicable to national universities until they became independent in 2004 but was applicable to patents generated in government research institutes. The implementation of the Japanese Bayh–Dole Act made it easier for private firms to obtain licenses for national inventions. It also gave incentives for university researchers to commercialize their inventions through patent fee reduction.

3.3. *Funding for start-ups*

To encourage more funding for start-ups, the Japanese government introduced several laws to encourage risk capital investments. In 1997, the Angel Tax Incentive program was implemented to reduce taxes on gains from angel investments and allowed losses from such investments to be deducted over 3 years instead of just the year they were incurred. During the same year, rules were changed for the first time to allow pension funds to invest in venture capital in Japan. This was analogous to the change of the "Prudent Man" rule in the US in 1979, which allowed US pension funds to begin investing in venture capital. In 1998, investors of venture capital funds in Japan could form Limited Liability Partnerships which placed their liability to the limit of their original investment.

Japan's capital market also faced regulatory changes. In 1998, the US NASDAQ announced that it would join with Masayoshi Son's SoftBank to open an exchange for venture business in Japan. In 1999, the Tokyo Stock Exchange opened Market of the High-Growth and Emerging Stocks (MOTHERS) to promote the listings of high-growth companies. Companies can be listed in MOTHERS without showing a profit and by meeting the minimum JPY500 million or approximately US$5 million market capitalization. The opening of new stock markets served to increase the opportunity for entrepreneurs to raise funds in the early stages of business and for venture capital investors to exit their investments.

The Japanese Commercial Code Law also had several revisions. In 2001, it liberalized the use of stock option schemes and allowed stock options to be issued. In addition, the minimum capital requirement to establish a stock company was reduced from JPY10 million (approximately US$100,000) to a mere JPY1, provided that the new company is established to start a new business and on the condition that the capital is increased to at least JPY10 million within 5 years of establishment. Such incentives were implemented to promote the establishment of start-ups.

4. Conditions and Present Status of Bioventures

The various reforms in Japan's innovation system discussed earlier influenced the emergence and growth of bioventures. By the end of 2009, the cumulative number of bioventures in Japan stood at 553 (see Figure 1). Although the creation of new bioventures was impressive, particularly from 1998 to 2006, in the past few years, the growth of new bioventures has slowed down considerably. Since 2004, the number of newly established bioventures has decreased each year. In 2008, there were only 14 new bioventures compared to 76 new bioventures in 2001 and 2004 (see Figure 2).

Of the 553 bioventures in Japan, only 20 are publicly listed. Listed bioventures represented about 3.6% of the total number of bioventures based on JBA's 2009 survey data (JBA, 2010). Even as listed companies, the financial performance of these bioventures was relatively weak compared to listed biotechnology firms outside of Japan. In 2009, average sale per listed bioventure was JPY1.25 billion or approximately US$13.4 million. Majority of the sales was derived from R&D support payments from their alliance partners or services rendered to their alliance partners. Market performance was not encouraging as well. As of June 2010, all the listed bioventures' market capitalizations were substantially lower than their market

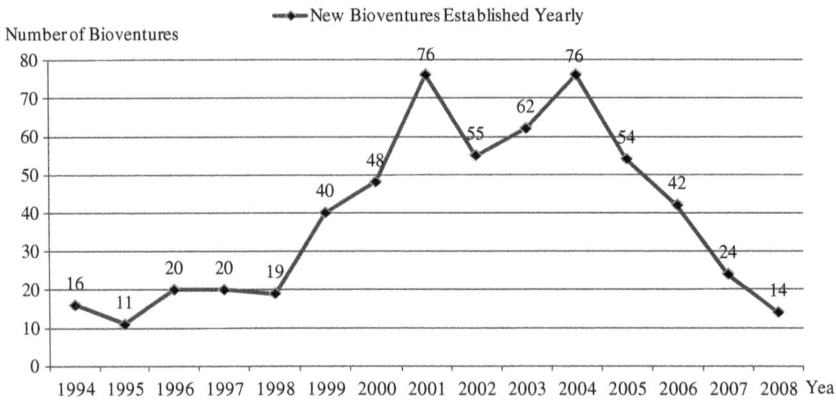

Figure 2. Number of new bioventures established (1994–2008).
Source: JBA (2009).

capitalizations at IPO except for Effector Cell Institutes, Nano Carrier, and Tella (see Table 1).

The performance of the listed bioventures in Table 1 provides a window into the state and condition of bioventures in Japan. If these so-called "more successful" bioventures are only making an average of US$13 million sales per year and have most of their market capitalizations wiped out after their IPO debut, one can only draw the assumption that the performance of the rest of the unlisted bioventures is not good. The question is, why are bioventures underdeveloped despite the various institutional reforms? What is the missing link to this puzzle? After all, when Japan's National Innovation System underwent various reforms and changes, many scholars are positive that such changes would encourage the growth of start-ups (Hane, 2002; Rowen and Toyoda, 2002; Odagiri, 2004; Lynskey, 2004, 2006; Schaede, 2008).

This chapter argues that such reforms are not sufficient for the development of bioventures. Missing in the picture is the lack of a sustainable funding system for bioventures. In other words, changes in the National Innovation System spurred the

Table 1. Financial performance and market capitalization of listed bioventures in Japan.

No.	Bioventure	IPO Date	Sales 2009 (US$ in millions)	Net Profit 2009 (US$ in millions)	Market Cap (at IPO)	Market Cap (6/30/2010)	Change in Market Cap (%)
1.	Anges MG	9/25/2002	6.26	−31.21	405.12	153.30	−62
2.	Trans Genic	12/10/2002	3.47	−6.78	133.12	91.92	−31
3.	Medibic Group	9/18/2003	2.84	−6.58	192.03	16.78	−91
4.	Medinet	10/8/2003	30.98	4.39	525.17	204.19	−61
5.	Oncotherapy Science	12/8/2003	35.56	1.58	1,427.28	385.40	−73
6.	Soiken	12/18/2003	21.15	−1.74	788.77	49.05	−92
7.	DNA Chip Research	3/18/2004	9.33	−3.63	174.08	14.09	−94
8.	Sosei Group	7/1/2004	1.62	−42.07	489.76	109.85	−78
9.	LTT Bio-Pharma	11/25/2004	13.47	−0.15	146.44	44.32	−70
10.	Effector Cell Institute	3/29/2005	3.32	−21.14	44.82	71.83	+60
11.	Pharma Foods International	6/12/2006	7.84	−2.22	163.59	17.39	−89
12.	GNI	8/31/2007	2.18	−14.59	56.71	28.63	−50
13.	J-Tec	12/21/2007	2.26	−11.75	73.00	69.04	−5

(*Continued*)

Table 1. *(Continued)*

No.	Bioventure	IPO Date	Sales	Net Profit	Market Cap (at IPO)	Market Cap (6/30/2010)	Change in Market Cap (%)
			2009 (US$ in millions)				
14.	Nano Carrier	3/5/2008	3.78	–5.61	32.45	32.67	+1
15.	Carna Biosciences	3/25/2008	7.34	–3.37	52.82	25.68	–51
16.	R-Tech Ueno	4/9/2008	64.04	10.00	192.29	74.78	–61
17.	JCL Bioassay	3/17/2009	26.58	2.77	19.44	17.08	–12
18.	Tella	3/26/2009	10.41	1.16	33.25	128.96	+288
19.	CanBas	9/17/2009	1.73	–2.38	119.28	15.05	–87
20.	D. Western Therapeutics Institute	10/23/2009	n/a	–4.19	68.23	32.52	–52
Average			13.38	–7.24	256.88	79.13	–36

Notes: The above amount is converted to US$ based on the following exchange rate — for 2009: JPY93.6 = US$1; for 2010: JPY87.8 = US$1; for Market Cap at IPO: JPY100 = US$1.

emergence of bioventures but did not sufficiently support their development.

5. Funding Impediments

Funding is important for the development of any start-up. However, when it comes to biotechnology start-ups, a supportive and sustainable system of funding is imperative. Unlike the other industries, the commercialization of biotechnology, especially in drug discovery and development, is a long, risky, and costly process. As Orsenigo (1989) noted, "the technical feasibility of the potential applications in biotechnology, the time required to develop them, and above all, the economic revenue that could be generated by innovations in this area are still extremely uncertain". Tufts Center for the Study of Drug Development estimated that a new drug generally takes 10–15 years from discovery and early research to approval. The average out-of-pocket cost per new drug was US$456 million (*in 2000 dollars*). The long and costly process is due to the extremely low percentage of success in drug candidates (DiMasi *et al.*, 2003).

In Japan, bioventures continue to face an uphill battle in procuring funds for their development. Japan's funding system is ill-equipped to nurture such young and risky start-ups. Although there seems to be various sources of funding, such sources of funding are either inaccessible or insufficient for bioventures. The issues of funding are further elaborated in what follows. This discussion is drawn based on a series of interviews conducted with bioventures (see Section 2).

5.1. *R&D funding*

The Japanese government increased its R&D funding for life sciences (including biotechnology) under the First Science and Technology Policy (1996–2000) and the Second Science and

Technology Policy (2001–2005).[1] In response to that, large amounts were sanctioned to grants-in-aid programs for supporting large numbers of individual basic research projects at universities (Nishizawa *et al.*, 2007).[2] However, most of the funds available under life sciences went toward supporting basic research at the universities and research institutes rather than developmental research.

Eight of the bioventures interviewed expressed that R&D funding from the government was inadequate. With the exception of three bioventures, the total amount of R&D funding received was approximately US$2 million per bioventure. The total amount of R&D funding is an aggregate number of grants received from the time of founding to the time the interview was conducted. In addition, most of the R&D grants were not given in the form of upfront payment but rather based on two-thirds of the R&D cost spent.

The bioventures interviewed also voiced that an application for the government R&D grants was a tiring and burdensome process. They commented that such burdensome paperwork was not commensurate with the amount of funding received. With regards to the funding allocation, the interviewed bioventures claimed that priority of funding and amount of funding were allocated based on the extent of collaborations

---

[1]In November 1995, Japan's Science and Technology Basic Law was implemented to provide the legal foundation for science and technology policies in accordance with a 5-year basic plan. The aim of the new law is to explore new frontiers of science and technology and to make greater contributions toward developing new technologies. Following Japan's Science and Technology Basic Law, the government doubled its R&D budget for life sciences (including biotechnology) from around US$2 billion in 1995 to more than US$4 billion in 2001 (Miyata, 2004; Collins, 2004).

[2] Grants-in-aid is awarded by the Ministry of Education, Culture, Sports, Science and Technology (MEXT) through screening by peer review to support creative and pioneering research aimed to develop "academic research" (researcher's creativity-driven research) across a wide spectrum of scientific fields, ranging from the humanities and social sciences to the natural sciences.

with universities. Hence, bioventures that collaborated with well-known university professors were more advantageous over bioventures that collaborated with less well-known university professors.

Only a handful of R&D funding programs released by the Japan's Council for Science and Technology go toward supporting developmental research. The amount of funding varies according to the ministry and their corresponding agencies and programs. For example, under the MEXT — "Local area innovation creation R&D" which intends to nurture university-oriented research results for commercialization — up to JPY26 million (approximately US$260,000) per R&D grant is available for 2–3 years. Under the Japan Science and Technology (JST) "Industry/university cooperation seeds innovation" program, JPY8 million (approximately US$80,000) per R&D grant for up to 1 year is available for proof of concept through feasibility studies. Another additional JPY50 million (approximately US$500,000) per R&D grant for up to 4 years is available for the practicality verification stage. Under the Ministry of Health, Labor and Welfare (MHLW), JPY100–300 million (approximately US$1–3 million) per R&D grant is available for the "Orphan Drug Development Research Project" and the "Investigator Oriented Clinical Trial".

5.2. *Angel investment and small business innovation research funding*

Angel investment is funding given to new ventures operating at the seed or start-up stage. Such investment provides the initial capital for ventures to formulate their businesses. In Japan, it is estimated that there are only about 360 angel investors (Kneller, 2007). Although a tax incentive to support angel investors was created in 1997, by 2008, the investment made by angel investors was just a little over US$80 million (The Nikkei, 2010). In comparison, the US has around 600,000 angel investors and invested an estimated US$23 billion (Shane, 2008). This indicates that the 1997 angel tax incentive program had apparently done little to promote angel investment in Japan.

Another form of funding which is usually available for start-ups is the Small Business Innovation Research (SBIR) program. In Japan, the Law for Facilitating Creation of New Business — known as the Japanese SBIR program — was implemented in 1999 to provide subsidies and debt guarantees to help SMEs to develop and commercialize new technologies. In 2005, the amount allocated for the Japanese SBIR was only US$349 million, about one-third the amount allocated for SBIR program in the US. Only 13% of the funding cases involved biomedical companies [Office of Pharmaceutical Industry Research (2007)]. Unlike the SBIR program in the US, there is no peer review system for the Japanese SBIR. The amount of funding varies from US$10,000 to as high as US$5 million and the period of assistance varies from 1 year to 5 years.

The effectiveness of the SBIR program in supporting the research activities of biotechnology start-ups in the US was noted by Lerner (1996) and Wallsten (2000). However, the same cannot be said of the Japanese SBIR program and its support on bioventures. One of the reasons is that the Japanese SBIR program lacks participating agencies such as the National Institutes of Health (NIH). The NIH contributed an average of US$350 million per year from 2000 to 2010 toward the US SBIR program for supporting start-up biomedical companies (NIH, 2010). The contribution from the NIH alone to the SBIR program was equivalent to the entire Japanese SBIR funding program.

5.3. *Venture capital funding*

Without having a lot of funding access to Angel investors and SBIR program, Japanese bioventures must rely on venture capital for their funding needs. However, Japan's venture capital system has not been developed long enough to provide an abundant supply of risk capital for bioventures. The venture capital system in Japan is modeled after the American venture capital system or "Silicon Valley model" after witnessing the success of its new technology-based industries. Prior to 1998, Japanese venture capital firms could not be legally structured as Limited Liability Partnerships (a common practice in the US and Britain). Thus, many were established as stock company subsidiaries or affiliates of larger securities companies, banks, insurance companies, or large established companies. Even after the establishment of the Limited Liability Partnerships in 1998, many of the old structures of venture capital firms remain. Such venture capital firms are used to giving "loans" rather than "equity investment". Although this ratio is now almost zero, in some venture capital firms the old attitude remains. Equity investments are often treated as functionally equivalent to loans and are evaluated the same way (Yonekura, 2001).

According to the OECD (2009), the amount of venture capital funding in Japan was one of the lowest among developed countries. Although a series of legislations and modifications to the investment system have been enacted to encourage risk capital investments since the late 1990s, the amount of venture capital funding in Japan remained small compared to the US and Europe (see Figure 3). In addition, the average venture capital investment was approximately US$1.13 million, whereas in the US, the average venture capital investment was approximately US$10.42 million (JVCA, 2007).

The amount of venture capital funding in Japan invested in the biotechnology field was ~11.6% per year from 1998 to 2008. This amount is small compared to the venture capital investment in other fields such as information technology (~40%), services (~27%), and manufacturing (~20%) during the same period (Venture Enterprise Center, 2002–2009).

The problem of venture capital funding in Japan lies in its supply of investors who are highly risk averse. The largest investors of venture capital funds in Japan are conventional financial organizations such as banks, securities houses, and insurance companies and large established corporations. In contrast, the largest investors of venture capital funding in the US are

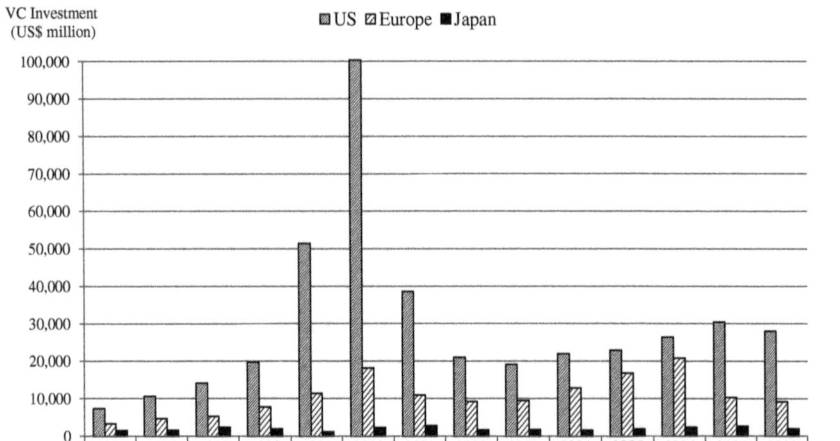

	1995	1996	1997	1998	1999	2000	2001	2002	2003	2004	2005	2006	2007	2008
US	7,373	10,590	14,104	19,658	51,395	100,36	38,524	20,943	19,058	21,897	22,874	26,322	30,422	28,010
Europe	3,380	4,680	5,330	7,800	11,407	18,157	10,932	9,245	9,492	12,875	16,770	20,800	10,400	9,230
Japan	1,511	1,644	2,427	2,004	1,157	2,301	2,814	1,742	1,813	1,650	1,968	2,444	2,790	1,933

Figure 3. Venture capital investment in Japan, the US, and Europe (1995–2008).

Notes: Venture capital investment here refers to the amount of venture capital invested in seed, start-up, expansion, and late stage only. Buyout investments are excluded from this figure. Yearly data are based on 12 months ending in December, including data from Japan. For the sake of simplicity, all the data are based on the following exchange rate: US$1 = JPY100; US$1.3 = 1 Euro. For more accuracy, please refer to the original currency available in the source of data.

Sources: Venture Enterprise Center (2002–2009); EVCA (2005, 2009); NVCA (2010).

pension funds. The contribution from Japanese pension funds remained limited, amounting to less than 3% of the total venture capital funding in Japan (see Table 2).

The highly risk-averse mentality of venture capital firms in Japan is reflected in their investment strategy. The majority of them practice portfolio investment rather than "true venture capital" style investment (Schaede, 2008). Their investment strategy is to invest small amounts in many companies and invite other venture capital firms to make similar investments. By doing so, the risk of a failed investment sullying the reputation of an investment manager will be limited. It is not

Table 2. Sources of venture capital funding in Japan (2001–2008).

Year	2001	2003	2005	2007	2008
Sources of VC funding	**Amount expressed in percentage**				
Bank, trust	28.70	35.00	17.60	12.00	15.20
Security company	2.40	6.60	4.70	5.60	4.30
Insurance	3.30	5.30	8.80	6.70	11.70
Corporations	23.10	12.70	20.10	24.00	18.90
General partner	6.00	15.90	21.50	13.90	36.60
Pension	2.00	2.40	0.00	1.20	2.40
Individual	7.90	0.30	14.40	14.60	5.50
Foreign VCs	3.30	1.10	1.50	13.40	0.20
Others	23.3	20.70	11.40	8.60	5.20
Total	100.00	100.00	100.00	100.00	100.00

Source: Venture Enterprise Center reports from 2002 to 2009.

uncommon for venture capital firms to have hundreds of such small-scale investments because of their investment strategy. They typically do not seek a position in the bioventures' Board of Directors and are often reluctant to do so because it is too time consuming. It is not uncommon for a bioventure to have more than 25 venture capital firms investing in them as well.

Another distinctive investment strategy of Japanese venture capital firms is the practice of *yoko narabi*. This is a Japanese term which literally means "do as others do". The rationality of *yoko narabi* is to avoid social embarrassment by adhering strictly to the group's norm, rules, and expectations. In order not to appear inferior to other companies, they "match each other's move and try to do the same thing" (Yoshimura and Anderson, 1997). In the case of venture capital funding, *yoko narabi* refers to how a venture capital firm copies another venture capital firm's move. If a venture capital firm invests in a bioventure, the rest of the venture capital community tends to follow because they do not want to miss out on the opportunity if the investment turns out to be good. On the contrary, if the investment fails, they minimize their risk by investing as a group. Due to the *yoko narabi* practice, most venture capital firms are less inclined to conduct their own extensive due diligence. They prefer to depend on the lead venture capital firm's evaluation or other venture capital firms who have already invested in the bioventure. This leads to fewer numbers of venture capital "specialists" or "professionals" who are truly competent in assessing biotechnology investments.

5.4. *Public equity funding*

Many biotechnology start-ups in the US, Canada, and Europe obtain their funding from public equity particularly through an IPO. There are two important reasons why an IPO needs to occur. First, an IPO provides the point of entry that gives start-ups expanded access to equity capital, allowing them to emerge and grow (Fama and French, 2004). Second, all the money invested by a venture capital firm needs to have an exit and the stock market provides one of the most common exits to venture capital investment. Without such exits, venture capital money will not flow back to the system for investments in new companies (Gompers and Lerner, 2001).

Japan lacks a vibrant IPO market for its biotechnology start-ups. Currently, there are only 20 listed bioventures compared to more than 350 listed biotechnology companies in the US. The average amount of funding procured from IPO for the 20 listed bioventures from 2002 to 2009 was JPY2,697 million or approximately US$27 million (see Table 3). In addition, the amount of funding from IPO was smaller compared to the amount of IPO funding obtained from the US and Europe during the same period (see Table 4).

The Japanese stock market failed to provide a favorable environment to encourage the listing of bioventures. One of the main reasons lies in the profile of its investors. Emerging

Table 3. Number of bioventure IPOs and amount of funding from IPOs (2002–2009).

Year	**2002**	**2003**	**2004**	**2005**	**2006**	**2007**	**2008**	**2009**
IPO by bioventures (from all stock exchanges in Japan)	2	4	3	1	1	2	3	4
Total amount of IPO funding (US$ million)	60.58	170.95	128.00	38.00	28.29	39.00	22.27	27.41
Average amount of IPO funding per bioventure (US$ million)	30.29	42.74	42.27	38.00	28.29	19.50	7.42	6.85

Notes: The original amount of funding is recorded in JPY. The amount reflected here is converted to US$ based on the following exchange rate: US$1 = JPY100.
Source: TSE (2010).

Table 4. Comparison of biotechnology IPOs between Japan, US, and Europe.

Year	Japan		Europe		US	
	Average amount of IPO funding (US$ million)	Number of biotech IPOs	Average amount of IPO funding (US$ million)	Number of biotech IPOs	Average amount of IPO funding (US$ million)	Number of biotech IPOs
2004	42.27	3	51.88	8	59.99	28
2005	38.00	1	38.90	21	48.15	13
2006	28.29	2	32.76	25	47.20	20
2007	19.50	3	48.10	21	56.27	22
2008	7.42	3	37.00	3	6.00	1

Sources: Ernst & Young (2005, 2006, 2007a, 2007b, 2008, 2009) and TSE (2010).

stock markets in Japan for high-growth companies such as MOTHERS, JASDAQ, and Hercules do not have a large participation from institutional investors. In 2007, the biggest group of investors for the MOTHERS, JASDAQ, and Hercules exchanges were individual investors with 76.3%, 78.9%, and 78.5% investment, respectively. Institutional investors account for less than 9% for each of the exchanges. On the contrary, during the same year, the biggest group of investors for the NASDAQ Stock Exchange in the US were institutional investors with 77% investment and individual investors accounting for only 6% investment (see Table 5).

Another reason is the tightening of listing requirements for Japan's emerging stock markets such as MOTHERS since 2005. Bioventures are still not required to show profitability in order to be listed. However, an additional requirement calls for drug discovery and development bioventures to have at least two drugs in the clinical trial stage and the drugs to be accompanied by a licensing or cooperative research agreement with one or more pharmaceutical companies.

The lack of participation by institutional investors is among the main reasons that caused wide swings in the market capitalization of the existing listed bioventures. Individual investors

Table 5. Investor profile in Japan's emerging markets and US NASDAQ stock exchange.

	Japan			US
Exchanges	**MOTHERS**	**JASDAQ**	**Hercules**	**NASDAQ**
Type of investors		**Unit in percentage**		
Institutional investors	8.7	8.0	8.7	77.0
Foreign investors	14.8	12.6	12.6	12.0
Individual investors	76.3	78.9	78.5	6.0
Others	0.2	0.5	0.2	5.0

Sources: Tokyo Stock Exchange, Osaka Stock Exchange, and NASDAQ Stock Exchange websites.

are small-time investors with limited cash, and they tend to trade based on rumors and news rather than rationality. Individual investors are unable to provide the same kind of investment amount and volume driven by institutional investors. Due to their low holding power, individual investors who have been scorched by declining stock prices are unable to invest more. According to Robbins-Ruth (2000), for the biotechnology sector, the support of institutional investors is needed to balance out the short-term trading of hedge funds, Internet-based day traders, and the general public. As indicated in Table 1 earlier, market capitalization of 18 out of the 20 listed bioventures has decreased substantially since the day they were listed. Thus, there is little attraction for bioventures to seek funding from Japan's capital market.

6. Conclusion and Implication

In the last decade, Japan has created a plethora of biotechnology start-ups known as bioventures. The emergence and the development of bioventures are important because they are a critical source of biotechnology innovation. The discussion of this chapter is limited to the funding impediment confronting bioventures in Japan. There could be other impediments to explain the underdeveloped state of bioventures such as entrepreneurship, mobility of researchers, university–industry linkages, and alliances. However, this chapter maintains that funding is the real issue hindering the development of bioventures. The development of bioventures is threatened by the lack of a sustainable system of funding that caters to high-risk technologies, long gestation periods, and high capital intensity.

Since the late 1990s, Japan's innovation system has underwent many changes, but funding of start-ups such as bioventures has remained a big impediment. For example, there is a general increase in R&D funding from the government, but as a science-based industry, biotechnology requires not only funding in basic research but also substantial funding in the developmental stage. Without funds for commercialization, bioventures are unable to produce proof-of-concept products or to conduct early clinical trials. Another example is angel investment. The low amount and low number of angel investors indicate that the current angel tax incentive program has done little to promote angel investment. Likewise, more attention should be given to promote venture capital funding. The 1997 investment rule that allowed pension funds to invest in venture capital is ineffective since the contributions from pension funds in Japan remained tiny, amounting to less than 3% of the total venture capital funding.

A vicious cycle has emerged among bioventures because the current funding system is not sustainable. The lack of R&D funding from the government and angel investors drove bioventures to seek venture capital funding at an early stage. However, many of the Japanese venture capital firms could only provide a small amount of investment. After a short period of time, bioventures must look for more capital. Going for an IPO becomes their last resort for funding, but even after the IPO, bioventures continue to struggle with funding. Many of the listed bioventures were at the premature stage of development when they had their IPO. They required more funding for their R&D before they could license out their products to their partners to generate any income of their own. The lack of funding led to delays in milestones and sales projections which plunged their share prices and erased their market capitalization. The chain of negative events discouraged new investments in bioventures, and the vicious cycle became more entrenched.

Unlike the case of Japan, the biotechnology industry in the US and certain European countries such as the UK prospered, thanks to an abundance of R&D funding from the government, high levels of venture capital investment, and a vibrant capital market. In 2008, the US had 1,754 biotechnology companies, of which 371 were publicly listed. These listed biotechnology companies had a total revenue of US$66 billion. Besides the US, the UK holds the next biggest biotechnology industry. In

2008, the UK had 777 biotechnology companies, of which 56 were publicly listed with combined revenues of approximately US$6.6 billion (Ernst & Young, 2009). In contrast, during the same year, total revenues from biotechnology companies in Japan amounted to only approximately US$870 million (JBA, 2009). In addition, during the last few years, there was a furry of M&A activities involving biotechnology companies. Lured by decreasing pipelines, patent expirations, and international competition, larger pharmaceutical companies or mega biotechnology companies were acquiring smaller biotechnology companies in the US, the UK, and Germany. However, none of the M&A deals involved Japanese bioventures as acquisition targets. Interestingly, Japanese pharmaceutical companies were some of the active acquirers of biotechnology companies, but they do not see Japanese bioventures as having a significant value to them due to their immature pipelines and technologies.

If the past is any indication of the future, the prospect of bioventures in Japan is at stake. Japan has successfully created a plethora of bioventures. However, the aim here should not merely be to create a large number of small businesses but to create large, sustainable, globally competitive biotechnology companies. Since funding from venture capital is particularly vital for the development of such bioventures, one possible solution is to increase the amount of venture capital funding. According to the *Wall Street Journal*, the Japanese Government Pension Investment is the largest single-pension fund in the world with assets totaling JPY123 trillion ($1.433 trillion). Roughly 67.5% of the fund's assets are invested in domestic bonds, including government and corporate bonds, 12% in Japanese stocks, 10.8% in overseas shares, and 8.3% in foreign bonds. The yield on the 10-year Japanese government bond is 1.075% (*The Wall Street Journal* Asia, 2010). If a mere 1% of the fund's assets is invested into venture capital, this would equal US$14.3 billion, more than seven times the total amount of venture capital investment made in Japan in 2008. Assuming some portion of the funding goes into biotechnology, bioventures would benefit from the increase in risk capital for their development.

Increasing the amount of venture capital funding for biotechnology is the first important step of many other steps needed to boost the biotechnology industry in Japan. That alone is a massive challenge because it calls for a change of mind-set to accept higher risks and a change in the old ways of doing business. There will be resistance to change because institutions and organizations exist within a complex, intertwined web of relationships with each system deeply rooted in its own idiosyncrasies, history, culture, and social patterns. However, change is very much needed if Japan wants to cultivate its bioventures to build a successful biotechnology industry.

Appendix A. Key Findings from Interviews with Japanese Bioventures

	Medinet Co. Ltd. (Interview date: 12 February 2010)
Founded	1995
Founder	Yoshiji Kimura and Koji Egawa
Business	Personalized medicine and immune-cell therapy
Origin of core technology (professor)	University of Tokyo (Koji Egawa)
R&D funding	Various R&D grants including Tokyo SME Agency, JST under MEXT and MHLW. Approximately US$3.5 million received in total R&D funding
Angel and venture capital	None from angel or venture capital during the early days. Approximately US$10 million private placement from venture capital prior to IPO
Public equity	Obtained US$42 million from IPO on 8 October 2003

(Continued)

(*Continued*)

	NanoCarrier Ltd. (Interview date: 26 October 2009; 1 and 20 January 2010)
Founded	1996
Founder	Ichiro Nakatomi
Business	Drug delivery system using nanoparticles
Origin of core technology (professor)	University of Tokyo (Kazunori Kataoka) Tokyo Women's Medical University (Teruo Okano)
R&D funding	Various R&D grants from Tokyo SME Agency, METI, JST under MEXT and MHLW. Approximately US$5–6 million received in total R&D funding
Angel and venture capital	US$2 million in 1999, US$5.7 million in 2001, US$16.3 million in 2004, US$3.4 million in 2006, and US$11.8 million in 2007. Approximately US$39 million in total
Public equity	Obtained US$6.4 million from IPO on 5 March 2008

	AnGes MG Inc. (Interview date: 24 and 25 December 2009; 20 August 2010)
Founded	1999
Founder	Ryuichi Morishita
Business	Drug discovery and development based on gene therapy
Origin of core technology (professor)	Osaka University (Ryuichi Morishita)
R&D funding	Various R&D grants from government agencies and ministries such as NEDO, MEXT, and MITI. More than US$10 million received in total R&D funding

(*Continued*)

(*Continued*)

Angel and venture capital	Small amount of angel investment during the early years. Approximately US$9.4 million private placement from venture capital prior to IPO
Public equity	Obtained US$35 million from IPO on 25 September 2002. Follow-up funding of US$58 million in October 2003 and US$73 million in March 2007

	M's Science Corporation (Interview date: 9 February 2010)
Founded	2000
Founder	Shiro Mita
Business	Drug discovery and development (central nervous system disorders and cancer)
Origin of core technology (professor)	Santen Pharmaceuticals and Nagoya University (Yukihiro Nishiyama)
R&D funding	Mainly from NEDO under MEXT. Approximately US$1.9 million in total R&D funding
Angel and venture capital	US$2.5 million in 2001, US$5.8 million in 2003, US$20.2 million in 2004, US$7 million in 2007, and US$8 million in 2008. Approximately US$44.5 million in total
Public equity	Not applicable because the company is not listed

	aRigen Pharmaceuticals, Inc. (Interview date: 20 February 2009; 21 July 2010)
Founded	2001
Founder	Gensuke Tokoro
Business	Drug discovery and development focusing on infectious diseases
Origin of core technology (professor)	In-licensed from universities in Japan. Details are not disclosed

(*Continued*)

(*Continued*)

R&D funding	Mainly from NEDO under MEXT. Approximately US$1.5 million received in total R&D funding
Angel and venture capital	Various stages since early days. Details are not disclosed. More than US$40 million in total
Public equity	Not applicable because the company is not listed

	Nobelpharma Co. Ltd. (Interview date: 9 February 2010)
Founded	2003
Founder	Jin Shiomura
Business	Drug development based on orphan drugs, off-label use pharmaceuticals, and pediatric pharmaceuticals
Origin of core technology (professor)	In house
R&D funding	Mainly from MHLW (R&D grant for orphan drug designation). Approximately US$1.8 million in total R&D funding
Angel and venture capital	None
Public equity	Not applicable because the company is not listed

	Oncolys Biopharma (Interview date: 3 December 2009)
Founded	2004
Founder	Yasuo Urata
Business	Drug discovery and development focusing on cancer and infectious diseases

(*Continued*)

(*Continued*)

Origin of core technology (professor)	Okayama University Hospital (Toshiyoshi Fujiwara) and in-licensed compounds from Yale University
R&D funding	Mainly from JST, NEDO under MEXT and Kobe City. Approximately US$1.5 million in total R&D funding
Angel and venture capital	US$5 million in 2004, US$26 million in 2006, and US$8 million in 2008. Approximately US$39 million in total
Public equity	Not applicable because the company is not listed

	PeptiDream (Interview date: 17 March 2010)
Founded	2006
Founder	Hiroaki Suga
Business	Drug discovery based on peptide therapeutics
Origin of core technology (professor)	University of Tokyo (Hiroaki Suga)
R&D funding	Some R&D funding from JST under MEXT. Details are undisclosed
Angel and venture capital	35% capital came from venture capital (University of Tokyo Edge Capital)
Public equity	Not applicable because the company is not listed

References

Braguinsky, S., Honjo, Y. and Nagaoka, S. *et al*. (2010). Science-based business: Knowledge capital or entrepreneurship ability? Theory and Evidence from a survey of biotechnology start-ups. *IIR Working Paper No. 10-05*. Hitotsubashi University.

Collins, S. (2004). *The Race to Commercialize Biotechnology: Molecules, Market and the State in Japan and the US*, Routledge, London.

DiMasi, J., Hansen, R. and Grabowski, H. (2003). The price of innovation: New estimates of drug development costs, *Journal of Health Economics*, 22(2), 151–185.

Ernst & Young (2005). *Beyond Borders: Global Biotechnology Report 2005*, Ernst & Young, London.

Ernst & Young (2006). *Beyond Borders: Global Biotechnology Report 2006*, Ernst & Young, London.

Ernst & Young (2007a). *Beyond Borders: Global Biotechnology Report 2007*, Ernst & Young, London.

Ernst & Young (2007b). Europe Supplement to *Beyond Borders: Global Biotechnology Report 2007*, Ernst & Young, London.

Ernst & Young (2008). *Beyond Borders: Global Biotechnology Report 2008*, Ernst & Young, London.

Ernst & Young (2009). *Beyond Borders: Global Biotechnology Report 2009*, Ernst & Young, London.

EVCA (2005). *Employment Contribution of Private Equity and Venture Capital in Europe*. European Private Equity & Venture Capital Association, Brussels.

EVCA (2009). *EVCA 2009 Yearbook*. European Private Equity & Venture Capital Association, Brussels.

Fama, E. F. and French, K. R. (2004). New lists: Fundamentals and survival rates, *Journal of Financial Economics*, 73(2), 229–269.

Gambardella, A. and McGahan, A. M. (2010). Business-model innovation: General purpose technologies and their implications for industry structure, *Long Range Planning*, 43(2), 262–271.

Gompers, P. and Lerner, J. (2001). The venture capital revolution, *Journal of Economic Perspectives*, 15(2), 145–168.

Grabowski, H. and Vernon, J. (1994). Innovation and structural change in pharmaceuticals and biotechnology, *Industrial and Corporate Change*, 3, 435–449.

Hane, G. (2002). *Opportunity to Outcome — Progress and the Paradox of Past Success in Japan's Evolving Venture Environment*. The MIT Japan Program.

JBA (2002). Biotechnology Strategy Guidelines. Biotechnology Strategy Council. Available at: http://www.jba.or.jp/jabex/pdf/BT%20Strategy%20Guideline%20%28translated%20by%20JETRO%29.pdf.

JBA (2009). *2008 Bioventures Statistic Report* [2008 nen baibencha toukei chousa houkokushou] (in Japanese). Japan Bioindustry Association, Tokyo.

JBA (2010). *2009 Bioventures Statistic Report* [2009 nen baibencha toukei chousa houkokushou] (in Japanese). Japan Bioindustry Association, Tokyo.

JVCA (2007). The Supply of Venture Capital [Bencha kyapitaru wo tsujite shikin kyoukyuu] (in Japanese). Available at: http://www.meti.go.jp/committee/materials/downloadfiles/g71025a04j.pdf.

Kneller, R. (1999). Intellectual property rights and university–industry technology transfer in Japan, in *Industrializing Knowledge — University–Industry Linkages in Japan and the United States*, The MIT Press, Boston.

Kneller, R. (2007). *Bridging Islands: Venture Companies and the Future of Japanese and American Industry*, Oxford University Press, New York.

Kneller, R. (2010). The importance of new companies for drug discovery: Origins of a decade of new drugs, *Nature Reviews Drug Discovery*, 9, 867–882.

Kondo, M. (2009). University–industry partnerships in Japan, in *21st Century Innovation Systems for Japan and the United States: Lessons from a Decade of Change: Report of a Symposium*, National Academies Press.

Lerner, J. (1996). *The Government as Venture Capitalist: The Long-run Impact of the SBIR Program*. National Bureau of Economic Research (NBER).

Lerner, J. (1999). Small business, innovation and public policy, in *Are Small Firms Important?* Academic Publishing, London.

Lynskey, M. J. (2004). Bioentrepreneurship in Japan: Institutional transformation and the growth of bioventures, *Journal of Commercial Biotechnology*, 11(1), 9–37.

Lynskey, M. J. (2006). Transformative technology and institutional transformation: Coevolution of biotechnology venture firms and the institutional framework in Japan, *Research Policy*, 35(9), 1389–1422.

Malerba, F. (2004). *Sectoral Systems of Innovation*, Cambridge University Press, Cambridge.

Miyata, M. (1994). Towards a new era in biotechnology, *Science and Technology in Japan*, 50, 10–13.

Motohashi, K. (2005). University–industry collaboration in Japan: The role of new technology-based firms in transforming the National Innovation System, *Research Policy*, 34, 583-594.

NIH (2010). SBIR and STTR: Awards and total funding, by phase. NIH Budget website. Available at: http://report.nih.gov/budget_and_spending/index.aspx.

Nikkei Biotechnology (2009). *2009 Nikkei Biotechnology* [2009 Nikkei Baio Nenkan] (in Japanese). Nikkei BP, Tokyo.

Nishizawa, M., Negishi, M. and Shibayama, M. (2007). Evaluation of Japanese universities' research activity based on the number of awards of Grants-in-aid for Scientific Research from 1998 to 2002 and in 2003, *Progress in Informatics*, 4, 79–101.

NVCA (2010). PricewaterhouseCoopers/National Venture Capital Association MoneyTree Report. Available at: https://www.pwcmoneytree.com/MTPublic/ns/index.jsp.

Odagiri, H. (2004). Advance of Science-Based Industries and the Changing Innovation System in Japan. *COE/RES Discussion Paper Series*, No. 64. Hitotsubashi University, Tokyo.

Odagiri, H. (2006). Co-Evolution of the National Business System and the National Innovation System in the Age of Science-Based Innovation, with an Application to Biotechnology. *COE/RES Discussion Paper Series*, No. 129. Hitotsubashi University, Tokyo.

Odagiri, H. and Nakamura, Y. (2002). Biotechnology-Related Start-up Firms in Japan: Lessons from a Survey Study [*Nihon no baio bencha kigyou igi to jinou*] (in Japanese). National Institute of Science and Technology Policy, Tokyo.

OECD (2009). *OECD Biotechnology Statistics 2009*, OECD Publishing, Paris.

Office of Pharmaceutical Industry Research (2007). *Future of Pharmaceutical Industry*. Office of Pharmaceutical Industry Research, Tokyo.

Orsenigo, L. (1989). *The Emergence of Biotechnology*, Frances Pinter, London.

Rowen, H. S. and Toyoda, M. A. (2002). From Keiretsu to Startups: Japan's Push for High Tech Entrepreneurship. The Walter H. Shorenstein Asia Pacific Research Center. *Working Paper*, Stanford University,

Schaede, U. (2008). *Choose and Focus: Japanese Business Strategy for the 21st Century*, Cornell University Press, New York.

Shane, S. (2008). The Importance of Angel Investing in Financing the Growth of Entrepreneurial Ventures. *Working Paper*, No. 331. Small Business Administration Office of Advocacy.

The Nikkei (2010). *Lack of Venture Capital Choking Bio Start-ups.* December 9, 2010. The Nikkei.

The Wall Street Journal Asia (2010). *Japan Weighs More Risk in Pension.* September 18, 2010. *The Wall Street Journal* Asia.

TSE. (2010). *Mothers Exchange Monthly Report* — May 2010. Tokyo Stock Exchange, Tokyo.

Venture Enterprise Center (2002). *2002 Venture Capital Investment Report,* [2002 bencha kyapitaru nado toushi doukou chousa houkoku] (in Japanese). Venture Enterprise Center, Tokyo.

Venture Enterprise Center (2003). *2003 Venture Capital Investment Report* [2003 bencha kyapitaru nado toushi doukou chousa houkoku] (in Japanese). Venture Enterprise Center, Tokyo.

Venture Enterprise Center (2004). *2004 Venture Capital Investment Report* [2004 bencha kyapitaru nado toushi doukou chousa houkoku] (in Japanese). Venture Enterprise Center, Tokyo.

Venture Enterprise Center (2005). *2005 Venture Capital Investment Report* [2005 bencha kyapitaru nado toushi doukou chousa houkoku] (in Japanese). Venture Enterprise Center, Tokyo.

Venture Enterprise Center (2006). *2006 Venture Capital Investment Report* [2006 bencha kyapitaru nado toushi doukou chousa houkoku] (in Japanese). Venture Enterprise Center, Tokyo.

Venture Enterprise Center (2007). *2007 Venture Capital Investment Report* [2007 bencha kyapitaru nado toushi doukou chousa houkoku] (in Japanese). Venture Enterprise Center, Tokyo.

Venture Enterprise Center (2008). *2008 Venture Capital Investment Report* [2008 bencha kyapitaru nado toushi doukou chousa houkoku] (in Japanese). Venture Enterprise Center, Tokyo.

Venture Enterprise Center (2009). *2009 Summary of Venture Business Survey and Prospect Report* [2009 bencha bijunesu no kaitou to tenbou — youyaku ban] (in Japanese). Venture Enterprise Center, Tokyo.

Wallsten, S. J. (2000). The Effects of Government-Industry R&D Programs on Private R&D: The Case of the Small Business Innovation Research Program. *Rand Journal of Economics*, 31, 1: 82–100.

Yin, R. K. (1984). *Case Study Research: Design and Methods*. Newbury Park: Sage Publications.

Yonekura, S. (2001). Venture capital system and venture business, in *Innovation Management Manual [Inobeshon manejimento nyumon] (in Japanese),* Hitotsubashi University: Institute of Innovation Research. Nikkei Publishing, Tokyo.

Yoshimura, N. and Anderson, P. (1997). *Inside the Kaisha: Demystifying Japanese Business Behavior*, Harvard Business Press, Boston.

Zucker, L. G. and Darby, M. R. (1994). The organization of biotechnology science and its commercialization in Japan, in *1994–1995 — Biotechnology Studies*, Volume VI, Institute of Social Science and Research, University of California Los Angeles.

Zucker, L. G. and Darby, M. R. (1996). *Star Scientists, Institutions and the Entry of Japanese Biotechnology Enterprises*. National Bureau of Economic Research.

Zucker, L. G. and Darby, M. R. (2001). Change or die: The adoption of biotechnology in the Japanese and U.S. pharmaceutical industries, *Comparative Studies of Technological Evolution*, 7, 85–125.

Chapter 3

Systems Engineering Approaches for Improving Reusable Medical Equipment Reprocessing Processes

James C. Benneyan* and Claire Massero†

Healthcare Systems Engineering Institute, Northeastern University, MA, USA

**j.benneyan@northeastern.edu*
†cmassero@bwh.harvard.edu

Abstract

Hospital reusable medical equipment (RME) include any items that are intended to be reprocessed and reused indefinitely, including surgical instruments, dental equipment, endoscopes, and others. Such equipment represent a significant portion of a hospital's inventory costs and recently have generated significant patient cross-contamination concerns due to reprocessing cleaning failures. This chapter discusses recent applications of industrial and systems engineering (ISyE) methods within healthcare organizations to help manage, understand, and improve RME processes, including quality control, reliability, patient safety, facility layout, queueing networks, and inventory management models. Several examples demonstrate the value of these approaches for improved reprocessing management of RME technology.

Keywords: RME, safety, queueing networks.

1. Introduction

1.1. *Motivation*

This chapter summarizes applications of industrial and systems engineering (ISyE) methods to reusable medical equipment (RME) reprocessing processes in order to improve their overall safety, quality, cost, flow, utilization, and scheduling. RME and related technologies used throughout healthcare present significant cost, logistical, and patient safety concerns. RME is defined as "any medical equipment designed by the manufacturer to be reused for multiple patients" (Department of Veterans Affairs, 2009) and comprises a significant portion of hospital inventory costs. Examples include surgical tools, dental equipment, endoscopes, laryngoscopes, anesthesia face masks, ob/gyn equipment, and others.

Figure 1 and Table 1 illustrate examples of common RME items. An average hospital owns hundreds of reusable instruments, some costing many thousands of dollars. Safety and quality of RME cleaning processes are also important concerns, with a number of recent incidents putting patient health at risk. As one of several examples, a miscommunication and human error within the Veterans Affairs (VA) healthcare system in 2008 resulted in 10,716 veterans being notified of possible viral infection risks (Daigh, 2009) due to an incorrect connector used to link cleaning solution to endoscopes during reprocessing (VHA Warning System, 2004). While causality is unclear, of those

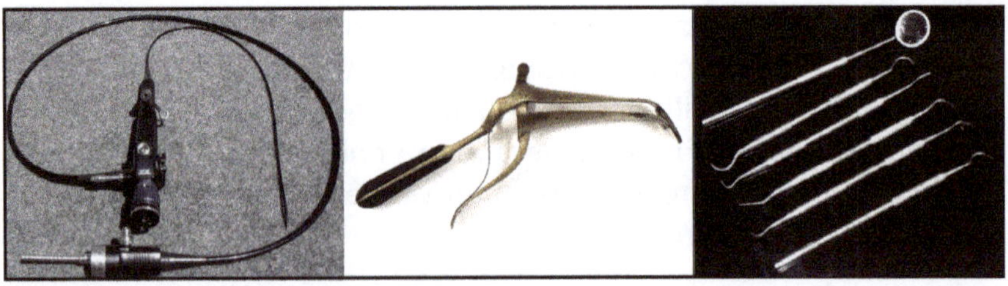

Figure 1. Examples of RME: Endoscope, laryngoscope, and dental tools.

Table 1. Examples of typical RME items within a typical mid-sized hospital.

Department/ Location	**Typical quantity***
Anesthesia	16
GI endoscopy	61
ENT endoscopy	52
Urology	24
Eye clinics	94
Bronchoscopy	21
Cardiology	4
Dental	9,980
Speech pathology	17
Specialty clinics	398
Sleep lab	249
OR	17
Primary care	199

Note: * quantities represent a typical 400-bed hospital.

notified, 28 patients subsequently tested positive for hepatitis B (6), hepatitis C (19), and HIV (3) (Associated Press, 2009).

In the private sector, similar incidents involving endoscopes and tools used for vaginal exams occurred in June 2010 at Palomar Hospital in San Diego, CA (Thomas, 2010). In 2005, Duke University's Health System reportedly operated on approximately 3,650 patients using surgical instruments that accidentally had been washed with hydraulic fluid due to a truly bizarre sequence of misplacement and confusion events (Duke, 2007). More recently, improper hand cleaning of dental equipment in July 2010 lead to more than 1,800 patients at the John Cochran VA Medical Center in St. Louis, MO, potentially being exposed to hepatitis and HIV (*CNN*, 2010). Over the past decade, roughly a dozen other RME patient safety concerns in public and private hospitals have been reported in the media. While such mistakes thankfully are rare, the health and liability consequences can be catastrophic. As in other industries, in such settings a variety of ISyE methods can help design ultra-reliable error-proof processes.

1.2. *General RME processes*

Figure 2 illustrates a typical process flow for reusable equipment, including transport to a reprocessing area, various cleaning and sterilization steps, quality control (QC), packaging and storage, and transport back to the point of use. Any reprocessing area typically has a large amount of cleaning and reprocessing equipment that technicians are expected to be expert in using correctly in handling different RME items. The RME items could come from any number of different care units throughout the hospital, including the surgical clinic, operating room, colonoscopy suite, respiratory devices, and others. While in this example all equipment is routed to a centralized reprocessing area (in this case the supply processing and distribution (SPD) area), in other

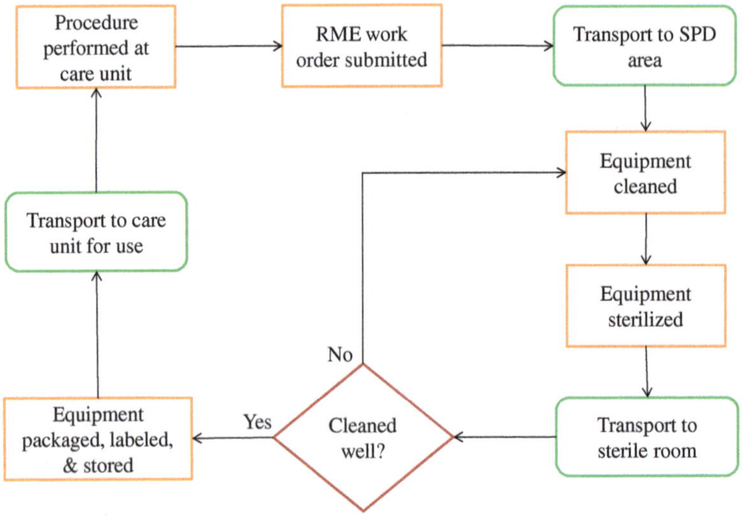

Figure 2. Typical flow of RME through SPD process.

facilities some of these functions may be decentralized and performed adjacent to where the RME items are used.

Figure 3 summarizes similar RME reprocessing logic from a 1980 study in a North Dakota hospital (Smalley, 1982). It is especially interesting to note that not much has changed over the

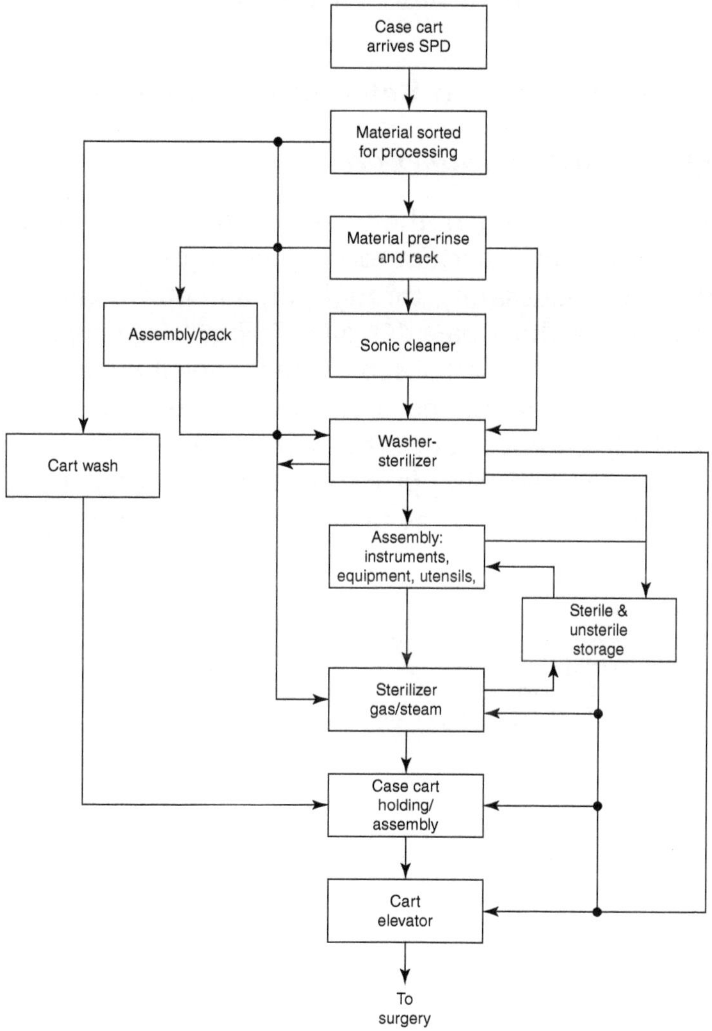

Figure 3. General reprocessing and cleaning process for RME.
Source: Adapted from Smalley (1982).

past 30 years in terms of general process logic, cleaning technology, and device design. The following sections therefore describe quality, safety, logistics, and flow methods that healthcare organizations can use to improve their reusable technology processes. In particular, recent uses of queuing networks, computer simulation, and redundancy optimization models are demonstrated for optimizing RME processes.

2. Quality, Safety, and Reliability Approaches

2.1. *Quality trilogy framework*

The use and integration of the three key legs of quality management (QM) play an important role in any industry to reduce variability and increase safety, throughput, and profitability. Figure 4 illustrates the three-part "Quality Trilogy" framework introduced by the QM expert Joseph Juran, consisting of an equal balance of (1) planning and prevention, (2) control and detection, and (3) improvement. The first phase, quality planning (QP), focuses on designing processes that do not fail in the first place by using tools such as failure modes and effects analysis

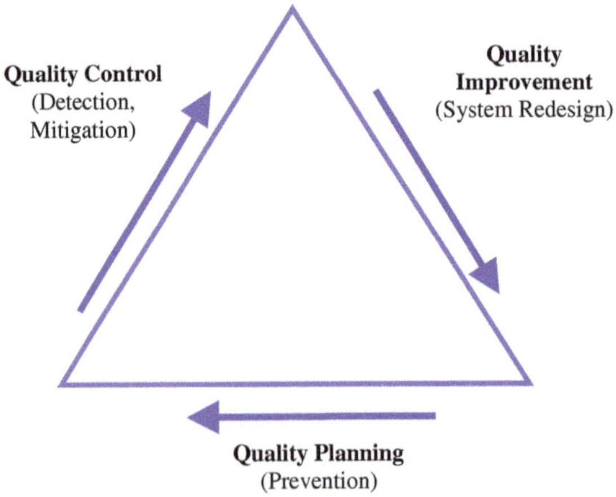

Figure 4. The Juran quality trilogy: Quality Planning, Quality Control, and Quality Improvement.

(FMEA), fault tree diagrams, deliberate redundant design, reliability analysis, and others. The second phase, quality control (QC), focuses on detecting and lessening problems soon after they occur, typically using statistical quality control (SQC), inspection sampling, and risk management methods. The third and final phase, quality improvement (QI), focuses on improving existing processes through data analysis, root cause analysis (RCA), and continuous process improvement methods such as Six Sigma and Lean.

This holistic view of process quality as an overall three-phase system was noted in a recent Senate hearing on the aforementioned VA endoscope reprocessing failure by Dr. Thomas Nolan, a healthcare improvement specialist, who stated "it is notable, however, that [QI efforts occurred only] *after* the fact. If instead they were an *input* to QP and system design, this would help accomplish one of the key goals of QM: *prevention* of defects through design of reliable systems" (Nolan, 2009). As Nolan indicated, healthcare currently tends to turn to quality methods only after a safety or other performance issue has occurred. Instead, QP and control methods such as FMEA and SQC should be used proactively rather than reactively to prevent such problems from occurring; in the ideal world, QI and system redesign are unnecessary. Table 2 lists

Table 2. Quality management methods within Juran's trilogy context.

Quality planning (QP)	Quality control (QC)	Quality improvement (QI)
Failure modes and effects analysis (FMEA)	Statistical quality control (SQC)	Data analysis
Fault tree diagrams	Acceptance sampling plans	Continuous QI
Forcing functions	Inspection	Six Sigma/Lean
Redundant design	Risk management	Root cause analysis
Critical path method	Cause–Effect diagram	Re-engineering
Design of experiments	Value stream maps	Pareto diagrams

some of the more common methods within Juran's framework, with several applications discussed in further detail in the remainder of this section.

2.2. *Statistical quality control*

Statistical quality control (SQC) methods are useful to accomplish two important functions, while accounting for natural process variability: (1) detecting process changes or verifying improvements, and (2) testing for and achieving standardized consistent processes. As an RME example of the first use, Figure 5 illustrates a control chart designed to detect an increase in the frequency of point-of-use flash sterilizations (Benneyan *et al.*, 2003), a general indicator of poor overall process quality often due to failures in the primary process.

Points on this graph above the upper threshold (the "upper control limit" in SQC terminology) indicated a statistically

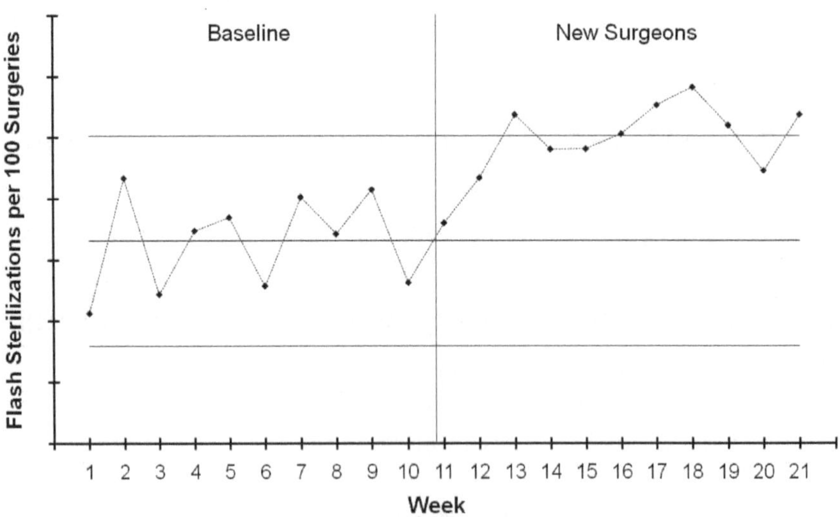

Figure 5. Quality control chart of the flash sterilization rate, detecting process deterioration due to untrained staff.
Source: Benneyan *et al.* (2003).

significant increase in failures to follow standardized procedures. Detection of such events in relatively real-time should immediately trigger (1) pre-designed contingency processes to mitigate or minimize harm and (2) QI activities to prevent similar events in the future, such as RCA and process redesign. While typically thought of in the context of detecting if processes deteriorate, such a chart is also useful to verify the effectiveness of improvement interventions, which would be indicated here by points below the lower control limit.

Prior to this passive monitoring activity, the second and equally important use of control charts is to test for and help achieve stable and standardized processes, which are critical for error prevention and efficient process flow. Figure 6 illustrates this concept in the context of RME items failing a QC inspection and needing to be re-cleaned, which in this example statistically is in a state of chaos — with data outside both control limits indicating an inconsistent, non-standardized, and poorly

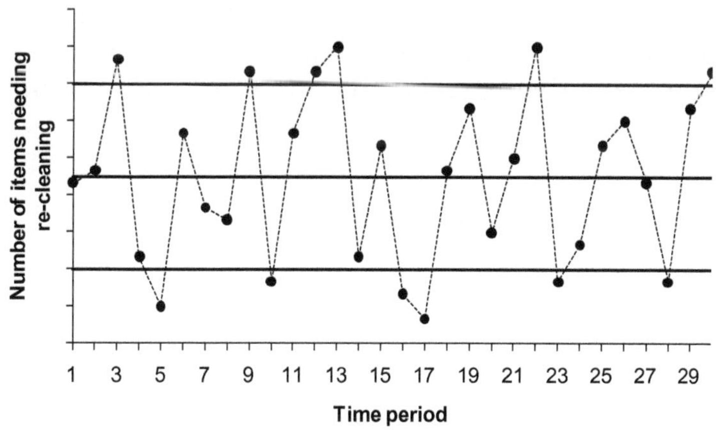

Figure 6. Control chart of QC failures: number of RME items needing to repeat cleaning steps, evidence of the lack of any standardized reprocessing process being followed consistently.

controlled process. The implications and liability associated with such processes are quite significant; specifically, in this example statistical evidence exists that no single process is being followed consistently and could be a cause for settlement. "Out of control" processes therefore have been identified as important areas requiring immediate remedial action and focused efforts to achieve standardized work processes.

Table 3 summarizes other RME applications of appropriate types of QC charts. Additionally, in any application more advanced exponentially weighted moving-average (EWMA) or cumulative-sum (Cusum) charts can be used, which can have greater ability to detect smaller sustained process changes than simpler Shewhart-type charts. Although not shown here, the operating characteristics and average run lengths should be examined to help determine appropriate chart types, sample sizes, and plotting frequency in order to detect process changes of practical significance (Benneyan, 2008). In some applications, it can also be helpful to identify surrogate measures of overall process quality, such as cleaning supply consumption, flash sterilizations, or training frequency.

Beyond QC charts, many other SQC methods exist that are useful in RME processes, including inspection models, error-proofing, redundant design, and others, as discussed in what follows.

2.3. *Reliability and safety methods*

Several reliability engineering methods are useful for preventing RME process failures, including FMEA, forcing functions, redundant cleanings or inspections, and others. To facilitate designing inspection processes, two quality engineering methods in particular are helpful for deciding what amount of inspection is best: (1) Deming's k_1/k_2 inspection cost model to decide when inspections should or should not occur, and (2) multiple inspection probability cost models to optimize the number of

Table 3. Possible RME statistical control chart applications.

Application	Process measure	Type of SPC chart*	Notes
Reprocessing times	Average, standard deviation of reprocessing times.	*X-bar* and *S* charts (for total time and times for each step)	If skewed distributions, may need transformation to normality.
Reprocessing delays	Time until initial cleaning, and delays between steps.		
QC failures	Fraction of items failing QC per month	*p* chart	If rate is fairly high (>5%)
	Number of items between QC failures.	*g* chart	If rate is fairly low (<1%)
Expedited items	Number of items or days between expedites.	*p* or *g* chart	Use *p* chart if rate is fairly high (>5%)
Near misses (including visual detections)	Number of items or days between near misses.		
Flash sterilizations	Monthly information per 100 surgeries.	*u* chart	*c* chart acceptable if the denominator is fairly constant.
Training or audit failures	Monthly number of inspection demerits or training issues.		

Note: * in each case, these can be Shewhart, EWMA, or Cusum chart versions.

redundant inspections. Applications of these methods to RME reprocessing are described here.

FMEA is a structured reliability method to help identify potential process failures of high consequence and actions for preventing or minimizing the effects of such failures. In the case of RME, this approach can help identify potential process failures and develop prevention and contingency plans. For example, in several recent RME analysis projects, in each particular setting each work step was studied to identify all potential failure modes, focusing on those with the largest risk priority number, including determining where forcing functions or redundant designs should be developed.

Forcing functions are deliberate process designs that eliminate any possibility of error by forcing the correct action to occur, particularly in systems involving routine actions prone to human error. Examples include mechanisms and geometries such as requiring cash to be taken from an ATM machine before returning a bank card, a clutch to be fully depressed to prevent starting a car in gear, or a floppy disk to be correctly oriented to allow insertion into a computer drive (see Figure 7). Healthcare examples include tube connectors that can only be coupled with the correct source, doors that only open when anti-bacterial hand cleaning gel is dispensed, or gravity-activated endoscope case latches that can only be opened when positioned in the intended orientation. Similar forcing functions to prevent RME reprocessing errors can include cleaning tube geometry that cannot be misoriented, endoscope timeouts that render equipment inoperable if stored for too long, or cleaning devices that cannot function unless the correct chemicals are present.

Examples of redundant design in RME reprocessing to raise the overall reliability of a process can include multiple cleanings of equipment or multiple staff inspecting each piece of equipment for debris. As Figure 8 illustrates, the reliability of an

(a)

(b)

(c)

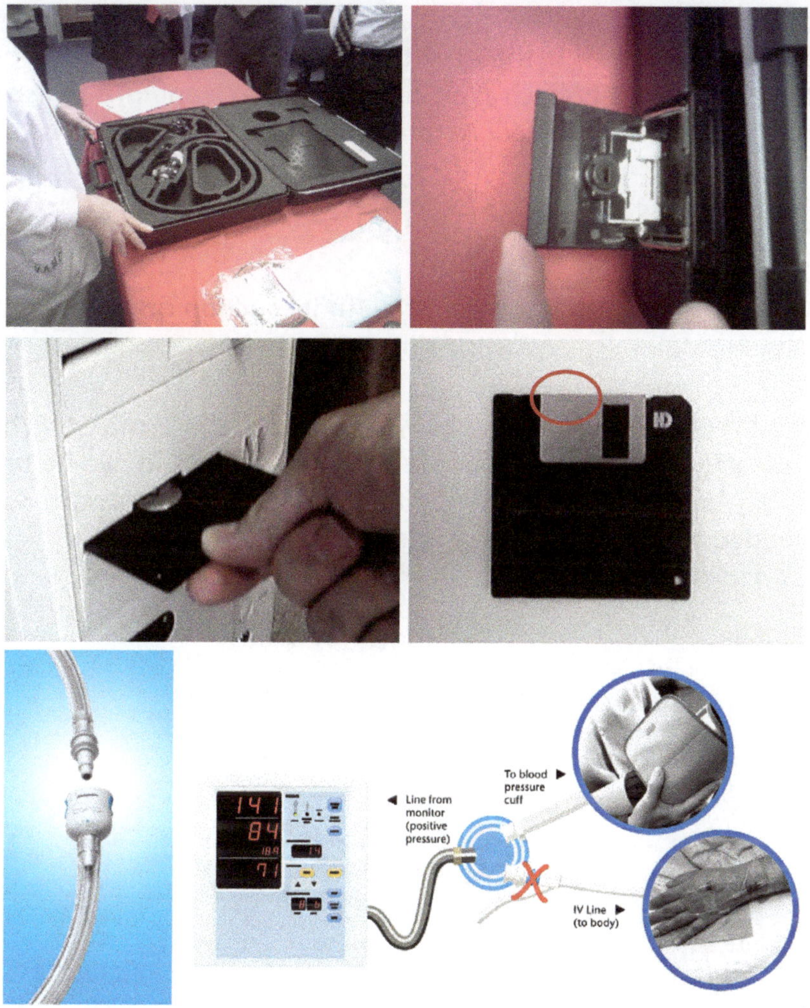

Figure 7. Forcing function examples: (a) Gravity-activated latch on endoscope case prevents dropped equipment from opening upside down causing breaks. (b) Floppy disk can only be inserted when oriented correctly due to a beveled corner to keep from breaking the drive. (c) Gas tubes that cannot be connected to a wrong source due to different connector diameters.

overall process can be made arbitrarily high via independent redundancy, even if the quality of each individual step is low. If the same activity (such as an inspection or a cleaning) is repeated n multiple times, the failure rate of the overall process, R, is

$$R = 1 - \prod_{i=1}^{n} (1 - p_i), \tag{1}$$

where p_i is the failure rate of the ith inspection or cleaning, or

$$R = 1 - (1 - p)^n, \tag{2}$$

if all repeated inspections have the same failure rate p. While the latter assumption may not strictly hold, Eq. (2) can be used as an initial approximation of the number of inspections, n, needed to achieve a specified reliability level R,

$$n = \frac{\log(1-R)}{\log(1-p)}, \tag{3}$$

or this can be found iteratively via Eq. (1).

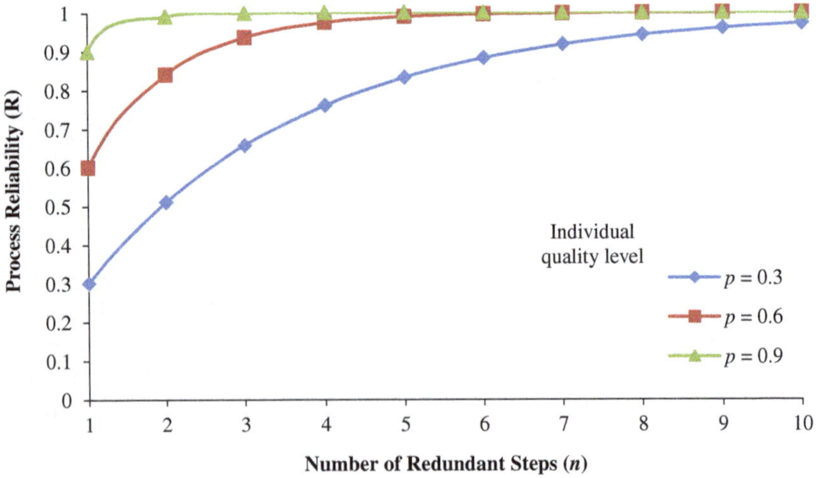

Figure 8. Illustration of the general benefit of redundancy on overall system quality.

While redundant design can improve overall process reliability based on the reliability concept of parallel series, high-quality individual steps can result in poor overall process quality based on the concept of serial systems (Figure 9). This figure also illustrates the fundamental design principles that high-quality systems can accomplish using low-quality subsystems and vice versa. Figure 10 illustrates this general concept, where the overall process reliability is given as

$$R = (1 - p)^n, \tag{4}$$

where R, p, and n have the same definitions as above. This approach also aligns with the lean simplification concept that less complex processes perform better, so it tends to be appealing within healthcare organizations following lean process improvement approaches.

Optimal redundant design extends the above ideas to best balance the number of redundant inspections, overall process

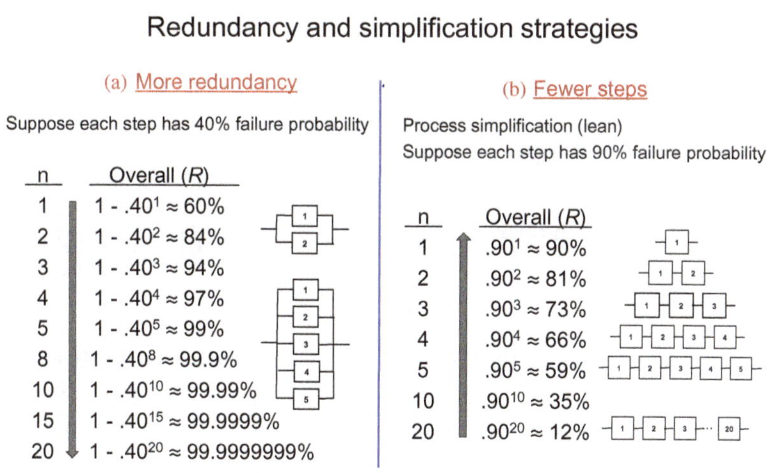

Figure 9. Reliability improvement strategy concepts of high and low overall process quality via (a) parallel redundancy and (b) serial complexity.

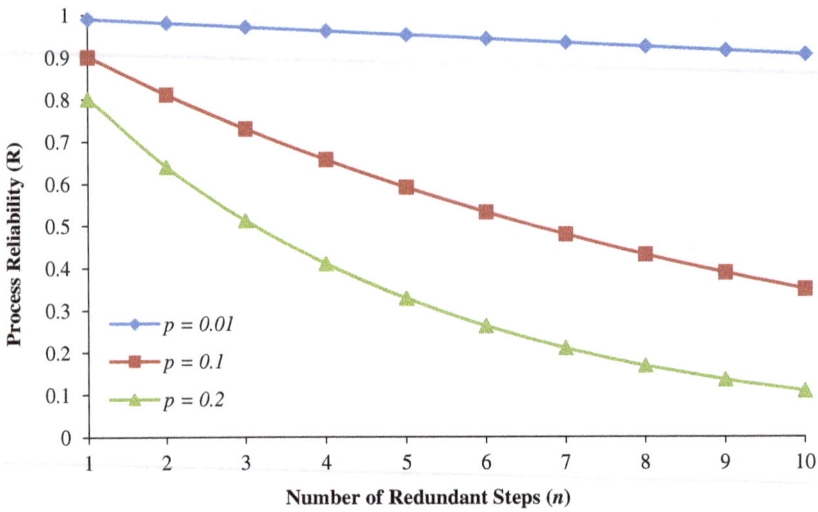

Figure 10. Illustration of decrease in reliability as complexity increases.

reliability, and cost. Since each inspection step costs time and money, the overall fraction of accepted items that are dirty (p') and the overall cost of J multiple inspections or cleanings of each item can be shown to be

$$p' = \frac{p\beta^J}{p\beta^J + (1-p)(1-\alpha)^J} \tag{5}$$

and

$$E(C) = \frac{k_1\left[\frac{p\alpha(1-\beta^J)+(1-p)(1-\beta)[1-(1-\alpha)^J]}{\alpha(1-\beta)}\right] + k_2 p\beta^J + k_3(1-p)[1-(1-\alpha)^J]}{(1-p)(1-\alpha)^J + p\beta^J}, \tag{6}$$

where k_1 is the average inspection cost per unit, k_2 is the average cost of accepting a dirty item, and k_3 is the average cost of rejecting a clean item per unit (Benneyan, 1997; Maleyeff *et al.*, 2003). The α and β terms denote Type I and Type II error probabilities, respectively, p is the non-conformance rate, and J is the number of inspections.

With respect to RME, until the primary processes can be improved, these models quickly identify the optimal amount of over-design in each reprocessing step. For example, Figure 11 illustrates the optimal number of QC inspections and the approximate potential savings for each of the four general types of RME cases summarized in Table 4. As is the case here, in most realistic cases one to four inspections typically are optimal (Benneyan, 1997). Case 4 represents a realistic case in many RME contexts for which the failure cost of an undetected non-sterile item (k_2) is very high compared to the inspection and re-cleaning costs (k_1 and k_3). The number of optimal inspections here is two with a savings per piece of \$56.08 and reducing the outgoing failure rate from 0.05 to 0.00011, illustrating the significant immediate benefits of optimizing redundant design. Moreover, applying this model to all reprocessing across a large integrated network could save well over \$1 million annually (e.g., 100 items per facility each reprocessed 50 times per year across 10 facilities results in a savings of roughly 50,000 × \$56 = \$2.8 million). As sensitivity analysis, Case 3 has a minimum cost at four inspections only due to very high p and β

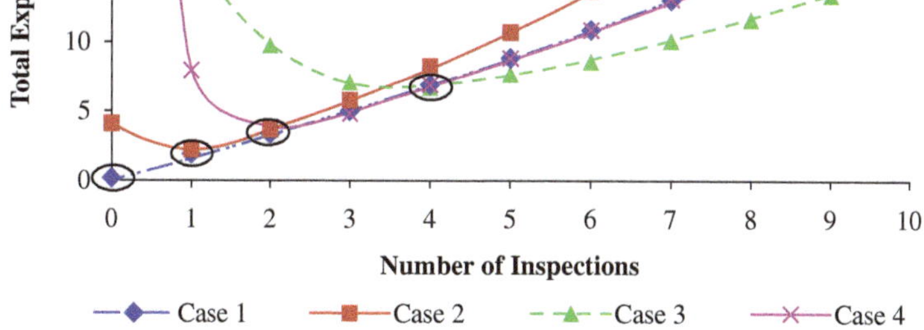

Figure 11. Optimal number of redundant RME inspections.

Table 4. Example applications and immediate benefits of optimal multiple redundancy model (savings per piece indicate the difference between optimal and zero inspection).

Parameter	Meaning	Case 1	Case 2	Case 3	Case 4
k_1	Inspection cost	\$1	\$1	\$1	\$1
k_2	Failure cost	\$3	\$20	\$100	\$6,000
k_3	Rejection cost	\$10	\$5	\$1	\$5
p	Non-conformance rate	0.05	0.2	0.3	0.01
α	Type I error rate	0.05	0.1	0.05	0.05
β	Type II error rate	0.1	0.05	0.4	0.1
Optimal inspections		0	1	4	2
Savings per piece		n/a	\$1.81	\$23.11	\$56.08
Optimized outgoing defect rate		0.05	0.0137	0.01329	0.000112
k_1/k_2 versus p		$0.33 > 0.05$	$0.05 < 0.2$	$0.01 < 0.3$	$0.00017 < 0.01$
Inspect? (yes/no)		No	Yes	Yes	Yes

values. Also note that while in some cases it may be difficult to identify exact k_2 costs, it is fairly easy to identify lower bounds for which additional inspections would or would not be warranted (Benneyan, 2008).

Related to the above, Deming's k_1/k_2 inspection cost model identifies where inspection should be conducted throughout the process, if at all (Deming, 1986), selecting between no inspection, partial sampling, and 100% inspection. From a practical standpoint, it can be shown mathematically that 100% inspection should occur everywhere in the process that $p > k_1/k_2$, where p, k_1, and k_2 are defined as above. For example, in the Case 1 setting in Table 4, $k_1/k_2 = \$1/\$3 = 0.33 > p = 0.05$, so no QC inspection should be performed, whereas for Case 3, $k_1/k_2 = \$1/\$100 = 0.01 < p = 0.3$, so that at least one inspection of every item should be performed. In many RME safety settings, these two approaches (deciding whether to inspect at all and the optimal amount of redundancy) should be applied immediately until other improvements can be realized.

Other risk analysis methods also can be helpful for RME safety problems, such as to help assess the relative benefits of different process designs and levels of inspection. To our knowledge, however, no exploratory work has been conducted in this area with respect to RME. In particular, while the above approaches are all based on expected values (and thus relate to long-term population average consequences), more individual patient-centric methods based on variances should be explored. Most simply, these might include mean variance, stochastic dominance, desirability function, and Monte Carlo models (Ok *et al.*, 2008). These approaches often can help identify the best process designs in the presence of competing criteria, uncertainties, and costs.

3. Logistics and Flow

3.1. *Process layout*

The physical layout of any process can significantly affect its performance, leading to better efficiency, throughput, operating costs, and profits. In other settings, for example, effective facilities planning can reduce manufacturing operating expenses by 10–30% (Tompkins and White, 1984), with Table 5 illustrating a few examples. Optimal reprocessing process layouts similarly can reduce unnecessary movement, activity, and time, with RME instruments more accessible and organized, shorter reprocessing times, and higher system efficiency. Several software programs exist to help develop optimal layouts, with some common ones including CRAFT, PLANET, and CORELAP (Tompkins and White, 1984), although it is also important to consider future volumes to optimize process layout over time.

Table 5. Examples of facility layout applications and resultant benefits.

Layout application	Benefit
McDonald's fast food chain	Designed a "Made for You" kitchen; $100 million savings per year in food costs.
Bayside Controls, automation manufacturer, Queens, NY	Increased sales in the past decade from $300,000 to $11 million due to layout change in cellular manufacturing.
Ernst & Young, Chicago accounting firm	30–40% of desks were empty at all times, developed "hotel program"; removed individual desks and instead consultants call ahead to reserve, saving office space.

Source: Heizer and Render (2004).

3.2. *Inventory models*

Reusable instruments generally are expensive and require considerable reprocessing supplies, so applying classic inventory control models can result in significant cost savings. In other settings, Table 6 summarizes several examples of benefits of traditional conventional economic order quantity or related methods that focus on re-order points and replenishment amounts. Items such as cleaning fluid and packaging materials, however, can benefit significantly from these methods. For RME items themselves, however, since a limited number of instruments arrive or depart the system (e.g., due only to new purchases and old equipment), these items are more amenable to modeling via closed and cyclic queuing networks, as described below. Such models can help study the anticipated effects of various process changes, staffing levels, and number of instruments in order to best balance competing criteria. For example, in many cases "no stock out" policies

Table 6. Applications of inventory methods in healthcare and non-healthcare settings.

Inventory application	Benefit
Mercy Medical Center (Wavemark, 2008)	25% reduction in inventory levels and net saving of $479,430 in 18 months.
Deere & Company, agriculture equipment producer (Hillier and Lieberman, 2010)	Improved on-time shipments that exceeded $1 billion in inventory reduction.
Time Inc., magazine publisher (Hillier and Lieberman, 2010)	Generated incremental profits over $3.5 million annually.
Solid structure timber producer (Gronalt and Rauch, 2008)	Reduced lost sales by ~20% using vendor-managed inventory policy.

may be desirable so that equipment always is available whenever needed. Additionally, some items have limits on the number of days before needing to be re-cleaned, irrespective of whether they have been used. Just-in-time policies can also be useful here, so that equipment is available at the exact time it is needed, with reduced inventory via improved scheduling and near-zero variability.

4. Queuing and Simulation

4.1. *Queuing networks*

Since new equipment rarely enters the system and old equipment rarely leaves, RME can be modeled as a closed queuing network where instruments flow sequentially from completion of use on a patient through all re-processing steps, to storage, and back to use in a procedure. As shown in Figure 12, each of the reprocessing operations (procedure, clean, sterilize, verify, package) is represented as a network of nodes connected by sequencing arcs, where $m = 5$ processes, $N = 10$ endoscopes, and the mean processing times are $t_1 = 3$, $t_2 = 2$, $t_3 = 1$, $t_4 = 0.5$, and $t_5 = 1$. Since this is a closed network, there is no arrival rate from outside the system.

Outputs of such models include utilization rates, queue wait times, server idle times, sojourn times (total cycle time of an item), number of entities in each queue, and others depending upon the precise purpose of the study. Inputs to such models include the arrival rate from one node to another, the duration of time for each activity, and the number of servers (staff or machines) available for each operation. By varying these inputs, one can study the effects of possible changes to the real system and trade-offs between service, cost, throughput, and delays. Within RME, these models have been used to study staffing levels, scheduling for staff and equipment, the number of instruments in the system, policy decisions (centralized versus decentralized), and idle equipment time after reprocessing. Examples of possible decisions include the number of servers at a process, process efficiency levels, the number of service facilities in a system, waiting space in queue, and entity priorities.

To provide some insight to the mathematics, the primary equations used in a closed queueing network are calculated iteratively in the order shown below and are based on the number

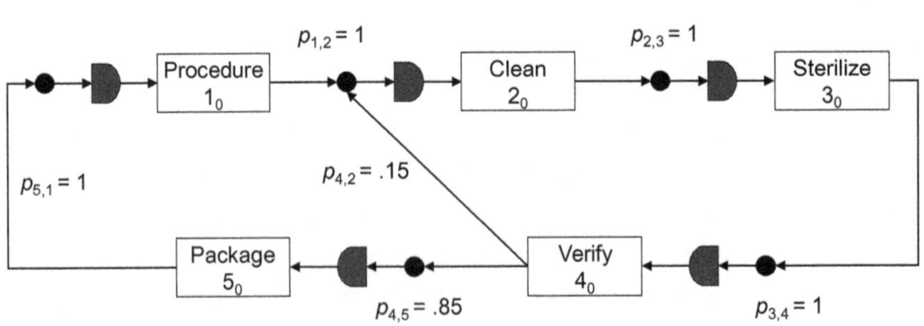

Figure 12. RME queueing network example.

of entities, N, in the system, where m is the number of processes, $p_{j,i}$ is the probability that an entity will move from process j to process i, and t_i is the processing time for each operation.

Relative arrival rate: $v_i = \Sigma_{j=1}^{m} p_{j,i} v_j \quad \text{for } i = 2,\ldots m \text{ and where } v_1 = 1$ (7)

Time at process i: $w_i(N) = t_i(1 + x_i(N-1)w_i(N-1)) \quad \text{for } i = 1,\ldots m,$ (8)

System throughput: $\lambda(N) = x_1(N) = N/\Sigma_{i=1}^{m} v_i w_i(N),$ (9)

Arrival rate at station i: $x_i(N) = \lambda(N)v_i \quad \text{for } i = 2,\ldots m,$ (10)

Number at process i: $n_j(N) = x_j(N)w_i(N) \quad \text{for } i = 1,\ldots m,$ (11)

Time in queue: $w_{qi}(N) = w_i - t_i \quad \text{for } i = 1,\ldots m,$ (12)

Number in queue: $n_{qi}(N) = x_i w_{qi} \quad \text{for } i = 1,\ldots m,$ (13)

Station efficiency: $\rho_i(N) = x_i t_i \quad \text{for } i = 1,\ldots m.$ (14)

Several software packages exist to help the analyst calculate these results (Snowdown and Ammons, 1988). Table 7 summarizes the results for the above example and input values, including for each process step the expected total time an item will spend there ($w_i(N)$), staff utilization rate ($\rho_i(N)$), expected number of items waiting in queue ($n_{qi}(N)$), and expected waiting time in queue ($w_{qi}(N)$).

Figures 13 and 14 summarize the impact of the number of items in the system on the utilization of staff (ρ_i) and mean number of items in queue ($n_{qi}(N)$) at each process step. In the case of the clinical procedure, the results for the number and time in queue equate to the number and time for which the item is kept in the storage rack before being used. Note that for all steps, more items in the system result in not only higher

Table 7. Example of RME queueing network results.

Measure	Procedure	Clean	Sterilize	Verify	Package
Average time at process i, $w_i(N)$	18.89 mins	6.84 mins	1.59 mins	0.62 mins	1.46 mins
Utilization, $\rho_i(N)$	0.97	0.76	0.38	0.19	0.32
Average number in queue, $n_{qi}(N)$	5.13 items	1.84 items	0.23 items	0.04 items	0.15 items
Average time in queue, $w_{qi}(N)$	15.89 mins	4.84 mins	0.59 mins	0.12 mins	0.46 mins

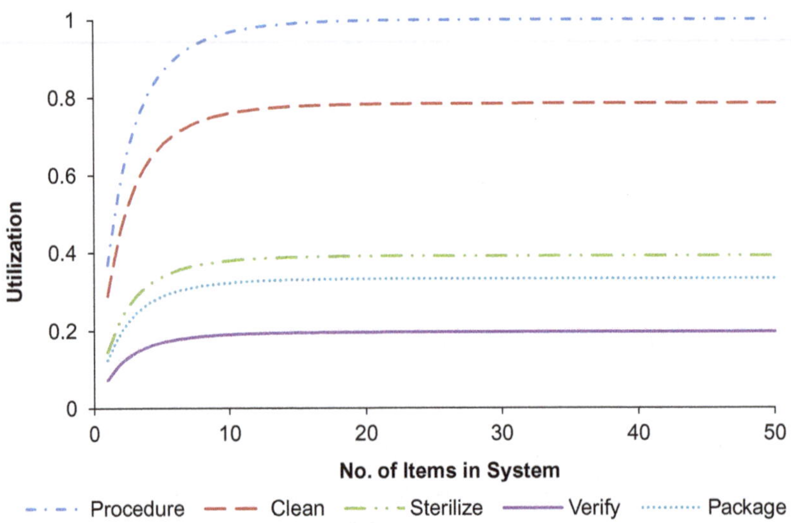

Figure 13. Queueing results for process utilization (ρ_i).

utilization by the individuals performing those activities but also more idle equipment, as would be expected. In this example, the individual performing the verification process has a very low utilization regardless of the number of items in the system, so it may be useful to further investigate staffing or process logic changes such as non-dedicated resources. This example also illustrates the common situation in which a system

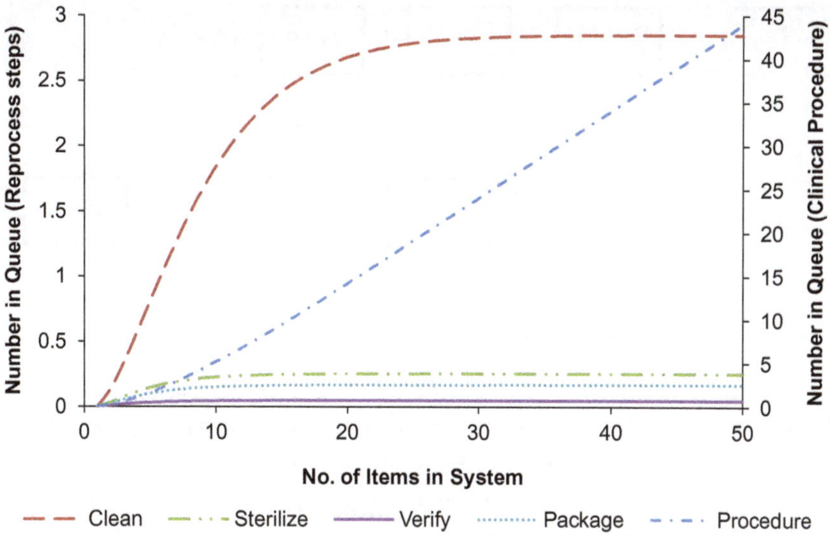

Figure 14. Expected number in queue at process *i* (n_{qi}).

simultaneously asymptotes at some point to both high utilization and high congestion — in this case, somewhere between 10 and 20 items in the system.

4.2. *Simulation*

Similar to queueing, computer simulation can be used to evaluate possible process changes but can also capture more complex process logic and distributional assumptions. Figure 15 illustrates a high-level RME simulation model using the Arena modeling software (Kelton *et al.*, 2010), based on the same assumptions. More detailed models can also be developed to capture microprocess logic specifics.

Table 8 compares RME queuing and simulation results using the same arrival and process assumptions as mentioned previously, based on 25 replications of 365 days each. As expected, the two models produce similar results with all simulation confidence intervals containing their true queuing results.

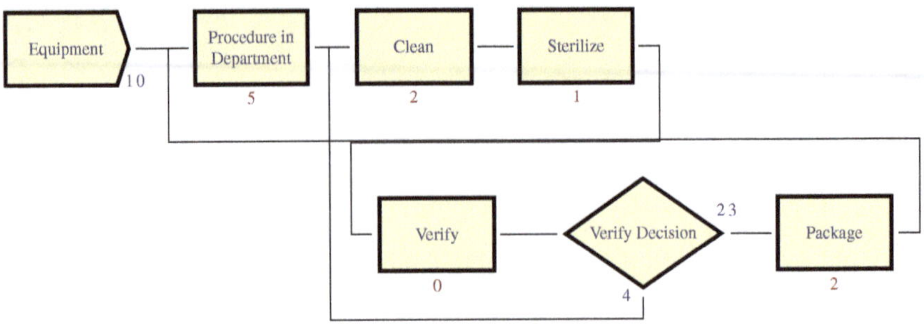

Figure 15. Simulation model of the RME process.

However, queuing networks can become inaccurate or intractable when the system becomes more complex or involves non-exponential distributions, demand patterns, resource schedules, and different equipment types.

For example, Table 9 compares the above results with those of all processing distributions that instead have the gamma distribution shape shown in Figure 16, with the shape parameter $\alpha = 3$ and the scale parameter β set such that each process mean equals that of the corresponding exponential distributions. For the utilization performance measure (ρ_i), the gamma-based model results in slight increases for all processes. The number (n_{qi}) and time (w_{qi}) in queue, however, decrease for all processes aside from clinical procedure, which increases for both measures. More generally, these results illustrate how more complex simulation results can differ from simpler queueing approximations.

Simulation also is useful for testing changes in process logistics, such as the number of resources available, resources being pooled or dedicated, or processing priorities for different types of equipment. For example, the current RME model assumes each process has one dedicated staff, whereas Table 10 illustrates the impact of pooling some number (1–4) of resources on a first-come first-served (FCFS) priority basis for the cleaning, sterilizing, verifying, and packaging processes. (The clinical

Table 8. Comparison of queueing and simulation model results (simulation is including 95% confidence intervals).

Measures	Method	Procedure	Clean	Sterilize	Verify	Package
Utilization, $\rho_i(N)$	Queueing	0.97	0.76	0.38	0.19	0.32
	Simulation	0.97 ± 0.00	0.76 ± 0.01	0.38 ± 0.00	0.19 ± 0.00	0.32 ± 0.00
Average number in queue, $n_{qi}(N)$	Queueing	5.13	1.84	0.23	0.04	0.15
	Simulation	5.14 ± 0.06	1.82 ± 0.06	0.23 ± 0.01	0.04 ± 0.00	0.15 ± 0.01
Average time in queue, $w_{qi}(N)$	Queueing	15.89	4.84	0.59	0.12	0.46
	Simulation	15.93 ± 0.24	4.80 ± 0.14	0.60 ± 0.02	0.11 ± 0.00	0.47 ± 0.02

Table 9. Simulation results for the RME process.

Distribution	Procedure	Clean	Sterilize	Verify	Package
Exponential	3 (9)	2 (4)	1 (1)	0.5 (.25)	1 (1)
Gamma	3 (3)	2 (2)	1 (1)	0.5 (.5)	1 (1)
Exponential	0.97 ± 0.00	0.76 ± 0.01	0.38 ± 0.00	0.19 ± 0.00	0.32 ± 0.00
Gamma	1.00 ± 0.00	0.79 ± 0.01	0.39 ± 0.00	0.20 ± 0.00	0.33 ± 0.00
Exponential	5.14 ± 0.06	1.82 ± 0.06	0.23 ± 0.01	0.04 ± 0.00	0.15 ± 0.01
Gamma	6.24 ± 0.05	0.96 ± 0.04	0.05 ± 0.00	0.01 ± 0.00	0.04 ± 0.00
Exponential	15.93 ± 0.24	4.80 ± 0.14	0.60 ± 0.02	0.11 ± 0.00	0.47 ± 0.02
Gamma	18.75 ± 0.24	2.43 ± 0.10	0.13 ± 0.01	0.02 ± 0.00	0.13 ± 0.00

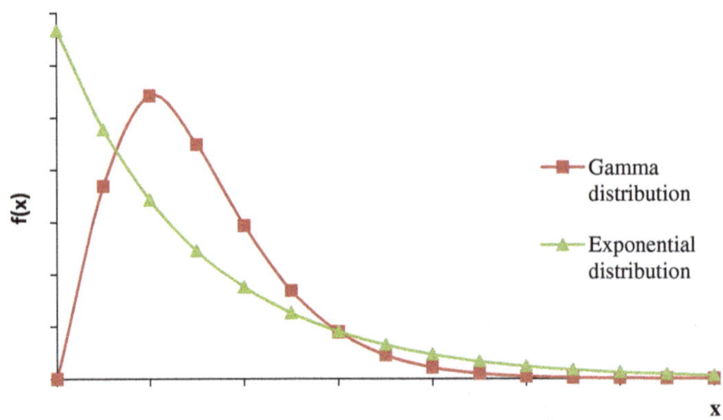

Figure 16. Illustration of exponential and gamma distribution shapes used in simulation.

procedure itself always uses its own dedicated resource, i.e., specially trained doctors or nurses.)

Note that pooling the same number (four) of reprocessing resources as originally used in the dedicated resource model significantly improves delays and throughput and that significant staff reductions can still produce roughly the same or better total turnaround times. These models have also been used to compare the FCFS results with those where sequential

Table 10. Time at process *i* using pooled resources for reprocessing processes.

Reprocessing resources	Clinical procedure	Reprocessing step				
		Clean	Sterilize	Verify	Package	Total
Dedicated	18.94 ± 0.26	6.80 ± 0.15	1.61 ± 0.03	0.61 ± 0.01	1.47 ± 0.02	9.94
4 Pooled	24.60 ± 0.21	2.06 ± 0.02	1.06 ± 0.01	0.56 ± 0.01	1.06 ± 0.01	4.74
3 Pooled	23.67 ± 0.21	2.29 ± 0.02	1.30 ± 0.02	0.80 ± 0.01	1.28 ± 0.02	5.68
2 Pooled	19.34 ± 0.29	3.58 ± 0.04	2.64 ± 0.03	2.10 ± 0.03	2.52 ± 0.03	10.84
1 Pooled	8.21 ± 0.28	10.52 ± 0.11	9.64 ± 0.10	8.76 ± 0.10	9.12 ± 0.11	38.02

priority for available reprocessing staff is given first to cleaning, sterilizing, verifying, and then packaging.

5. Discussion

Efficient and safe management of reusable medical technology is a growing concern. This chapter described several systems and industrial engineering techniques that have been used to help understand, improve, and optimize such processes. In particular, in our work we have found redundancy optimization and SQC to be particularly useful to address safety issues and methods such as queuing, simulation, and inventory methods to have value in improving efficiencies. In each setting at different facilities, some unique modeling and implementation issues have existed that need to be addressed. Availability of good data can be a barrier, although to some extent sensitivity analyses can help address this.

A more important limitation can be the development of the type of interdisciplinary team of healthcare and engineering personnel who are often needed to conduct these types of studies. Forming such teams often requires cross-education, patience, and relationship building. In our experience, education and implementation can often be a greater challenge than the analyses themselves. Appreciation also is critical of the investment of time, effort, and staff skills set required to develop and use models such as those described here. For example, basic methods such as FMEA and standard control charts can be taught to many frontline non-engineering staff. However, more advanced technical methods, such as queuing, inventory control, and redundancy optimization, typically require an experienced engineer with either undergraduate or masters level training. Once built, however, these models can help explore many process improvement concepts quicker and more economically than could be done directly.

References

Associated Press (2009). 3 Receive HIV from VA Contamination. *The Washington Times*. Retrieved August 3, 2010, from www.washingtontimes.com/news/2009/apr/18/va-confirms-3-positive-for-hiv-in-follow-up-tests.

Benneyan, J. C. (1997). *Optimal Inspection Policies in the Presence of Inspection Error*. Doctoral Dissertation (University of Massachusetts Amherst), UMI Press, Ann Arbor MI.

Benneyan, J. C. (2008). Design, use, and performance of statistical process control charts for clinical process improvement, *International Journal of Six Sigma*, 219–239.

Benneyan, J. C., Lloyd, R. C. and Plsek, P. E. (2003). Statistical Process Control as a Tool for Research and Healthcare Improvement. *Quality and Safety in Health Care*, 458–464.

CNN Wire Staff (2010). *VA Hospital May Have Infected 1,800 Veterans With HIV*. Retrieved September 13, 2010, from CNN News: www.cnn.com/2010/US/06/30/va.hospital.hiv.

Daigh, J. (2009). Statement by the Assistant Inspector General for Healthcare inspections. Subcommittee on oversight and Investigations Committee on Veterans Affairs U.S. House of Representatives on Endoscopy Procesures at the VA: What Happened, What Has Changed?

Deming, W. E. (1986). *Out of the Crisis*, Massachusetts Institute of Technology, Cambridge, MA.

Duke University Health System (2007). *Duke University Health System Hydraulic Fluid Quality Assurance Follow-up Program*. DukeMedicine.

Gronalt, M. and Rauch, P. (2008). Vendor managed inventory in wood processing industries — A case study *Silva Fennica*, 101–114.

Heizer, J. and Render, B. (2004). *Principles of Operations Management*, 5th edition, Pearson Education, Inc., Upper Saddle River.

Hillier, F. S. and Lieberman, G. J. (2010). *Introduction to Operations Research*, 9th edition, McGraw-Hill, New York.

Kelton, W. D., Sadowski, R. P. and Swets, N. B. (2010). *Simulation With Arena, 5th Edition*, McGraw-Hill, New York.

Maleyeff, J., Kaminsky, F. C. and Farris, J. P. (2003). Minimum cost 100% inspection systems with inspection error, *Quality Engineering*, 557–563.

Nolan, T. (2009). Submitted testimony to the U.S. Senate Committee of Veterans Affairs Quality Management Hearing.

Ok, Z., Benneyan, J and Isaacs, J. (2008). Risk analysis modeling of production costs and occupational health exposure of SWNT manufacturing, *Journal of Industrial Ecology, Nanotechnology*, 12(3):411–434.

Smalley, H. E. (1982). *Hospital Management Engineering: A Guide to the Improvement of Hospital Management Systems,* Prentice-Hall, Inc., New Jersey.

Snowdown, J. L. and Ammons, J. C. (1988). A survey of queueing network packages for the analysis of manufacturing systems *Manufacturing Review*, 14–25.

Thomas, D. (2010). *Patients May Have Been Exposed to Viruses in Colonoscopies, Trans-Vaginal Ultrasounds*. Retrieved September 15, 2010, from the Examiner: www.examiner.com/news-in-san-diego/patients-may-have-been-exposed-to-viruses-colonoscopies-trans-vaginal-ultrasounds.

Tompkins, J. A. and White, J. A. (1984). *Facilities Planning*, John Wiley & Sons, Inc., New York.

Veterans Health Administration Warning System (2004). *Patient Safety Alert.* VA Central Office.

Wavemark (2008). *RTIM: Real Time Inventory Management, A White Paper Case Study on the use of RTIM for Tracking High-Value, Consumable Medical Devices.* Retrieved July 2010, from Wavemark: www.wavemark.net.

Part 2

Organizational Perspectives

Chapter 4

R&D Management in the Japanese Pharmaceutical Industry

Jörg Mahlich

University of Vienna, Department of Economics, Vienna, Austria

joerg.mahlich@univie.ac.at

Abstract

We analyze how Japanese pharmaceutical firms internationalized their research and development (R&D) investments during the 1980s and 1990s. In order to tap into foreign knowledge bases, they heavily invested in setting up R&D canters abroad. However, knowledge transfer, evidenced by international patent applications, was very limited during the early phase of globalization. As a response, Japanese firms have shifted their R&D strategy toward a better organizational integration of their foreign units.

Keywords: R&D management, Japan, globalization, pharmaceutical industry.

1. Introduction

In many industries, Japanese companies are eye to eye with their western rivals, and in the automotive industry, Toyota has even surpassed General Motors (GM) as the world's biggest car manufacturer. In many other industries, Japanese companies have become global leaders as well. Examples include firms like Nitto Denko or Japan Synthetic Rubber that supply sophisticated material components for LCD displays (Schaede, 2008). One outlier is the Japanese pharmaceutical industry, and it is the only high-technology sector where Japan runs a trade deficit. The limited presence of Japanese firms on international markets is also reflected by the fact that there are no Japanese firms among the leading pharmaceutical companies (Table 1).

The market share of Japanese pharmaceutical firms at the end of the 1990s in Europe reached only 1.3% and was a mere 1.9% in the United States (US). The reason for the weak performance in international markets lies in the failure of Japanese companies to come up with a sufficient number of innovative new drugs. To substitute for their weak own product pipeline, around 50% of their products are licensed from western firms (Okada and Kawara, 2004). The poor innovative performance of Japanese pharmaceutical firms is also mirrored by the assessment of the US Food and Drug Administration (FDA). Between 1998 and 2004, the FDA has approved 168 new active substances from which only six were of Japanese origin. Moreover, for four of the six new drugs the FDA perceived no major therapeutic gain compared to drugs which had already been on the market (Mahlich, 2007a). Even Japanese authorities are concerned about the competitive situation of the industry. The Ministry of Health and Welfare concludes in a strategy report: "The drug discovery environment of Japan's market is regrettably no longer internationally attractive. [...] The disappearance of Japanese companies from the domestic and global marketplace would be inevitable in 10 years unless R&D efforts were redoubled" (PhRMA, 2004).

Why are Japanese pharmaceutical companies less innovative in comparison to their international competitors? One major reason for the low competitiveness is the strict price control policy adopted by the Japanese government (Thomas,

Table 1. Top 10 pharmaceutical companies in 2008.

Rank	Company	Country	Pharmaceutical turnover (million USD)	Profit margin (pharmaceutical operating profits in % of pharmaceutical sales)	Pharmaceutical R&D (as % of pharmaceutical sales)
1	Pfizer	US	44,170	49.3	18.0
2	Sanofi-Aventis	France	40,562	15.9	16.6
3	GlaxoSmithKline	UK	37,810	31.1	18.1
4	Novartis	China	33,888	25.6	18.9
5	Roche	China	33,316	36.2	22.0
6	AstraZeneca	UK	33,601	28.9	16.4
7	Johnson & Johnson	US	24,567	31.0	20.7
8	Merck	US	23,619	41.6	20.3
9	Eli Lilly	US	19,285	−6.7	19.9
10	Wyeth	US	19,025	35.0	16.4
18	Takeda	Japan	14,050	20.5	31.3
20	Astellas	Japan	9,367	25.9	16.5
22	DaiichiSankyo	Japan	8,135	10.3	22.0
23	Eisai	Japan	7,383	12.4	20.5
25	Otsuka	Japan	6,564	n/a	20.1

Source: Scrip Pharmaceutical League Tables, 2009.

2001; Mahlich, 2007b, 2010). In order to control healthcare expenditures, the Japanese Ministry of Health, Labor and Welfare biannually cuts the drug prices significantly. These price cuts do ease pressure on the public health bill but have significant impacts on the drug market. Because of the essential price cuts, the average life span of a drug is significantly shorter than elsewhere. Shorter drug life cycles in turn reduce payback periods of investments. For this reason, the development of risky breakthrough medicines is commercially not very attractive. In regulatory regimes that drive down the originator price over the life cycle, it pays to launch minor pseudo-new versions of old molecules to obtain a higher regulated price (Danzon and Chao, 2000).

Abstracting from the macroeconomic drivers mentioned above, we want to focus in this chapter on innovation management and the management of foreign R&D laboratories in particular. We argue that Japanese firms have heavily invested in the establishment of foreign R&D centers of excellence during the 1980s and 1990s but have failed to take full advantage of them. We hypothesize that this was because foreign R&D centers were too autonomous and knowledge flows to the headquarters were insufficient. Only recently have Japanese pharmaceutical firms adopted a more integrative R&D management strategy, which von Zedtwitz and Gassmann (2002) labeled the "integrated network approach".

2. Internationalization of R&D

Internationalization of multinational corporation's R&D activities is a rather new phenomenon, and R&D was traditionally located in close proximity to the firms' global headquarters. Only during the last decade or so, growth in international R&D expenditures has outpaced the increase of domestic R&D investments (Kurokawa *et al.*, 2007). Majority-owned affiliates of foreign companies located in the United States, for instance, invested $29.9 billion in R&D. Between 1999 and 2004, R&D by these affiliates increased 2.1% on an annual average rate basis after adjusting for inflation. This compares with a mere increase of 0.2% of overall industrial R&D in the United States (National Science Board, 2008).

The same trend can also be observed for Japan. Although being a latecomer in internationalizing corporate R&D, Japanese firms perform around 4% of their R&D expenditures abroad, up from 0.5% in 1989 (OECD, 2006). Despite this remarkable growth rate, the current degree of internationalization is still far behind other developed countries. In general, Japanese multinationals seem to differ from American and European firms in their reluctance to internationalize their R&D operations (Belderbos, 2003; Patel, 1995; Bartlett and Ghosal, 1991). In 2002, the ratio of foreign to total R&D expenditures was only 4% in Japan compared to 27% in Germany or 17% in USA (Figure 1). On the contrary, a mere share of 4% of Japanese R&D translates into a quite large amount in absolute terms as Japan has one of the highest R&D ratios of all industrialized

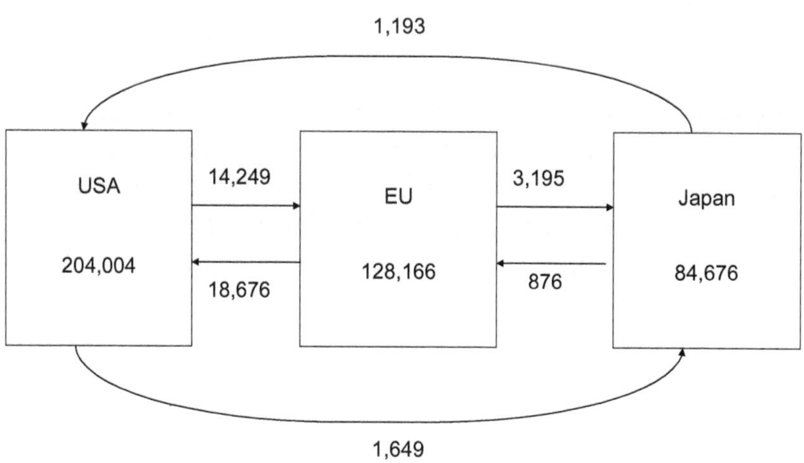

Figure 1. R&D investments in and among the United States, European Union, and Japan in 2003 in million USD.
Source: OECD (2008).

countries.[1] According to METI estimates, Japanese firms invested more than US$3.5 billion in foreign R&D in the year 2002 alone. Around 46% of the outward R&D investments went to USA, 28% to Europe, and 22% to Asian countries (Bartnik, 2009).

Nonetheless, Japanese R&D laboratories abroad seem to be smaller in size than those of their Western rivals (Kiba, 1998). Hence, the output of overseas R&D units measured in patents is extremely low — though increasing — in the Japanese case. In the late 1980s, only 1% of Japanese patents originated abroad, compared with 8% for US and more than 30% for European multinationals (Patel, 1995). This number increased to around 2% in the early 1990s (Belderbos, 2001). In a more recent study, Iwasa and Odagiri (2004) suggest that between 1998 and 2003 around 6% of Japanese USPTO patents were based on inventions abroad, which is still significantly lower than the share for Western firms (van Zedwitz and Gassmann, 2002). This pattern is explained by Japan's strong domestic inter-firm networks, which are difficult to transfer abroad and which have constrained Japanese-owned firms from internationalizing their R&D (Cantwell and Zhang, 2006). Historically, Japanese firms have given priority to manufacturing excellence and process innovation that requires intensive collaboration with suppliers and communication between different firm units (Odagiri and Yasuda, 1996). This specific form of industrial organization makes a strong degree of geographic proximity among headquarters and R&D units inevitable (Belderbos, 2003). An alternative explanation refers to the "latecomer hypothesis" of Vernon (1979), who states that R&D functions are transferred abroad at a later stage of internationalization. Because Japanese firms were relatively late in establishing international R&D centers, they have not gained sufficient experience in operating decentralized networks (Belderbos, 2001; Westney, 1996).

[1]Japan's R&D expenditure as percentage of GDP is 3.3% compared with 2.5% for Germany and 2.6% for the USA (OECD, 2007).

Two main motivations for the internationalization of corporate R&D have been identified in the literature. One is to augment its own knowledge base by getting access to foreign know-how. The other is to exploit its knowledge base abroad in order to adapt technologies and products to local markets and environments. The former motive leads to the establishment of R&D facilities close to universities, while the latter type leads to the establishment of laboratories close to the existing manufacturing plants (Kuemmerle, 1999). The knowledge-exploiting motive dominates in the early phase of R&D internationalization, and the knowledge-augmenting motive gains importance in the later stages of internationalization (Belderbos, 2002; Florida, 1997; Geybadze and Reger, 1999). Most of the R&D flows into the United States is motivated by the knowledge-augmenting purpose. Frost (2001) demonstrates that foreign R&D is driven by the desire to gain knowledge from diverse institutional contexts. Analyzing patent citation behavior, he finds that foreign R&D subsidiaries in the US tend to cite US patents in technological fields in which the United States has a proven technological advantage.

This applies in particular for Japanese pharmaceutical firms. Granstrand (1999) and Kurokawa *et al.* (2007) surveyed R&D executives and concluded that the most important motive for Japanese pharmaceutical firms for establishing research centers abroad was getting access to foreign knowledge bases. This observation is in line with interviews conducted by Kiba and Collinson (1998), who discovered that Japanese R&D managers rated the quality of basic science in the US and Europe higher than that of Japan. The quality of basic research in Japan is also reflected in an analysis of the ISI Web of Knowledge that has calculated the impact factor of scientific publications from researchers based in Japan (ISI, 2003).[2] According to this analysis, Japanese researchers seem to publish their papers in low-impact journals.

[2] The impact factor of a journal reflects the number of current year citations to the source items published in that journal during the previous 2 years.

Compared to the world average, the impact factor of publications of Japanese origin is up to 60% lower (in computer sciences). For molecular biology, which is relevant for pharmaceutical research, it is almost 20% below the world average. Table 2 supports this argument. It shows that Japan is only second to the USA in terms of the total number of scientific papers. However, measured by citation per paper, Japan slumps to rank 36, although it is debatable to what degree the number of citations and the impact factor of a journal can serve as a quality measure.

Some scholars argue that the cultural environment shapes a country's propensity to innovate. Using Hofstede's (1980) typology, Shane (1992, 1993), for instance, found that scientists from more individualistic and non-hierarchical countries were more productive (measured in patents per capita) than scientists from other societies. According to Hofstede, the Japanese culture is characterized by a high degree of uncertainty avoidance (i.e., the extent to which the members of a culture feel threatened by uncertain situations) and power distance, which can be defined as the extent to which the less powerful members of institutions and organizations within a country accept that power is distributed unequally. On the contrary, Japan scores low in the individualism index, which is high in societies in which everyone is expected to look after themselves and their immediate family. This cultural setting has to a certain degree shaped Japanese competitive performance. Japan has developed a competitive advantage in efficient production

Table 2. Scientific output of scientific articles by Japanese researchers in 2003.

Total for Japan	Papers	Citations	Citations per paper
Number	784,945	6,522,893	8.31
Rank for Japan among the 145 top performing countries	2	4	36

Source: ISI (2003).

technologies and incremental innovation. Breakthrough innovations on the contrary are difficult to achieve under such cultural circumstances (Pudelko and Mendenhall, 2009). As cultural factors are stable even in the long run, they constitute path dependencies. In contrast, path-dependent processes lead to the development of firm- or country-specific capabilities and core competencies that cannot be replicated easily. However, as Leonard-Barton (1992) argued, core competencies may easily turn into core rigidities in dynamic environments. Institutions then find themselves locked in by choices made in the past. When global demand shifts toward breakthrough instead of incremental innovations, countries like Japan will find themselves in difficulties. A deep-rooted institutional change is then needed to regain competitiveness.

Such a change toward a more innovative culture is a difficult and long-term endeavor at the industry level as well. To foster their innovative performance and to acquire the necessary competencies needed in today's drug-making industry, Japanese pharmaceutical firms have set up R&D facilities in countries like the US which are at the forefront of scientific research. Dunning and Narula (1995, p. 43) call this behavior "strategic asset-seeking R&D". Other taxonomies of foreign R&D are, for instance, from Gupta and Govindarajan (1991), who distinguish the magnitude of transactions (extent of knowledge transfer) and the directionality of transactions (provider or receiver of knowledge). Depicted on a matrix, one can derive four roles: global innovator (high outflow, low inflow), integrated player (high outflow, high inflow), implementer (low outflow, high inflow), and local innovator (low outflow, low inflow). Building on Gupta and Govindarajan (1991), Ambos and Reitsperger (2004) come up with a slight modification of the taxonomy, which is based on the dimensions "technological mandate" and "task-related interdependence". The dimension "technological mandate" refers to Kuemmerle's (1999) distinction between knowledge-exploiting versus knowledge-enhancing tasks (Figure 2).

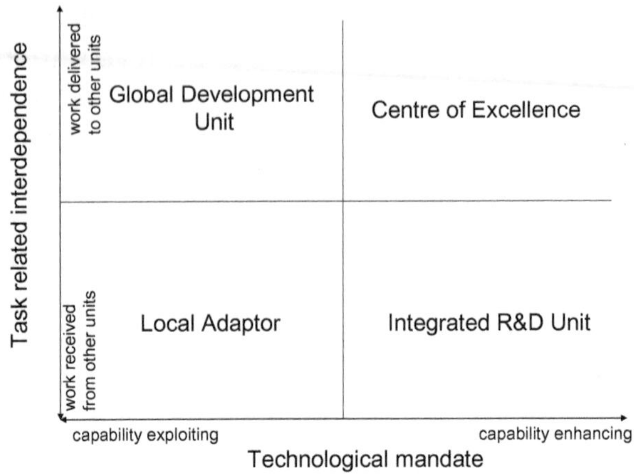

Figure 2. Typology of R&D units.
Source: Ambos and Reitsperger (2004).

According to the taxonomy of Ambos and Reitsperger (2004), most R&D centers of Japanese pharmaceutical firms can be considered as centers of excellence as their intention is to augment the company's knowledge stock by linking up with foreign knowledge bases.

An example is Eisai, which led the way in 1987 with the establishment of a basic research laboratory in Massachusetts, US. Fujisawa founded a research center in Edinburgh, UK, only 2 years later, and Yamanouchi followed in 1990 with a facility in Oxford, UK. Table 3 provides a list of foreign R&D laboratories of major Japanese pharmaceutical firms.

USA is the favorite location for pharmaceutical R&D centers and many foreign R&D laboratories have been set up through an acquisition. For instance, Japan's biggest pharmaceutical player Takeda internationalized its R&D by acquiring research-intensive biotech firms in the UK and the US (Cambridge, San Diego, and San Francisco) in close proximity to the leading universities. Examples are the purchase of San Diego-based Syrrx in 2005, the acquisition of the Cambridge University spin-off Paradigm Therapeutics in 2007, and the recent US$9 billion

Table 3. Internationalizing of R&D in Japanese pharmaceutical companies, 1987–2008.

Company	Country	City	Foundation	Acquisition	Activity
Daiichi Sankyo	UK	London	1993		Clinical development
	DE	Munich	1990	Luitpold Pharma	Clinical development
	US	New Jersey	2004		Clinical development
	US	San Diego	1998		Basic research
Kyowa Hakko	DE	London			Clinical development
	US	Princeton	2002		Clinical development
Eisai	US	New Jersey	2002		Clinical development
	US	North Carolina	1997		Clinical development
	UK	London	1990		Basic research
	US	Massachusetts	1987		Basic research
Astellas	US	North Carolina	2006	Dynogen to establish Urogenix	Basic research
(Fujisawa)	US	Illinois	1996		Basic research and clinical development
	UK	Edinburgh	1989–2007		Basic research
	NL	Leiderdorp	1991	Gist Brocades	Clinical development
	DE	Munich	1988	Klinge	Clinical development

(*Continued*)

Table 3. (*Continued*)

Company	Country	City	Foundation	Acquisition	Activity
(Yamanouchi)	US	California	1997		Clinical development
	UK	Oxford	1990–2002		Basic research
Takeda	US	Cambridge	2008	Millennium	Basic research
	US	Illinois	2004		Clinical development
	US	New Jersey	1994–2004		Clinical development
	UK	London	1998		Basic research and clinical development
	DE	Frankfurt	1992–1998		Clinical development
	US	San Diego	2005	Syrrx	Basic research
	US	San Francisco	2007		Basic research
	SG	Singapore	2007	Paradigm Therapeutics	Basic research
	UK	Cambridge	2007	Paradigm Therapeutics	Basic research

Source: Company reports.

offer to the shareholders of Boston- based Millennium Pharmaceuticals in 2008, which would eventually become Takeda's biggest acquisition in its corporate history. With this deal, Takeda further enhances its knowledge base in leading-edge biotechnology and cancer research. On the contrary, the two UK laboratories of Astellas had been closed for 12 and 18 years after their establishment as they probably fell short of expectations. Astellas, which emerged from the merger of Yamanouchi and Fujisawa in 2005, instead consolidated basic R&D in the US, mainly in Illinois (ARIA — Astellas Research Institute of America). Table 3 also shows that many R&D centers are clustered around high-rank universities and research centers to secure access to scientific talent (cf. Florida and Kenney, 1994).

3. Management of Foreign R&D Activities: Autonomy vs. Integration

We presented evidence that the internationalization of R&D has increased significantly during the last 10–15 years mainly because firms wanted to access foreign knowledge bases. However, the management of a set of geographically dispersed R&D laboratories is a big challenge as it is difficult to integrate knowledge inputs from different countries to eventually come up with new product innovation. It is therefore not clear to what degree an international R&D strategy leads to an increase in corporate performance. Fors (1997), for instance, could not establish a correlation between productivity and overseas R&D intensity for a sample of Swedish firms. According to Gassmann, Reepmeyer, and von Zedwitz (2004), international R&D is associated with three significant problems: lack of face-to-face time, cultural differences, and lack of trust. Lack of face-to-face time makes it difficult to transfer tacit knowledge that is embedded in people.

One central issue of the management of R&D subsidiaries is the degree of headquarter control expressed, for instance, by the degree of direct supervision, the existence of integrated planning systems, or the utilization of report systems (Ambos and Schlegelmilch, 2007). Both autonomy and integration are associated with costs and benefits. The costs of the centralization approach are due to the high transaction costs of across-border decision-making. Additionally, there are opportunity costs of not exploiting local resources and ignoring local market needs (Boutellier *et al.*, 2000; Bartnik, 2009). The cost of the autonomy approach is due to possible duplication of overhead costs and not achieving a critical mass.

How do Japanese firms manage their foreign subsidiaries? Many scholars state that Japanese firms seem to maintain a relatively strong headquarter control including overseas R&D operations (Reger, 1999; Bartlett and Ghosal, 1991; Gassmann and van Zedwitz, 1999), others have arrived at contrasting conclusions (Krieger and Salomon, 1992). Bartnik's (2009) results suggest that domestic R&D units of Japanese firms are controlled to a stronger degree than overseas R&D units, which enjoy a relatively high degree of local decision-making autonomy. To find the right balance of autonomy and integration for those centers of excellence is a big challenge for the R&D management. On the one hand, creation of new knowledge requires a certain degree of organizational and operational freedom. On the other hand, integration is needed to fully take advantage of this new knowledge. For R&D units of German firms, Ambos and Schlegelmilch (2007) established a positive relationship between cultural distance and centralization. Centralization was also significantly correlated to the degree of interdependence and the functional form. Using a one-dimensional taxonomy that only relates to the technological mandate (local adaptor, international adaptor, and international creator), they found that international adaptors and international creators are more likely to have a low level of autonomy compared to local adaptors. Eventually,

German firms use a more centralized coordination mechanism, the more important the unit's output is for the entire firm. This seems to be different for Japanese firms. While empirical support is scarce, there is at least anecdotal evidence that Japanese firms do not intervene in the operational business of their centers of excellence. Rather, the opposite seems to be true. A R&D manager quoted by Asakawa (2001) describes the situation as follows: "Our lab has been protected by top management [···] and it created the Chinese wall between HQ and our lab to make sure we don't get brainwashed by the R&D headquarters". The president of Sankyo's US activities confirms that "the secret to success is to delegate the responsibility to local people with experience, and that's what Sankyo is trying to do" (Koberstein, 2002). This approach was regarded the silver bullet in the 1990s. Academics like Ghoshal (1986) and Birkinshaw *et al.* (1998) also showed that the creation of innovation in subsidiaries was associated with high autonomy. However, they also point to the pitfalls of subsidiary autonomy as autonomy might also indicate a lack of integration that may limit the chances of gaining recognition for specialized resources. Japanese pharmaceutical companies probably learned exactly this the hard way. Their foreign R&D centers enjoyed a high degree of autonomy, which offered scientists a comfortable and attractive working environment. At the end of the day, however, they failed to come up with new innovations due to a lack of recognition and integration.

To test this statement, we checked a few patent applications of a Japanese pharmaceutical firm (Takeda) and a German firm (Boehringer Ingelheim).

Figure 3 displays a typical patent application from Boehringer Ingelheim in contrast to a patent application from Japan's biggest player, Takeda, which is based in Osaka (Figure 4). A patent application does not only reveal the name of the firm that files the application (applicant) but also the names and addresses of the individual researchers who were

(12) INTERNATIONAL APPLICATION PUBLISHED UNDER THE PATENT COOPERATION TREATY (PCT)

(19) World Intellectual Property Organization
International Bureau

(43) International Publication Date
28 August 2003 (28.08.2003)

PCT

(10) International Publication Number
WO 03/070278 A1

(51) International Patent Classification⁷: **A61K 45/06**, 31/415, A61P 25/28

(21) International Application Number: PCT/EP02/01722

(22) International Filing Date: 19 February 2002 (19.02.2002)

(25) Filing Language: English

(26) Publication Language: English

(71) Applicant: BOEHRINGER INGELHEIM INTERNATIONAL GMBH [DE/DE]; Binger Strasse 173, 55216 Ingelheim am Rhein (DE).

(72) Inventors: YUSUF, Salim; 48 Woodend Drive, Carlisle, ON L0R 1H2 (CA). **ANDERSON, Craig**; 17 Cambria Road, Devonport, Auckland (NL). **SLEIGHT, Peter**; 32, Crown Road, Wheatley, Oxfordshire, OX33 1UL (GB). **HILBRICH, Lutz**; Hasengartenstrasse 20, 65189 Wiesbaden (DE).

(81) Designated States *(national)*: AE, AG, AL, AM, AT, AU, AZ, BA, BB, BG, BR, BY, BZ, CA, CH, CN, CO, CR, CU, CZ, DE, DK, DM, DZ, EC, EE, ES, FI, GB, GD, GE, GH, GM, HR, HU, ID, IL, IN, IS, JP, KE, KG, KP, KR, KZ, LC, LK, LR, LS, LT, LU, LV, MA, MD, MG, MK, MN, MW, MX, MZ, NO, NZ, PH, PL, PT, RO, RU, SD, SE, SG, SI, SK, SL, TJ, TM, TR, TT, TZ, UA, UG, UZ, VN, YU, ZA, ZW.

(84) Designated States *(regional)*: ARIPO patent (GH, GM, KE, LS, MW, MZ, SD, SL, SZ, TZ, UG, ZM, ZW), Eurasian patent (AM, AZ, BY, KG, KZ, MD, RU, TJ, TM), European patent (AT, BE, CH, CY, DE, DK, ES, FI, FR, GB, GR, IE, IT, LU, MC, NL, PT, SE, TR), OAPI patent (BF, BJ, CF, CG, CI, CM, GA, GN, GQ, GW, ML, MR, NE, SN, TD, TG).

Published:
— *with international search report*

For two-letter codes and other abbreviations, refer to the "Guidance Notes on Codes and Abbreviations" appearing at the beginning of each regular issue of the PCT Gazette.

Figure 3. Patent application of Boehringer Ingelheim showing the international origins of the inventors.

responsible for the innovation (inventors). While Boehringer's invention was by a group of researchers based in California, New Zealand, United Kingdom, and Germany, Takeda's researchers were from Amagasaki and Hyogo, both in the immediate vicinity of Osaka.

To present a slightly broader picture, we also checked all patent applications by Boehringer Ingelheim and Takeda in the year 2004 at the European patent office (Table 4). Although there is a clear home bias for Boehringer Ingelheim, the patent share of researchers residing outside Germany reaches almost 40%. At Takeda on the contrary, only one researcher has its domicile outside Japan. We also examined the geographical

(19) Europäisches Patentamt
European Patent Office
Office européen des brevets

(11) **EP 1 857 457 A3**

(12) **EUROPEAN PATENT APPLICATION**

(88) Date of publication A3:
05.12.2007 Bulletin 2007/49

(43) Date of publication A2:
21.11.2007 Bulletin 2007/47

(21) Application number: **07075609.3**

(22) Date of filing: **23.02.2005**

(51) Int Cl.:
C07D 413/14 ***(2006.01)*** ***A61K 31/4245*** ***(2006.01)***
A61P 9/12 ***(2006.01)***

(84) Designated Contracting States:
AT BE BG CH CY CZ DE DK EE ES FI FR GB GR HU IE IS IT LI LT LU MC NL PL PT RO SE SI SK TR
Designated Extension States:
AL BA HR LV MK YU

(30) Priority: **25.02.2004 JP 2004048928**
07.01.2005 US 31057

(62) Document number(s) of the earlier application(s) in accordance with Art. 76 EPC:
05719737.8 / 1 718 641

(71) Applicant: **Takeda Pharmaceutical Company Limited**
Osaka 541 (JP)

(72) Inventors:
- **Kuroita, Takanobu**
Katano-shi
Osaka 5760016 (JP)
- **Sakamoto, Hiroki**
Amagasaki-shi
Hyogo 6610001 (JP)
- **Ojima, Mami**
Amagasaki-shi
Hyogo 6610002 (JP)

(74) Representative: **Lewin, John Harvey**
Takeda Euro IP Department
Arundel Great Court
2 Arundel Street
London WC2R 3DA (GB)

(54) **Benzimidazole derivative and its use as AII receptor antagonist**

(57) The present invention relates to a medicament comprising a compound represented by the formula (I)

Figure 4. Patent application of Takeda showing the Japanese location of the inventors.

allocation of scientific publications written by researchers affiliated to pharmaceutical firms. The results for Takeda, Boehringer Ingelheim, Glaxo SmithKline, Pfizer, and Merck are depicted in Table 5.

The home bias for publications is much smaller than that for patents, but it is still significant for Japanese and American firms. In both cases, more than 80% of the scientific publications emerge from domestic R&D centers. In contrast, European

Table 4. The residence of inventors for patents granted to Boehringer Ingelheim and Takeda in 2004.

Company	Country	Patents
Boehringer Ingelheim	Canada	5
	Germany	30
	USA	8.75
	Austria	2.15
	UK	0.25
	New Zealand	0.25
	Switzerland	0.33
	Japan	1.4
	Mexico	0.7
		49
Takeda	Japan	43.66
	USA	0.33
		44

Source: Own calculations.

firms such as Boehringer Ingelheim or Glaxo SmithKline generate a much higher share of their research output abroad, first of all in North America. While both US and Japanese firms are less international in terms of their research output, the nature of the home bias of Japanese and American firms is very different. If it is true that the quality of basic science pertaining to the pharmaceutical industry (i.e., biotechnology and genetic engineering) is better in North America than in Japan, then the incentive for home base augmenting R&D centers abroad is much lower for American firms than for Japanese firms. Therefore, Japanese firms are either underrepresented in the US or the productivity of Japanese R&D centers in the US is low. A low productivity in turn might be a consequence of a lack of integration.

Table 5. Geography of publication output (2004).

Takeda (JP)		Boehringer Ingelheim (DE)		GSK (UK)		Pfizer (US)		Merck (US)	
Location	**Pub.**	**Location**	**Pub.**	**Location**	**Pub.**	**Location**	**Pub.**	**Location**	**Pub.**
Kyoto (JP)	4	Leval (CA)	25	Research Triangle Park (US)	58	La Jolla (US)	15	Rahway (US)	172
Osaka (JP)	28	Ridgefield (US)	19	Collegeville (US)	14	Ann Arbor (US)	64	West Point (US)	194
Tsukuba (JP)	6	Richmond (US)	1	King of Prussia (US)	37	Cambridge (US)	3	Montreal (CA)	4
Lincolnshire (US)	6	Biberach (DE)	13	Madrid (ES)	7	New London (US)	5	Harlow (UK)	32
London (UK)	1	Vienna (AT)	8	Verona (IT)	12	Groton (US)	145	Lyon (FR)	3
		Kawanishi (JP)	7	Beckenham (UK)	1	Amboise (FR)	3	Rom (IT)	6
				Greenford (UK)	8	Sandwich (UK)	28	Tsukuba (JP) Banyu	21
				Welwyn (UK)	1	Nagoya (JP)	5	Hoddesdon (UK)	3
				Stevenage (UK)	22	Tokyo (JP)	8	Madrid (ES)	5
				Harlow (UK)	39			Pomezia (IT)	11
				Tsukuba (JP)	1				
Total	45		73		200		276		451
Home share	84%		38%		45%		84%		82%

Source: Mahlich (2006).

4. New R&D Management Approach

We argued that the difficulty of managing foreign centers of excellence is to find the right balance of autonomy and integration. A high degree of autonomy enhances knowledge flows between the subsidiary and its local environment such as universities and research organizations, which is vital for knowledge creation. During the early phase of R&D globalization (late 1980s until beginning of this decade), foreign R&D laboratories were given a high degree of freedom and headquarters have not intervened in the operational business of their foreign centers of excellence. While a certain level of independence and autonomy is important to foster creativity and for the emergence of entirely new ideas, this approach bears the risk that the foreign R&D unit becomes too self-centered and does not contribute to the overall corporate success. Kurokawa *et al.* (2007), for instance, found that the performance of Japanese R&D laboratories in the US measured in patents and publications is inversely correlated with the degree of autonomy of the subsidiary. Autonomy is therefore a kind of double-edged sword and Japanese firms are aware that the integration of their foreign R&D centers of excellence was not sufficient. Japanese pharmaceutical firms are therefore undergoing significant changes with regard to the management of their foreign laboratories.

In the course of this strategic shift, R&D units are consolidated (mainly in the US) and R&D personnel are exchanged more frequently between the Japanese and the international laboratories. This move was in line with the findings of the management literature. Bresman *et al.* (1999), for instance, analyze knowledge transfer in international acquisitions and find that both the intensity of communication and the frequency of visits and meetings are positively and significantly related to the degree of knowledge transfer. Moreover, the impact of the latter variable was higher in terms of both significance and magnitude. This result confirms the reasoning of innovation theorists, who differentiate between knowledge and information. Information is factual (Saviotti, 1998) and codified, while knowledge has an interpretative role and encompasses both cognitions and problem-solving heuristics (Dosi, 1998). Therefore, knowledge can be considered as "tacit" (Polanyi, 1967) and "local" (Saviotti, 1996). While the transfer of information is easy and almost free in the era of e-mail and Internet, knowledge transfer requires face-to-face contacts and the exchange of personnel. The intelligent utilization of information and communication technologies is also crucial in this respect (Howells, 1995). Hacievliyagil *et al.* (2007) show how pharmaceutical companies, such as Eli Lilly, use virtual knowledge brokers to ease information flows between subsidiaries and the headquarters.

The shift toward a higher degree of integration is also reflected in the changing organizational structure of many R&D departments. Takeda, for instance, has adopted the R&D management structure of Merck, where R&D management decisions are made by an interdisciplinary international committee instead of a single R&D executive based in Japan. Daiichi Sankyo introduced a similar committee (Global Executive Meeting of Research and Development) in the year 2005. This international and inter-functional committee aims at integrating the global R&D network of Daiichi Sankyo and is headed by the global R&D director based in the US. To put a subsidiary in charge of the global R&D management is a big step forward and is still very uncommon for Japanese firms. Many Western pharmaceutical firms have made this move already a few years ago and have relocated their R&D management to the US, which is apparently home to the world's leading scientists in the disciplines relevant to the drug business. Swiss drug maker Novartis, for instance, concentrates the lion's share of its basic research efforts in the "Novartis Institutes for BioMedical Research (NIBR)" that is headquartered in Massachusetts, USA.

The trend to relocate R&D management responsibilities abroad affects not only basic research investment decisions but also clinical development. Because legal deregulation has made it easier to use international clinical data for drug approval applications in Japan, many firms conduct their clinical trials outside Japan. Sankyo's R&D director states: "Although the ability to conduct clinical research is slowly improving in Japan, many of the resources will still be in the West, where there are many experienced investigators, a favorable regulatory environment, and an array of contract resources. It means that we can develop drugs faster in the United States than we can anywhere else" (Koberstein, 2002). To utilize and leverage foreign resources is therefore the key to the success of Japanese pharmaceutical companies.

5. Conclusions

We tried to offer an explanation as to why the Japanese pharmaceutical companies have a low innovation level. Not neglecting institutional factors such as price regulation or general healthcare policies, which are outside the firm's discretion, we focused on R&D management issues in this chapter. We saw that Japanese R&D still has a strong home bias and Japanese firms have been latecomers in internationalizing their R&D efforts. In the early phase of R&D internationalization, firms established satellite R&D centers abroad, which were only loosely connected to the R&D headquarters in Japan. While the high degree of autonomy might have fostered the regional linkages with universities and other local R&D centers, knowledge transfer to the headquarters was not sufficient. For this reason, Japanese R&D management shifted recently to a more integrative approach, whereby coordination between international R&D centers is stronger than before. This goes together with the dislocation of formal decision-making authority to the subsidiaries.

References

Ambos, B. and Reitsperger, W. (2004). Offshore centres of excellence: Social control and success, *Management International Review*, 44(2), 51–65.

Ambos, B. and Schlegelmilch, B. (2007). Innovation and control in the multinational firm: A comparison of political and contingency approaches, *Strategic Management Journal*, 28, 473–486.

Asakawa, K. (2001). Organizational tension in international R&D management: The case of Japanese firms, *Research Policy*, 30, 735–757.

Bartlett, C. A. and Ghoshal, S. (1991). Managing innovation in the transnational corporation, in Christopher, A., Bartlet, Y. D. and Gunnar, H. (eds.), *Managing the Global Firm*, Routledge, London and New York.

Bartnik, R. (2009). *Organizing International Innovation: R&D Mandates and Coordination Patterns in Japanese Multinational Corporations*, Metropolis, Marburg.

Belderbos, R. (2001). Overseas innovations by Japanese firms: An analysis of patent and subsidiary data, *Research Policy*, 30(2), 313–332.

Belderbos, R. (2003). Entry mode, organizational learning, and R&D in foreign affiliates: Evidence from Japanese firms, *Strategic Management Journal*, 24(3), 235–259.

Birkinshaw, J. M., Hood, N. and Jonsson, S. (1998). Building firm-specific advantages in multinational corporations: The role of subsidiary initiative, *Strategic Management Journal*, 19, 221–242.

Bresman, H., Birkinshaw, J. and Nobel, R. (1999). Knowledge transfer in international acquisitions, *Journal of International Business Studies*, 30(3), 439–462.

Boutellier, R., Gassmann, O. and von Zedwitz, M. (2000). *Managing Global Innovation, Uncovering the Secrets of Future Competitiveness*, Springer, Berlin.

Cantwell, J. and Zhang, Y. (2006). Why is R&D internationalization in Japanese firms so low? A path-dependent explanation, *Asian Business & Management*, 5, 249–269.

Cohen, W. M. and Levinthal, D. A. (1989). Innovation and learning: Two faces of R&D, *The Economic Journal*, 99, 569–596.

Danzon, P. and Chao, L.-W. (2000). Does regulation drive out competition in pharmaceutical markets? *Journal of Law and Economics*, 43, 311–357.

Dosi, G. (1998). The contribution of economic theory to the understanding of a knowledge-based economy, in Neef, D., Siesfeld, G. A. and Cefola, J. (eds.), *The Economic Impact of Knowledge*, Butterworth-Heinemann, Boston and Oxford.

Dunning, J. and Narula, R. (1995). The R&D activities of foreign firms in the United States, *International Studies of Management and Organization*, 25, 39–73.

Florida, R. and Kenney, M. (1994). The globalization of Japanese R&D, the economic geography of Japanese R&D investment in the United States, *Economic Geography*, 70, 305–323.

Fors, G. (1997). Utilization of R&D results in the home and foreign plants of multinationals, *Journal of Industrial Economics*, 45, 341–358.

Frost, T. (2001). The geographic sources of foreign subsidiaries' innovations, *Strategic Management Journal*, 22, 101–123.

Gassmann, O. and von Zedtwitz, M. (1999). New concepts and trends in international R&D organization, *Research Policy*, 28(2–3), 231–250.

Gassmann, O., Reepmeyer, G. and von Zedwitz, M. (2004). *Leading Pharmaceutical Innovation*, Springer, Berlin.

Ghoshal, S. (1986). *The Innovative Multinational: A Differentiated Network of Organizational Roles and Management Processes*, Doctoral Dissertation, Harvard Business School, Boston, MA.

Granstrand, O. (1999). Internationalization of corporate R&D: A study of Japanese and Swedish corporations, *Research Policy*, 28, 275–302.

Gupta, A. and Govindarajan, V. (1991). Knowledge flows and the structure of control within multinational corporations, *The Academy of Management Review*, 13(4), 768–792.

Hofstede, G. (1980). *Culture's Consequences: Institutional Differences in Work Related Values*, Beverly Hills.

Howells, J. (1995). Going global: The role of ICT networks in research and development, *Research Policy*, 24(2), 169–184.

ISI (2003). *Essential Science Indicators*, Philadelphia.

Iwasa, T. and Odagiri, H. (2004). Overseas R&D, knowledge sourcing, and patenting: An empirical study of Japanese R&D investment in the US, *Research Policy*, 33, 807–828.

Kiba, T. and Collison, S. (1998). R&D performance in Japanese companies: A relative evaluation of overseas-based and domestic R&D, *Science and Public Policy*, 25(4), 227–238.

Koberstein, W. (2002). Sankyo Pharma, Pharmaceutical Executive, July.

Kuemmerle, W. (1999). 'Foreign direct investment in industrial research in the pharmaceutical and electronics industries — Result from a survey of multinational firms', *Research Policy*, 28, 179–193.

Kurokawa, S., Iwata, S. and Roberts, E. (2007). Global R&D activities of Japanese MNCs in the US: A triangular approach, *Research Policy*, 36, 3–36.

Leonard-Barton, D. (1992). Core capabilities and core rigidities: A paradox in managing new product development, *Strategic Management Journal*, 13, 111–125.

Mahlich, J. (2007a). Die japanische Pharmaindustrie, in Moerke, A. and Wieczorek, I. (eds.), *Japans Zukunftsindustrien*, Springer, Berlin.

Mahlich, J. (2007b). The Japanese pharmaceutical industry in transition: Has higher research orientation resulted in higher market value? *Asian Business & Management*, 6(1), 75–94.

Mahlich, J. (2010). Patents and performance in the Japanese pharmaceutical industry: An institution-based view, *Asian Pacific Journal of Management*, 27(1), 99–113.

National Science Board (2008). *Science and Engineering Indicators 2008*, National Science Foundation, Arlington, VA.

Odagiri, H. and Yasuda, H. (1996). The determinants of overseas R&D by Japanese firms: An empirical study at the industry and company levels, *Research Policy*, 25, 1059–1079.

OECD (2006). *Science, Technology and Industry Outlook*, Paris.

OECD (2007). *Science and Technology Scoreboard*, Paris.

OECD (2008). *Recent Trends in the Internationalization of R&D in the Enterprise Section*, Paris.

Okada, Y. and Kawara, A. (2004). *Research Productivity in the Japanese Pharmaceutical Industry-Economies of Scale, Economies of Scope and Spillovers*, Hitosubashi University, Working Paper.

Patel, P. (1995). Localized production of technology for global market, *Cambridge Journal of Economics*, 19, 141–153.

PhRMA (2004). *Industry Profile*, Washington, D.C.

Polanyi, M. (1967). *The Tacit Dimension*, Garden City.

Pudelko, M. and Mendenhall, M. (2009). The contingent nature of best practices in national competitiveness: The case of American and Japanese innovation processes, *European Management Journal*, 27(6), 456–466.

Reger, G. (1999). How R&D is coordinated in Japanese and European multinationals, *R&D Management*, 29(1), 71–88.

Saviotti, P. P. (1996). *Technological Evolution, Variety and the Economy*, Cheltenham.

Saviotti, P. P. (1998). On the dynamics of appropriability of tacit and of codified knowledge, *Research Policy*, 26(7–8), 843–856.

Schaede, U. (2008). *Choose and Focus: Japanese Business Strategies for the 21st Century*, Cornell University Press, Ithaca.

Shane, S. (1992). Why do some societies invent more than others? *Journal of Business Venturing*, 7, 29–46.

Shane, S. (1993). Cultural influences on national rates of innovation, *Journal of Business Venturing*, 8, 59–73.

Thomas, L. G. (2001). *The Japanese Pharmaceutical Industry: The New Drug Lag and the Failure of Industrial Policy*, Cheltenham.

Vernon, R. (1979). The product lifecycle hypothesis in a new institutional environment, *Oxford Bulletin of Economics and Statistics*, 41, 255–267.

Westney, E. (1996). Japanese multinationals in North America, in Lorraine, E. (ed.), *Multinationals in North America*, Calgary.

von Zedtwitz, M. and Gassmann, O. (2002). Market versus technology drive in R&D internationalization: Four different patterns of managing research and development, *Research Policy*, 31(4), 569–588.

Chapter 5

Analyzing Co-Opetition Strategy Through Patents in the Stent Market

Kuei-Kuei Lai[*,**], Fang-Pei Su[†,††], Calvin S. Weng[‡,‡‡],
Mei-Lan Lin[§,§§] and Chiau-Ling Chen[¶,¶¶]

[*]*Graduate School of Business Administration,
National Yunlin University of Science and Technology,
Douliou, Yunlin, Taiwan*

[†]*Graduate School of College, Department of Management Information Systems,
National Yunlin University of Science and Technology,
Yung-Ta Institute of Technology & Commerce, Taiwan*

[‡]*Graduate School of Business Administration, Department of Finance,
National Yunlin University of Science and Technology, Takming College,
Taiwan*

[§]*Department of Business Management, Far-East University,
Hsin-Shih, Taiwan*

[¶]*Chunghwa Picture Tubes, Taoyuan, Taiwan*

[**]*laikk@yuntech.edu.tw*

[††]*uffpsu@ms9.hinet.net*

[‡‡]*calvinweng@mail.takming.edu.tw*

[§§]*melianab@ms17.hinet.net*

[¶¶]*g9222722@yuntech.edu.tw*

Abstract

Technology innovation and its evolutionary path can be explored by patent analysis. Therefore, for those firms which need a large investment and high business performance, such as those that manufacture stents, integrating patent information with business strategy is the critical issue. The competition among stent manufactures is intensifying because of the increase in global demand. From the resource-based view, adopting a co-opetition strategy is the essential way for the firms to maintain a sustainable competitive advantage. In the last decade, patents have become a major tool of the co-opetition strategy. This chapter applies patent data in USPTO during 1984–2005 and constructs patent indicators by patent information to verify the process of technology evolution. On these grounds, we can understand the relative technological position and technological strength of the major manufactures in this industry and also monitor their changes in position and business performance to examine the relationship between each firm's technology strategy and business strategy.

Keywords: Patent strategy, co-opetition strategy, stent.

1. Introduction

Patent information can represent the technology's capability and the competitive advantage of a company. By collecting or monitoring the patent development of a certain field in technology, an analyst is able to get crucial business information, understand the technological specialties of the companies, and explore a certain industry's technological trajectory and strategic planning of the company. Therefore, patent analysis is not only an important activity for patent management but also an analysis tool for patent, technology, and business strategies.

In the last few years, several articles have been devoted to the study of patent analysis. Mogee applied his patent analysis results to the technology analysis and planning of a corporation (Mogee, 1991). Berkwitz (1997) analyzed how to make proper patent strategies to achieve and maintain competitive advantages under the process of technology development, while Hufker and Alpert (1994) discussed the various situations for applications of patent strategy from a managerial perspective. Since it is very difficult to get valid information from competitors, these articles show a discrepancy between the perceived importance and the actual level of information available on the competitor's R&D strategies. Ernst, on the contrary, applied patent information on the analysis and research of the mechanical engineering industry and proposed two types of patent portfolios — company level and technological level — as core analysis methods and then accordingly applied the results to determine how many research resources were needed in strategic R&D planning (Ernst, 1997, 1998). The patent strategy for any company should fit its technology strategy, which is a critical success factor for a business strategy in high-tech industries. Therefore, it's of critical importance for a company to make coordinated efforts among the patent, technology, and business strategies (Berkowitz, 1993).

Judging strategy planning from a company's resource perspective, one can arrive at two different standpoints, resource based and resource dependent, and study how to gain a competitive advantage both from the inside and outside of the company, respectively. The resource-based view is internally focused; it emphasizes that a company should gain a competitive advantage through the building and application of its core competency. Patent information is the indicator of a company's technology capability. Patent information can be used to not only determine an industry's technology trend but also judge the strength and technology categories of a company by its patent volume and categories. Therefore, if one analyzes the technology core competency of a certain company from the resource-based view, the quality and quantity of its patents are very representative. A great-fit portfolio of patents can be the best indicator of a company's core competency. On the contrary, the resource dependence theory studies how a company uses various methods to lower its dependence on resources from other companies, and as a result, gains other companies' dependence instead, increasing its independence and competitive advantage. Thus, patent information can be used to provide technology information to decision-makers as the basis for seeking external partners for technology resources, and accordingly choosing the right business strategy.

The above two viewpoints are based on the concepts of competition and cooperation, respectively. At the early stage, the two were considered mutually exclusive extremes. Now, the combined use of both competition and cooperation is already being viewed as an indispensable strategy for a company to achieve success. Brandenburger and Nalebuff proposed the concept of "co-opetition" and emphasized that both competition and cooperation have the same importance in the market. They believed that competition and cooperation do not exist exclusively in the market, nor do they take turns to exist in the market; instead, they co-exist (Brandenburger and Nalebuff, 1996).

The application of such a co-opetition strategy can be clearly observed in the market of interventional cardiology medical device companies. The invention of the Percutaneous Transluminal Coronary Angioplasty (PTCA) in 1977 has replaced Coronary Artery Bypass Graft surgery (CABG) to become the mainstream multi-vessel treatment for Coronary Artery Disease (CAD). The FDA approved the first Bare Metal Stent (BMS) by Johnson & Johnson. Although the combined application of PTCA and BMS can lower the recurrence rate of a vessel's in-stent restenosis, the long-term use of BMS will cause inflammation and fibrous scarring, which in turn will cause the vessel to become infected once again. Therefore, the lowering of the recurrence rate of a vessel's in-stent restenosis became an important research direction for the industry.

The world's first Drug-Eluting Stent (DES), Cypher™, made by Cordis, which is a subsidiary under Johnson & Johnson, was approved by the FDA in 2003, and it became the first such product in the US market. The product was proven to lower by around two-thirds the in-stent restenosis of a vessel. Therefore, within a few short months, it grabbed 58% of the BMS market by the end of 2003. Drug-eluting stents have strongly penetrated the traditional BMS market and have made a huge market impact that ended in the complete collapse of the BMS market.

The manufacturers of BMS had sensed the potential of this technology and had started R&D on such technology years before, but did not beat Cordis' DES product to the market. Many other competitors are nevertheless still working hard to gain the competitive edge. Boston Scientific is the biggest competitor, having produced its own DES called Taxus™. Guidant, the leading BMS manufacturer, is also developing its own DES product called Achieve™, which is already in its final clinical trial stage. Another wave of high competition will begin at any moment.

Since DES was a new innovation, its manufacturer tried to use patent infringement to block competition. Within a year of the DES's introduction, there were many lawsuits between the major manufacturers. The cross-suits by Cordis, Boston Scientific, and Guidant, the leading BMS manufacturer, have become the most visible cases in the industry. However, the dynamic environment of such a co-opetition situation changes very rapidly. The federal court judged in August 2003 that Guidant had to compensate Cordis US$425 million, which caused a financial crisis for the company. On February 2, 2004, Boston Scientific and Guidant reached a settlement over the infringement lawsuits and also an agreement on the cross-license. However, immediately afterward, on February 24, 2004, Cordis, one of their biggest competitors, not only showed good intentions to Guidant but also agreed to work together with Guidant and granted Guidant the right to sell Cordis products, in addition to many other agreements to share technologies.

How did Guidant emerge from under the tremendous pressures of R&D schedule delays and the loss of a patent lawsuit that almost led to the loss of its market share to become the hot partner of Cordis and Boston Scientific? From Table 1, one

Table 1. Year 2002 BMS market share (%) by major manufacturers (prior to the production of DES).

Company	Global market share (%)	US market share (%)
Guidant	38	44
Cordis/Johnson & Johnson	28	27
Boston Scientific	13	12
Medtronic	16	14

Source: Industrial Economics & Knowledge Center of Industrial Technology Research Institute. (http://www.iek.org.tw, 2005/12/08).

can tell that Guidant had 44% BMS market share before the production of DES. Guidant still leads the markets in BMS surgery-related supporting technology and devices, such as the balloon used in angioplasty and PTCA. The clinical trial results of the effectiveness of both the dug-eluting stents — Cypher™ of Cordis and Taxus II™ of Boston Scientific — had no visible difference; there is little chance for Cordis to block Boston Scientific by using a patent lawsuit.

In addition, it will take a long time for the lawsuits between Boston Scientific and Guidant to come to an end. Therefore, Boston Scientific and Cordis both decided to turn their averse relations with Guidant into friendship and work together with Guidant. What kind of strategy would each use, based on its own resources and advantages to leverage Guidant and to edge out the other? From this co-opetition situation among the stent manufacturers, it is clear that the technology positioning and patent strategies are not the only factors for success. It is more critical to use patents as strategic weapons, while leveraging the existing advantages, technologies, or any other functional strategies to fight effective business battles in such a dynamic environment.

Patents are viewed as one of the most important tools for co-opetition. Therefore, this chapter aims to use patent analysis to construct patent indicators for monitoring the integrated technology development of the interventional cardiology medical device industry and the research activities by its major manufacturers. As a result, one can assess the technology strategy and business strategy connections through the patent strategy. In order to achieve the above research goals, this chapter is divided into three parts. The first part describes the research method, including research subjects, patent searching strategy, and the patent indicators for patent portfolio analysis. The second part explains the patent portfolio analysis of the technology capabilities of the stent industry and its major manufacturers. The third part includes the results of the patent analysis and the discussion of the implications for management.

2. Methodology

2.1. *Search strategy and dataset*

The United States of America is the most important country for stent research and production. The United States Patent and Trademark Office (USPTO) was used as the research population for the patent data search. The patent search was done based on interviews with experts and industrial leaders and studies on related topics.

This study used "stent" as the keyword in the claim field using LearningTech Corp.'s Patent Guider 1.0 (2005). The initial search resulted in 2,366 pieces of information, which ended up as 2,334 valid pieces after filtering out the obsolete and invalid patents. The 2,334 patents belonged to 587 assignees after sorting and matching the registered company names with the updated assignees. Lastly, the authors used the number of patent grants, and the number of patents was cited as the final search criterion. The information was then sorted based on the average rank of the citation rate and the number of patent grants, with the 10 companies with the smallest average

Table 2. The final list after applying the searching strategy.

Company	Number of patents	Rank of number of patents	Total citation rate	Rank of total citation rate	Average of the two ranks
Medtronics, Inc.	114	3	22.64	3	3
Cordis Neurovascular, Inc.	112	4	21.759	4	4
Cook, Inc.	47	6	40.468	2	4
Corvita Corp.	20	10	47	1	5.5
Schneider (USA)	47	7	20.021	5	6
Impra, Inc., a subsidiary of C.R. Bard, Inc.	32	8	19.063	6	7
Medinol Ltd.	49	5	14.796	10	7.5
Guidant Corp.	328	2	10.835	16	9
Iso Stent, Inc.	18	11	16.111	9	10
SCIMED Lifesystems, Inc.	339	1	7.333	21	11

number being the subjects for this study. The calculation process and results are listed in Table 2.

2.2. *Analysis of stent-related technology*

First of all, by looking at the technology life cycle (Figure 1), one can understand the correlations between patent application numbers and the number of assignees. Through the sections between the dots, one can determine the trend of technology development and accordingly understand the process of the related technology changes in the industry.

The emerging stage of stent-related technology was from 1976 to early 1990. The technology development reached its peak in the mid-1990s and ended, reaching the bottleneck stage, in 2001, when both the number of applications and assignees decreased. The decrease was due to the 20% failure rate caused by the BMS, which caused the side effect in in-stent

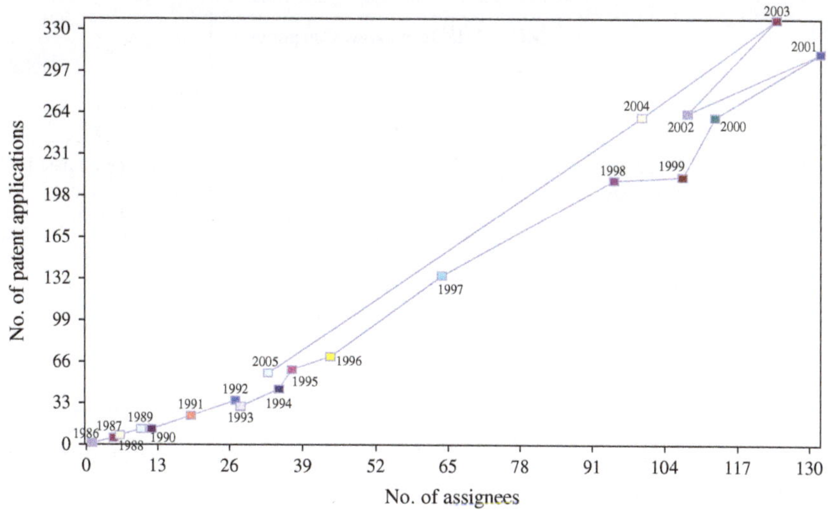

Figure 1. The technology lifecycle of stent-related technology.

restenosis. This led to the stagnation of revenue growth in 1999 and even slight regression in the revenue. By 2003, it was showing growth again, perhaps due to the appearance of DES, which caused the number of applications and assignees once more to increase, and then again in 2005, possibly due to the time lag between patent applications and technology development, which caused the decrease of both the number of applicants and number of assignees.

Because using the classification of UPC is too laborious, it will lead to over-estimation which will cause duplicated calculations for the same patent to occur, and because it's not easy to tell which products were applied by those technologies later, this study adopted the Patent Co-Citation Approach (PCA) (Lai and Wu, 2005) for its technology classification system and came up with three different major technology categories as the result of interviews with medical technology experts and cardiologists. Figure 2 shows the three major technology categories and their corresponding UPCs, which serve as the basis for the subsequent patent analysis.

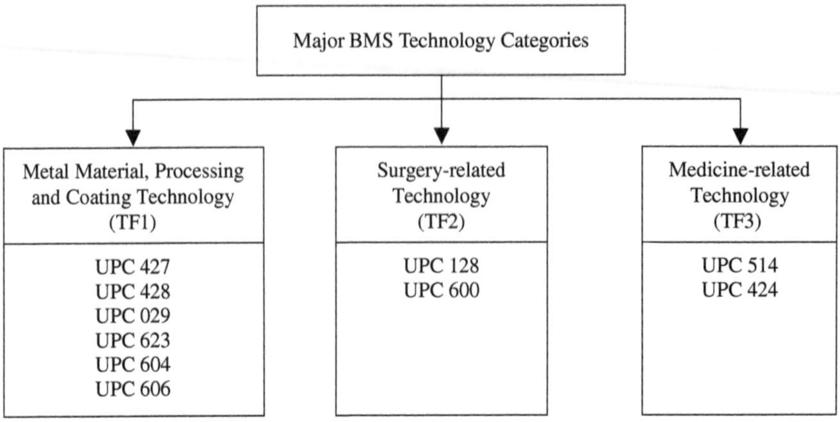

Figure 2. Major categories of stent-related technology and the corresponding UPCs.

2.3. *The construction of patent indicators*

The aim of this chapter is to study the field of technology and the major manufacturers of the stent industry. The study partially used an edited version of a two-dimensional patent portfolio by Brockhoff (1991). The indicators used were the following: the Relative Growth Rate (RGR), the Relative Development of Growth Rate (RDGR), and the Relative Patent Position (RPP) by Ernst (1998), and the Revealed Patent Advantage (RPA) by Schmoch (1995), to construct a three-dimensional patent portfolio analysis.

The use of those indicators will enable one to:

- make proper judgments about research companies' resource allocation and direction in the mainstream technology field;
- measure the differences in technology strengths or relative patent positioning between research companies and leading players;
- research the positioning of a company's patent portfolio and its adoptable research planning directions.

The four patent portfolio indicator instructions are detailed in what follows.

2.3.1. *Technology relative growth rate*

RGR represents relative growth rate. In this study, it is mainly used to measure the attractiveness of a certain technology field. If the RGR is high for that technology field, it means that that technology is growing quickly and with higher technology attractiveness.

The calculation of RGR is based on data from 1994 to 2004, as the total number of patent applications was not yet finalized for the year 2005. The number is the result of dividing the average rate of growth during the period by that of total technology fields' total in that year. This study assumed a zero growth rate for the years if the previous year had zero patent applications.

The calculation process and the results are listed in Table 3. One can see that the 10-year average growth rate for stent-related patent applications was 0.56 and concentrated on metal material, processing, and coating technology: the TF1 category. For the whole stent-related technology field, the relative growth rate of TF1 was 0.99, far higher than that of the other two technology categories. It's obvious that most of the stent manufacturers invested heavily in the TF1 category.

2.3.2. *Technology relative development growth rate*

RDGR indicates the relative development growth rate. It represents the mainstream technology patent applications in the last half period versus the first half period of the whole study window; it is also the measurement indicator of the technology's attractiveness. If the RDGR is higher in a certain technology field, it means that that particular technology had a higher growth rate in the recent years and more patent research was

Table 3. The growth rate, RGR, and RDGR of three major categories of stent manufacturers in 10 years.

	TF1		TF2		TF3		Total growth rate
Year	No. of Patents	Growth rate	No. of Patents	Growth rate	No. of Patents	Growth rate	
1994	7		0		0		
1995	26	2.71	0	0.00	0	0.00	2.71
1996	24	−0.08	3	0.00	0	0.00	0.04
1997	72	2.00	7	1.33	1	0.00	1.96
1998	95	0.32	17	1.43	0	−1.00	0.40
1999	82	−0.14	9	−0.47	1	0.00	−0.18
2000	104	0.27	16	0.78	2	1.00	0.33
2001	134	0.29	5	−0.69	5	1.50	0.18
2002	133	−0.01	2	−0.60	0	−1.00	−0.06
2003	180	0.35	3	0.50	2	0.00	0.37
2004	142	−0.21	3	0.00	5	1.50	−0.19
2005	26	−0.82	1	−0.67	1	−0.80	−0.81
Total no. of applications	999		65		16		
Average growth rate		0.55		0.23		0.20	0.56
RGR		0.99		0.41		0.36	
Average growth rate for the first 5 years		0.96		0.46		−0.20	
Average growth rate for the last 5 years		0.14		−0.002		0.60	
RDGR		0.14		−0.004		−3.00	

focused on that area. On the contrary, if the RDGR is lower in a certain technology field, then it means that that particular technology had negative growth or was in a stagnant stage and it was not a hot mainstream technology for the industry.

The study calculated each technology field's RDGR in the 5 years before 1999 and after 2000, per year. The calculation process and the results are listed in Table 3.

Ernst (1998) did not explain why the RDGR showed negative numbers, and the study will further explain this based on empirical data from the surgical and medicinal stent technology categories. If the RDGR rate was negative when the last half of the study period's average growth rate of applications numbers was negative and the first half's was positive, it meant that this technology field showed stagnation or regression in its development. It is very possible that it was facing a bottleneck stage or it was soon to be replaced by a new technology. This phenomenon can be validated by the data shown in TF2 where surgery-related technology showed slow growth in the 10-year period and its relative growth potential was close to zero. On the contrary, if the last half of the study period's average growth rate of application numbers was positive and the first half's was negative, it meant that this technology field was growing rapidly and had the potential to be the superstar of tomorrow that deserved close observation.

The above-mentioned phenomenon can also apply to the TF3 medicine-related technology field. One can find that although its RDGR was negative (–3) at the beginning, its last 5-year average growth rate was positive (0.6) and it had the fastest growth among the three categories. Therefore, one can conclude that coating medicines had a high growth in recent years. Combined with the continuous development of new medicines, coating medicines can either be applied to different diseases or be the target of co-opetition by other manufacturers of all three technology categories. The trend and development of the coating medicine field are worthy of close observation. Due to the above-mentioned validation and the application of theory to practices, the study herein modified Ernst's RDGR formula to make it more meaningful: The RDGR's absolute value will be positive when the last half of the study period's average growth rate of applications numbers was positive and the first half's was negative.

2.3.3. *Relative patent position*

RPP represents relative position. In this study, it is used to measure the relation between a certain company's number of patents pertaining to one technology with those of the leading technology companies. If the RPP value is close to 1, it means that the company's patent number is leading in that particular technology field. If the RPP is close to 0, then it means that there is a big gap between the company's technology capability and that of the leading companies.

The calculation process and the results are listed in Table 4. It shows that SCIMED Lifesystems, a subsidiary of Boston Scientific, is the leading company on a number of patents for both TF1 category's metal material, processing, and coating technology and TF2 category's surgery-related technology categories; it was also far ahead of others on patent numbers of TF3 category's medicine-related technology. On the contrary, Guidant is not only the benchmark company in TF3 technology but also its RPP is neck and neck with SCIMED, which is leading in TF1 technology. Therefore, one can conclude that although Guidant is behind in the new drug-eluting stent (DES) technology, it still has a very solid foundation that is worthy of attention.

The other point worth mentioning is that although Cordis is the leader in DES technology, its RPP does not hold any leading positions in the three technology categories. However, the fact that Cordis still demonstrates its competitive advantage in the market shows that it obviously has other core competencies. Those other core competencies may include the good relationship Cordis has with the Centers for Medicare and Medicaid Services (CMS) when its DES product was the first of its kind in the market, which decreased the time for other hospitals or doctors to adopt the new products (Lu, 2005). Cordis' better technology for lowering in-stent restenosis may also be their other core competency. Other companies can follow after or target Cordis for co-opetition.

Table 4. RPP for 10 companies on three major technology categories.

Company	SCIMED Life-systems Inc.	Guidant Corp.	Medtronics, Inc.	Cordis Neuro-vascular Inc.	Iso Stent Inc.	Medinol Ltd.	Schneider (USA)	Impra Inc.	Corvita Corp.	Cook Inc.	Total No. of patents
Technology											
TF1											
Total No. of patents	327	315	112	109	12	46	47	32	18	43	1061
RPP	1.00	0.96	0.34	0.33	0.04	0.14	0.14	0.10	0.06	0.13	
TF2											
Total No. of patents	16	9	16	8	9	6	0	2	2	1	69
RPP	1.00	0.56	1.00	0.50	0.56	0.38	0.00	0.13	0.13	0.06	
TF3											
Total No. of patents	5	7	2	2	0	0	1	0	0	0	17
RPP	0.71	1.00	0.29	0.29	0.00	0.00	0.14	0.00	0.00	0.00	
Average RPP	0.89	0.82	0.58	0.38	0.23	0.18	0.09	0.07	0.06	0.05	

2.3.4. *Revealed patent advantage*

RPA refers to revealed patent advantage. In this study, it is used to describe the technology strength of a company in the three major technology categories. Technology strength represents the scale of research of patent portfolio charts for the research companies. It can be used to judge the technology capabilities of the research companies. If the RPA is positive, it means that its relative technology capability is high. In order to get a positive PRA, the study added 100 to the respective RPAs from the three technology categories for the 10 companies, so that the RPAs were all between 0 and 200, in order to make a meaningful patent portfolio chart.

The calculation process and the results are listed in Table 5. The RPA results enable a company to understand its own technology development focus in all three categories. Take SCIMED Lifesystems, for example. Its internal technology focus resides in TF1 metal material, processing, and coating technology, while Guidant focuses more on the development of TF3 medicine-related technology development, and the RPA shows that Guidant has unbalanced development in the three technology categories.

3. Patent Portfolio Analysis

RGR and RDGR are used as the measurement indicators for technology attractiveness in Figures 3 and 4: RPP for the corresponding positioning between a company's technology development versus the patent numbers of the leading companies and RPA as the measurement indicator for a company's technology strength. The size of the circles represents the technology strength — the bigger the circle is, the stronger the technology strength. Together, they show the talent portfolio of the stent-related technology industry. This figure represents the integration of the three pieces of information. If the circles are big and moving toward the upper right, it means that the companies

Table 5. RPA for 10 companies on three major technology categories (after adding 100 to RPA).

Technology Category	TF 1			TF 2			TF 3			
	# (P1j)	P1j/ΣP1j	RPAij+100	# (P2j)	P2j/ΣP2j	RPAij+100	# (P3j)	P3j/ΣP3j	RPAij+100	Total (ΣPij)
Company										
SCIMED Lifesystems Inc.	327	0.94	101.57	16	0.05	73.75	5	0.01	96.89	348
Guidant Corp.	315	0.95	102.84	9	0.03	33.93	7	0.02	134.12	331
Medtronics Inc.	112	0.86	92.90	16	0.12	161.43	2	0.02	103.73	130
Cordis Neurovascular Inc.	109	0.92	99.02	8	0.07	111.07	2	0.02	112.51	119
Iso Stent Inc.	12	0.57	55.24	9	0.43	196.14	0	0.00	0.00	21
Medinol Ltd.	46	0.88	95.54	6	0.12	157.26	0	0.00	0.00	52
Schneider (USA)	47	0.98	105.68	0	0.00	0.00	1	0.02	132.79	48
Impra Inc.	32	0.94	101.73	2	0.06	97.76	0	0.00	0.00	34
Corvita Corp.	18	0.90	97.26	2	0.10	146.86	0	0.00	0.00	20
Cook Inc.	43	0.98	105.49	1	0.02	24.98	0	0.00	0.00	44
(ΣPij)	1061			69			17			1147
ΣPij/ΣΣPij	0.93			0.06			0.01			

are currently developing hot or innovative technology products and are generating many patents. In contrast, if the circles are smaller and are moving toward the lower left, it generally means that the companies' technologies have matured, their futures are limited, and their patents will also be relatively fewer. Figure 3 is the patent portfolio chart that is based on RGR, while Figure 4 is the patent portfolio chart that is based on RDGR.

The analysis of the three technology categories in the stent-related technology industry is carried out in what follows.

3.1. *Metal material, processing and coating technology* (*TF1*)

Comparing the three technology categories of stent-related technology, the RGR of the metal material, processing, and coating technology category (TF1) is higher than that of the other two and the RDGR of TF3 technology is also relatively higher than that of the other two, with better potential. It shows that the new-generation stent-related technology research is focused on drug-eluting technology.

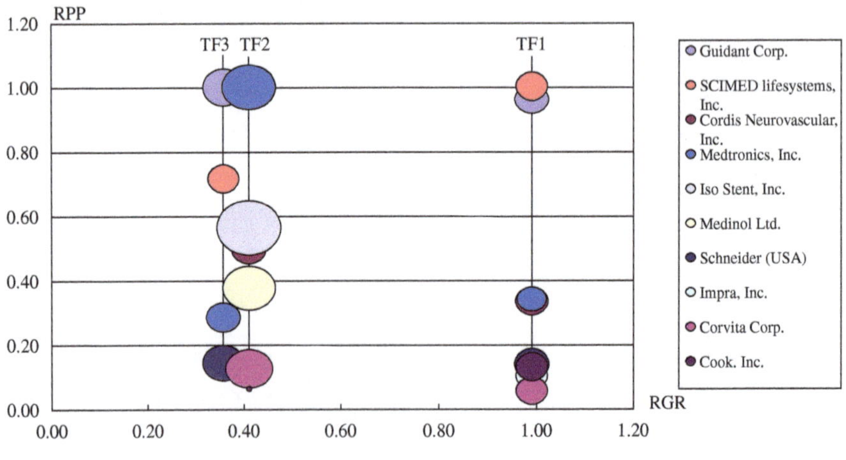

Figure 3. The patent portfolio with RGR as indicator.

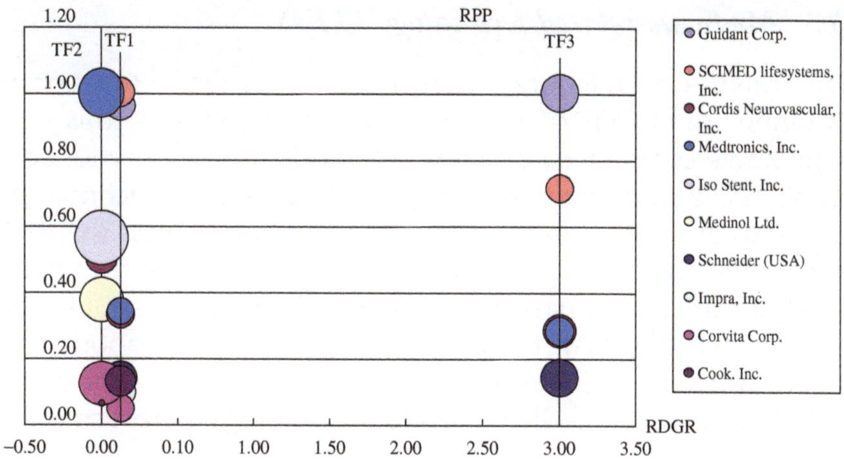

Figure 4. The patent portfolio with RDGR as indicator.

If one observes the circle sizes of the 10 companies, the technology strengths are about the same for all in the TF1 category, which means that their technology capabilities are almost equal. Cook and Schneider (USA) are the two with higher technology capabilities from the RPA point of view. Looking at RPP, all 10 companies have their own patents, with SCIMED Lifesystems leading with the most patents and Guidant ranking second in the number of patents.

3.2. *Surgery-related technology* (*TF2*)

The growth of surgery-related technology (TF2) has been slower in the past 10 years, with its RDGR being negative. One can conclude that the stent-related surgical technology has matured. From the TF2 circle sizes, it is clear that Iso Stent has the strongest technology, and Medtronics ranks second. SCIMED Lifesystems and Medtronics are the two benchmark companies with the most number of patents. Only Schneider (USA) has no patents in this category.

3.3. *Medicine-related technology (TF3)*

One can tell from Figure 4 that the RDGR of the TF3 category is higher than that of the other two categories. In this category, five companies, Iso Stent, Medinol, Impra, Corvita, and Cook, had zero patents and they scored a zero for technology strength and RPP. Among the other five companies, the RPP for Schneider (USA) is only 0.14, which is far behind that of the benchmark company Guidant. However, for both Guidant and Schneider (USA), their technology strength is about the same under the TF3 category. It is possible that Schneider (USA) has greater medicine-related technology expertise than Guidant.

4. Conclusion

Based on the above analysis, the results of the patent analysis for the 10 companies in the three technology categories are listed in Table 6.

The companies can figure out their own technology investment and technology capability positions based on the four situations mentioned subsequently and then start to plan their co-opetition strategies.

- When the relative patent positioning is minor (RPP≥0.5) and the technology capability is high (RPA≥100) between one company and the leading company, that company has a competitive advantage in that particular technology category, such as TF1, so that company should continue with its research and development. The co-opetition strategy can then focus on how to license its patents to outsiders and strengthen its marketing capability, perhaps by finding partners who can compliment its market assets in order to maintain its leading edge. The company also needs to make long-term plans with technologies that have future potential, such as TF3, in order to sustain its long-term growth.

Table 6. The correlation of RPP and technology capability of the 10 stent manufacturers.

		TF1 Metal Material, Processing, Coating Technology (Current technology with high attractiveness)	**TF2** Surgery-related Technology (Low technology attractiveness)	**TF3** Medicine-related Technology (Future technology with high attractiveness)
RPP≥0.5	RPA≥100	SCIMED Lifesystems Guidant	Medtronics Cordis Neurovascular Iso Stent	Guidant
	RPA<100		SCIMED Lifesystems Guidant	SCIMED Lifesystems
RPP<0.5	RPA≥100	Schneider (USA) Impra Cook	Medinol Corvita	Medtronics Cordis Neurovascular Schneider (USA)
	RPA<100	Medtronics Cordis Neurovascular Iso Stent Medinol Corvita	Schneider (USA) Impra Cook	Iso Stent Medinol Impra Corvita Cook

- When the relative patent positioning is minor (RPP≥0.5) but the technology capability is low (RPA<100) between one company and the leading company, that company should consider cutting down its technology investments in that particular field or try to get external resources to support that technology. SCIMED Lifesystems and Guidant lack R&D efficiency in the TF2 technology and they may consider working with external technology resources from or even mergers with companies like Medinol or Corvita that have high technology capability and higher RPP.
- When the relative patent positioning is large (RPP<0.5) and the technology capability is high (RPA≥100) between one company and the leading company, it means that that company owns important patent technology. Even if the number of patents it owns is not large, it is still good enough for a greater technological capability and R&D in that area should be continued. Schneider (USA), Impra, and Cook are the examples in TF1 that own important technology resources and can consider leveraging these technology resources for licensing or for strategic alliances.
- When the relative patent positioning is large (RPP<0.5) and the technology capability is low (RPA<100) between one company and the leading company, that company may consider giving up that technology field and finding a new direction like, harvesting its patents; selling the patents; or merging, licensing, or getting outside technology resources. Schneider (USA), Impra, and Cook are such companies in the TF2 category.

This study used patent indicators to analyze the stent-related technology industry. This study followed three major technology categories and their respective development trends and the companies that represented those categories and their technology capabilities and strengths. Biotech is an industry that requires a longer investment period, with higher costs and bigger risks. The laws that regulate the biotech industry are more rigid, as it may impact people's lives. In order to use its resources more effectively, the co-opetition concept should be one of the major foci when planning business strategies.

The analysis and discussion in this chapter will help decision-makers integrate patent and technology strategies while forming business strategies. They should leverage their competitive advantages to gain market shares and license externally and compensate for their weaknesses by seeking proper external technology resources through mergers, co-ownership, or alliances in order to maximize benefits.

References

Berkowitz, L. (1993). Getting the most from your patents, *Research Technology Management*, 36(2), 26–31.

Brandenburger, A. M. and Nalebuff, B. J. (1996). Co-opetition: A revolution mindset that combines competition and cooperation, *The Game Theory Strategy that's Changing the Game of Business*, Bantam Doubleday Dell Publishing Group, Inc., New York.

Brockhoff, K. (1991). Competitor technology intelligence in German companies, *Industrial Marketing Management*, 20, 91–98.

Ernst, H. (1997). The use of patent for technological forecasting: The diffusion of CNC-Technology in the machine tool industry, *Small Business Economy*, 9, 361–381.

Ernst, H. (1998). Patent portfolios for strategic R&D planning, *Research Policy*, 9, 361–381.

Hufker, T. and F. Alpert. (1994). Patents: A managerial perspective, *Journal of Product & Brand Management*, 3(4), 44–54.

Lai, K. K. and Wu, S. J. (2005). Using the patent co-citation approach to establish a new patent classification system, *Information Processing and Management*, 41, 313–330.

LearningTech Corp. (2005). Patent Guider v2.0. http://www.learning.com.tw.

Lu, Y. W. (2005). From the successful case of Cypher™. http://www.itis.org.tw.

Mogee, M. E. (1991). Using patent data for technology analysis and planning, *Research Technology Management*, 34(4), 43–49.

Schmoch, U. (1995). Evaluation of technology strategies of companies by means of MDS maps, *International Journal of Technology Management*, 10, 426–427.

Chapter 6

Success Factors for Strategic Partnerships in the Biotechnology Sector

Uwe Kehrel*,‡, Kai Klischan*,§ and Nathalie Sick†,¶

**Institute of Business Administration, Department of Chemistry and Pharmacy, University of Muenster, Germany*

†*Faculty of Engineering and IT, University of Technology, Sydney, Australia*

‡*u.kehrel@uni-muenster.de*

§*k.klischan@uni-muenster.de*

¶*Nathalie.Sick@uts.edu.au*

Abstract

Over half of all research-oriented partnerships in the biotechnology industry fail due to problems in inter-organizational relationships. The analysis of factors that determine the success of strategic partnerships can help companies reduce the high failure rates. Based on the resource-oriented and relationship-oriented approach, this chapter examines the influence of three structural factors and three dynamic factors on the success of strategic, research-oriented partnerships in the biotechnology industry. In the empirical analysis, data from 48 research collaborations by 28 companies were collected and analyzed. The results confirm the significant influence of the factors "complementary resources", "operational compatibility", "bilateral exchange of information", and "opportunistic behavior". On the basis of these findings, companies can identify approaches to influence the success of their own research collaborations. In particular, appropriate recommendations for action can be derived in the context of the structural design of partnerships and the dynamic exchange process.

Keywords: Biotechnology, research collaboration, strategic partnership, technology alliances, technology collaboration.

1. Introduction

In the period 1977–2010, about 71% of all research-oriented partnerships in the biotechnology industry failed before the product under development had reached the market (Havenaar and Hiscocks, 2012). It must be emphasized that only about 46% of failed partnerships were terminated due to unsatisfactory research results, while in about half the cases, the problems were based on inter-organizational relationships. Biotechnology companies, however, have to rely on numerous mutualistic partners, in the context of research as well as other partnerships along the value chain (Hagedoorn and Duysters, 2002). The company's success is therefore particularly dependent on the capabilities of the partner companies, the design of the respective partnerships, and ultimately on the success of the strategic partnerships (Baum *et al.*, 2000). The analysis of factors that explain the success of strategic partnerships in research-intensive industries such as the biotechnology industry can help companies reduce the high failure rates. Given the importance of strategic partnerships for biotechnology companies, empirically validated success factors can therefore lead to significant efficiency gains.

In previous academic works, the investigation of the success factors of inter-firm partnerships took place in the context of different theoretical approaches and different industry sectors (Duysters *et al.*, 1999; Gulati, 1998; Jiang *et al.*, 2008; Kale and Singh, 2007; Pekar and Allio, 1994; Taylor, 2005; Zollo *et al.*, 2002). However, many of the existing works use a single predominant theoretical approach or focus on factors that are of relevance at or after the formation of a strategic partnership (Deitz *et al.*, 2010; Mohr and Spekman, 1994). Frequently, no account is taken of the specificities that occur with regard to the measurement of success in partnerships. In addition, there are only a few studies which deal with the characteristics of research-intensive industries and in particular of the biotechnology industry (Al-Laham *et al.*, 2010; Baden-Fuller and Morgan, 2010; Baum *et al.*, 2000; Stuart, 2000; Zollo *et al.*, 2002). From the perspective of this chapter, these aspects can be an explanation of why the failure rate for partnerships in the biotechnology industry, despite the many years of scientific investigation of potential success factors, is still unsatisfactorily high.

The aim of this chapter is thus to derive factors from the resource-oriented approach as well as from the relationship-oriented approach and to verify empirically their impact on the success of strategic partnerships in the medical biotechnology industry. The derived factors relate to aspects that may be relevant both at and after the formation of the partnership. In summary, the following research question guides this work:

> What factors influence the success of strategic partnerships in the medical biotechnology industry from the perspective of the resource- and relationship-oriented approach?

The chapter is structured as follows: Section 2 deals with the basics of strategic partnerships in research-intensive industries. In this context, structure and aims of strategic partnerships along the value chain of the medical biotechnology industry are described. In Section 3, the hypotheses are derived in the light of the existing literature and an appropriate model is formulated, while Section 4 focuses on data and methods. In Section 5, the results of the empirical analysis are presented, while Section 6 summarizes discussion and implications. Section 7 continues with a summary of the results, making particular reference to the limitations of this work and the need for further research.

2. Strategic Partnerships in the Biotechnology Industry

2.1. *Strategic partnerships in research-intensive industries*

In research-intensive industries, access to the resources of the partner is the overriding motive for the formation of strategic partnerships (Das and Teng, 2000a; Hagedoorn *et al.*, 2000). According to the resource-oriented approach, valuable, difficult-to-imitate, and non-substitutable resources form a sustainable competitive advantage for companies (Hagedoorn *et al.*, 2000). The performance potential of a company is therefore a result of the strategic differentiation of its resource base compared to the competition. Thus, the resource-oriented approach concludes that access to capital, skills, expertise, and new technologies are important motives. The observation of new technologies in the context of partnerships can be regarded as a separate motive (Hagedoorn, 1993).

In research-intensive industries — in which the development and commercialization of advanced technologies are essential — access to new technological expertise is frequently mentioned in the literature as the main motive (Baum *et al.*, 2000; Mowery *et al.*, 1996). Companies face the long-lasting challenge of obtaining new knowledge from outside the company boundaries, in order to transform their own skills with it and apply these to the development of new products and services (Al-Laham *et al.*, 2010). Partnerships with other companies are viewed as an effective way to acquire the implicit knowledge of other companies (Al-Laham *et al.*, 2010; Hagedoorn *et al.*, 2000). In summary, it is argued in the resource-oriented approach that companies in research-intensive industries are able, by using strategic partnerships, to internalize the necessary resources to compete successfully (Hagedoorn, 1993). Partnerships, thus, enable companies in complex and capital-intensive performance processes to achieve their objectives more efficiently (Murphy, 1988).

In addition to the resource aspect, research and development (R&D) partnerships also offer the opportunity to reduce risk in R&D of new products. The high risk is reduced on the one hand by combining the expertise and, on the other hand, by reducing the resulting financial loss to the individual partner companies in the event of a failed development or commercialization (Mellewigt, 2003). Especially in high-tech industries, the capital requirements and risk profiles of R&D projects are high and rising (Mowery *et al.*, 1996). Strategic partnerships in this context are a good way to spread the risk and the cost to both partners (Glaister and Buckley, 1996).

Another important motive for strategic partnerships is to gain a time advantage during the value creation process (Hagedoorn, 1993). Strategic partnerships can thus lead to an earlier market entry, which makes it possible to establish strategic advantages over potential, challenging competitors in the market (McCutchen and Swamidass, 2004). According to this reasoning, strategic partnerships should be pursued if the strategic advantages of the "first-mover" effect outweigh the costs of the partnership.

The institutionalization and management of complex and research-intensive partnerships are extremely challenging (Douma *et al.*, 2000). Contrary to the hopes of being able to realize synergies quickly, many partnerships do not reach their initial goals (Deitz *et al.*, 2010). Das and Teng (2000b) and Spekman *et al.* (1996) assume a failure rate of approximately 60%. In this context, failure is defined as a material change or early termination of the strategic partnership, which was unplanned from the perspective of one or more partners (Das and Teng, 2000b).

2.2. *Overview of the biotechnology industry*

The biotechnology industry is heterogeneous and covers different disciplines, fields of application, and procedures. The focus of the study at hand is on companies in the medical biotechnology sector whose main business objective is in the application of biotechnological processes for the production and provision of medical products and services or the carrying out of R&D activities (Beuzekom and Arundel, 2009).

The value creation process in the pharmaceutical and biotechnology industry is complex, risky, time-consuming, and costly. The costs for the development of innovative therapies, from the initial idea in basic research to an approved, marketable drug, have risen steadily over the past decades (Morgan *et al.*, 2011). The average size of the R&D expenditure varies greatly, depending on the illness involved and the underlying success rates and cost of capital. A study by DiMasi and Grabowski (2007) on the average R&D expenditure per successfully developed biotechnologically active ingredient calculated the costs at approximately 613 million dollars. Taking the size of the capital costs over the entire development period into account, the absolute R&D expenses increased to 1,362 million dollars, of which 675 million dollars were spent on research and 687 million dollars were spent in the development phase (DiMasi and Grabowski, 2007).

2.3. *Strategic partnerships along the biotechnology value chain*

In scientific literature, the biotechnology value chain is often distinguished into inbound and outbound partnerships to

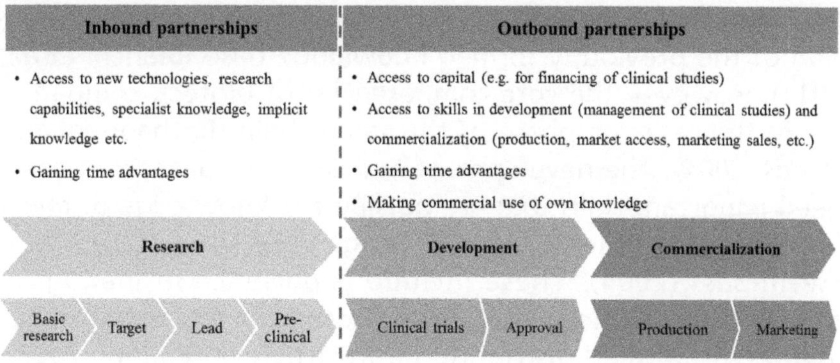

Figure 1. Different forms of partnerships assigned to the respective value chain steps in the biotechnology industry.
Source: Based on Baum *et al.* (2000), Bianchi *et al.* (2011) and Rothaermel and Deeds (2004).

categorize typical motives, partnership types, and partner companies more accurately (see Figure 1).

Inbound partnerships are particularly relevant in the research phase of the value chain, from basic research to pre-clinical studies (Bianchi *et al.*, 2011). The main motives for the formation of these strategic partnerships are to gain access to the new technologies, research capabilities, and expertise of other companies (Rothaermel and Deeds, 2004). However, in the research phase of the value chain, this knowledge is often still implicit, i.e., company-specific and difficult to transfer (Baum *et al.*, 2000). In contrast to licensing agreements or market-oriented transactions, strategic partnerships are therefore particularly suitable for obtaining access to the knowledge of other biotech companies. Acquiring a license in conjunction with an intensive partnership exchange relationship is also an effective way to ensure access to knowledge from the biotech company's perspective. Strategic partnerships with universities, research institutes, and other biotech companies can also ensure timely access to new ideas and research approaches thereby resulting in time-saving (Baum *et al.*, 2000).

Outbound partnerships are mainly sought by biotech companies in the second part of the value chain, after the clinical trial, and thus help with the development and commercialization of the previously formed knowledge base (Bianchi *et al.*, 2011). However, the core competencies of biotech companies are in the research phase of the value chain (Rothaermel and Deeds, 2004). The development and commercialization phases need important skills that are outside the knowledge of many biotech companies (Das and Teng, 1998; McCutchen and Swamidass, 2004). These include experience in managing clinical trials, sufficient production capacity, marketing skills, and an established distribution infrastructure (Villiger, 2009). McCutchen and Swamidass (2004) therefore found the following: "(···) Small biotech firms have limited capabilities. Small biotech firms need the capital and the downstream capabilities that larger firms possess, (···)". Large pharmaceutical companies have both the necessary knowledge as well as the necessary financial resources to support biotech companies in successfully developing a drug at this stage of the value creation process (Baum *et al.*, 2000).

From the view of the biotechnology company, one solution, at this stage of the value chain, can be a combination of an off-license of the product and a strategic partnership with a pharmaceutical company. Both the biotech company and the pharmaceutical company are bringing active knowledge into these partnerships (Al-Laham *et al.*, 2010). The off-license — through which a pharmaceutical company secures rights to the drug — allows biotech companies a direct commercialization of research results and ensures the continued funding of operating activities (Havenaar and Hiscocks, 2012).

However, the limitations of a biotech company's capital and knowledge for the development and commercialization phase lead to the fact that most strategic partnerships between biotech companies in the therapeutics market and pharmaceutical companies are already formed at the beginning of the first phase of the clinical trial. In a few cases, partnerships with pharmaceutical companies also come into being before the end of the pre-clinical phase, since the risk of failure there is still very high (Bianchi *et al.*, 2011). In about 20% of cases, biotechnology companies are able to independently develop the candidate drug by the end of the second clinical study (March-Chordà and Yagüe-Perales, 2011).

In summary, the observations on inbound and outbound partnerships show that biotechnology companies — due to the high complexity of the process and their own specialization in certain phases of the value chain — are dependent on many other companies and institutions to be able to successfully develop and market a new drug. The success of a biotechnology company is therefore particularly dependent on the capabilities of all the partner companies, as well as the design of the respective partnership (Baum *et al.*, 2000). McCutchen and Swamidass (2004) speak in this context of a "functional incompleteness" of smaller biotech companies.

3. Research Model

Compared to the intensive examination of success factors and the reasons for failure in strategic partnerships, there are few studies that feature the specific key performance indicators of a partnership (Zollo *et al.*, 2002). Gulati (1998) explains this in particular based on the difficulty of collecting relevant and comparable data on the success of strategic partnerships.

Many of the early empirical studies measuring the success of strategic partnerships use financial or quantitative measures, such as profitability, growth, or life of the partnership (Nielsen, 2007). The primary goal of strategic partnerships, however, is rather to generate growth in knowledge, to minimize risks, or to gain time advantages. For example, it is conceivable that a strategic partnership in terms of the original motives far exceeds the goals of its partners and is perceived by its stakeholders as very successful, even though the financial results or other objective measures might be negatively assessed (Geringer and Hebert, 1991). Ohmae (1989) holds in this context the following view: "Most of the time, the financials don't capture the real benefits of alliances". More quantitative measures such as the duration of the partnership are also unsuitable to measure the success of the partnership, as many inter-company relations can be terminated by mutual agreement as a success after very different time periods (Mohr and Spekman, 1994). It should also be noted that the high-risk profile of partnerships in research-intensive industries makes the use of financial ratios difficult (Glaister and Buckley, 1999). The subjective evaluation of a strategic partnership by the participants is therefore recognized as a meaningful measure of success (Huang *et al.*, 2009; Jiang *et al.*, 2008; Kale and Singh, 2007; Nielsen, 2007; Sarkar *et al.*, 2001; Saxton, 1997). Analogous to these findings, the perceived success of the partnership is taken as a measure in this chapter. A partnership will be perceived as successful when the benefits of a partnership are greater than the individual potential brought to the partnership and the individual expenses incurred for the organization and coordination of the partnership (Anderson and Narus, 1990; Balling, 1997; Gaister and Buckley, 1999).

In the literature on strategic partnerships, two theoretical frameworks have emerged to derive determinants of the success or failure of partnerships — the resource-oriented and the relational approach (Nielsen, 2007). Supporters of the resource-oriented approach focus on the structural factors of a strategic partnership, which should be taken into account *ex ante* (Sarkar *et al.*, 2001). Thus, the resource-based dependency between the partner companies, as well as the compatibility between their operations, is the key success factor in order to achieve the objectives in a partnership (Sarkar *et al.*, 2001). In addition to the resource-oriented approach, the dynamic (socio-psychological) factors of a strategic partnership are highlighted in the relational approach (Nielsen, 2007). Instead of looking at each partnership as a single transaction, the relationship-oriented approach focuses on the long-term cooperation between the partner companies (Saxton, 1997).

3.1. *Structural factors*

Previous studies suggest that the complementary resources of the partners are important for the success of the partnership (Sarkar *et al.*, 2001). From their theoretical derivation, based on transaction cost theory and the resource-oriented approach, Madhok and Tallman (1998) conclude that interfirm partnerships in which the partners bring complementary resources are likely to have above-average success. Sarkar *et al.* (2001) found in their study that complementary resources had a significant positive impact on the project's success. However, they have not demonstrated a significant impact on the strategic success of the partnerships they studied (Sarkar *et al.*, 2001). Suarez and García-Canal (2003) showed, in their empirical study of 72 international partnerships, a significant and clearly positive correlation between complementary resources and abnormal returns. Deitz *et al.* (2010) came recently to a similar result, based on a sample of 201 equity joint ventures. In their study, they have shown that complementary resources had a significant positive impact both on the stability of the joint venture as well as on the subjective evaluation of the joint venture by the respective partners. For strategic partnerships in the high-tech sector, complementary resource endowments between the partners are particularly important since businesses can operate in areas that they could not have dealt with independently (Sarkar *et al.*, 2001). It can therefore be inferred that more pronounced the success of the partnership is, the greater are the complementary resources brought in by the partners:

H1: *The perceived partnership success is positively influenced by complementary resources in the partnership.*

However, for successful collaboration, it might be useful for partnering companies not to be too far apart and having too different or complementary resources in order to have a common basis to communicate and exchange basic technical knowledge.

In this regard, Madhok and Tallman (1998) remarked that compatibility, or the congruence in organizational cultures and structures between alliance partners, has a positive effect on the potential for synergies and increases the ability of partners to raise this potential for synergies within the partnership. Mowery *et al.* (1996) also find, in their empirical study on 792 alliances, a positive relationship between a similar technological base in the expertise of the partners and the potential growth of knowledge, which was used as a measure of the success of the partnerships. With respect to companies in a high-tech sector, Fornahl *et al.* (2011) have also recently demonstrated that a large cognitive distance between the partner companies has a significantly negative effect on the number of registered patents and the success of the partnership. Thus, operational compatibility provides the ability to assess the value of the partner's new information, so as to be able to integrate and apply it in one's own company. A higher compatibility reduces the costs of coordination. It also allows the partner's behavior to be monitored and facilitates the management of expectations in the partnership (Sarkar *et al.*, 2001):

H2: *The perceived success of the partnership is positively influenced by operational compatibility of the partners.*

Compatibility between their operations includes the requirement for a relationship between the partner companies that is as free as possible from competitive considerations. Glaister and Buckley (1999) show, for example, in their study of 94 international partnerships, a significant negative correlation between the competitive situation in the partnership and the subjective assessment of the cost–benefit ratio of the partnership. Mowery *et al.* (1996) also measure a significantly negative relationship between the degree of market and product similarity and the knowledge transfer between two partner companies. Also, Park and Russo (1996) show that joint ventures fail most frequently when the partner companies are in direct competition with each other outside the partnership.

Accordingly, it can be assumed that in the high-tech sector, success-endangering effects are particularly likely to occur in partnerships between companies with a similar business model. In these horizontal partnerships, access to strategically relevant resources is very difficult to achieve (Balling, 1997). In vertical partnerships with companies that have different business models, success-endangering effects are less likely. Balling (1999) also points out that small businesses in particular are at risk of losing advantages in their strategic position in R&D partnerships, when they bring their R&D expertise into a partnership. This again illustrates the special relevance of the competitive relationship as a success factor in the high-tech sector:

H3: *The perceived success of the partnership is negatively affected by competition between the partners.*

3.2. *Dynamic factors*

Trust can be understood as a general assessment of the reliability and integrity of the partner company (Morgan and Hunt, 1994). Morgan and Hunt (1994) demonstrate in their study that a high level of trust leads, for example, to a reduction in uncertainty and strengthens the partnership. Trust in the partner promotes tolerance in the case of conflict and reduces friction between the partners (Mohr and Spekman, 1994; Nienaber and Schewe, 2014). Similarly, Deitz *et al.* (2010) showed that trust in strategic partnerships had a positive influence on the stability of the partnership. Anderson and Narus (1990) also confirmed that trust has a significantly negative impact on conflicts in the partnership and a significantly positive effect on the success of and satisfaction with the partnership.

The degree of complexity of strategic partnerships in research-intensive industries is extremely high. Trust is more important in complex partnerships, since it is hardly possible here to evaluate and monitor every piece of information that is exchanged between the partners (Nielsen, 2007). Only a sufficient level of trust can reduce the perceived need to monitor a partner company. Consequently, the trust of a high-tech company in its partner company promotes access to external knowledge and supports its ability to develop new skills in a mutual exchange with the partner. In a partnership related to research or development, trust acts to increase efficiency in the formation of new resources and allows the research-intensive companies to gain an above-average benefit from the partnership (Al-Laham *et al.*, 2010):

H4: *The perceived success of the partnership is positively influenced by trust in the partner.*

The strength of the bilateral exchange of information is another dynamic success factor that can be derived from the relationship-oriented approach. The bilateral exchange of information is defined as the degree of formal and informal communication of meaningful and timely information between the partner companies (Anderson and Narus, 1990).

A high bilateral exchange of information supports the management of the companies' expectations regarding their partner, improves the perception of the partnership, and helps to develop strategies on how to proceed with the partnership (Wittmann *et al.*, 2009). Only through the regular exchange of relevant information is it possible to align the interests and values of its partners and to reduce misunderstandings and uncertainty (Sarkar *et al.*, 2001). Where commitment to the operational exchange of information is deteriorating from the point of view of timeliness, formality and content, the likelihood of conflicts in the partnership also increases (Balling, 1997). Effective communication between the partners is therefore essential to gain the advantages of a partnership (Mohr and Spekman, 1994):

H5: *The perceived success of the partnership is positively influenced by bilateral information exchange between the partners.*

Strategic partnerships are inherently incomplete contracts in which property rights with respect to the results of the partnership are not always fully defined and clearly divided between the partners (Parkhe, 1993). In the context of strategic partnerships, it is regarded as opportunistic behavior if a company violates the mutual partnership agreement in order to be able to realize short-term gains to the detriment of its partner company (Parkhe, 1993). Opportunism, or the perception of opportunistic behavior, has the potential to have a negative influence on the performance and the success of a partnership (Luo, 2007). The perception of opportunism means that the partnership structures need to be adapted, with time-consuming effort. This adaptation eventually causes high transaction costs, for example, for the negotiation, monitoring, and enforcement of claims against the partner company. This enabled Parkhe (1993), in his empirical study on strategic partnerships, to demonstrate that the perception of opportunistic behavior has a significantly negative effect on both measurements of success used by him. Also, Delerue (2005), in her analysis of 87 partnerships, showed that opportunistic behavior had a strongly negative and significant effect on the perceived performance of the partnership:

H6: *The perceived success of the partnership is negatively affected by opportunistic behavior between the partners.*

3.3. *Control variable*

The success of a strategic partnership may also be influenced by the degree of partnership experience of both partners (Wittmann *et al.*, 2009; Zollo *et al.*, 2002). Partnership competence is defined in this context as "an organizational ability for finding, developing, and managing alliances" (Lambe *et al.*, 2002). This definition shows that both structural and dynamic aspects are included in the competency-based approach. Access to appropriate partner companies is dependent on experience with partnerships (Day, 1995). Therefore, companies with experience of partnership are better able to select appropriate partners, to conduct negotiations on the design of the partnership, and to determine the distribution of roles within the partnership. As Baum *et al.* (2000) found, this is especially true for the biotechnology industry: "(···) in biotechnology, a firm's success is widely held to depend on (···) its prior set of alliances". Second, the experience of similar partnerships has a positive effect on a company's ability to manage the partnership, to develop it, and to absorb new knowledge (Lambe *et al.*, 2002; Wittmann *et al.*, 2009). In research-intensive industries, these skills are particularly important (Al-Laham *et al.*, 2010). In order to check the validity of the hypothesis system that has been developed, "partnership experience" is considered as a control variable and included in the model.

4. Data and Methods

For the empirical study, a standardized questionnaire was developed. Before data collection, the reliability and validity of the questionnaire were pre-tested. The sample includes companies whose main business objective is the application of biotechnological processes for the production and delivery of products and services or the performance of R&D activities. The products, services, and R&D activities of these companies directly or indirectly aim to develop new drugs or new diagnostic methods. In this analysis, 207 companies in the medical biotechnology sector were considered in more detail. A total of 31 companies answered questions about one or more of their strategic partnerships with other companies. The proportion of actual respondents out of all the companies contacted was thus around 15%. A total of 51 questionnaires were completed by the 31 companies surveyed, of which three questionnaires were incomplete. These three questionnaires were not considered further. A total of 48 full questionnaires, which were answered by 28 companies, were finally included for the subsequent descriptive characterization of the data set and further analysis.

The variables, which were theoretically derived in Chapter 3, were operationalized in the context of the empirical analysis, where possible, by using scales that had been used in a similar context in the literature. For a detailed overview of constructs and items, see Table 1.

- **Operationalization of partnership success:** This work is based on perceived success in the partnership. Here, success is measured by three indicators on a five-point Likert scale, taking into account the objectives of partnerships in the biotechnology industry (Zollo *et al.*, 2002).
- **Operationalization of the structural factors:** The three structural factors which had been identified were covered by using a total of eight items on a five-point Likert scale. The factor "complementary resources" was measured with two indicators relating to the permanent value and dependence on the partner's resources (Sarkar *et al.*, 2001). Three indicators for the measurement of the factor "operational compatibility" were developed, based on Sarkar *et al.* (2001), and relate to technical, organizational, as well as employee compatibility between the partners. The operationalization of the factor "competitive relationship" follows the definition used by Abell (1980).
- **Operationalization of the dynamic factors:** The three structural factors which had been identified were covered by using a total of 13 items on a five-point Likert scale. The factor "trust" was measured with four items (Deitz *et al.*, 2010). For the operationalization of the "bilateral exchange of information" between the partnership companies, a scale from Sarkar *et al.* (2001) was used with three items that relate to the regularity, simplicity, and the degree of formality of the contacts. The six items of the factor "opportunistic behavior" ultimately come from Parkhe (1993) and are aimed at a behavioral assessment of the partner company by the biotech company.

Table 1. Operationalization of factors.

Construct	Item
Complementary resources (Sarkar *et al.*, 2001)	
CR_dependent	Both firms needed each other's resources to accomplish their goals and responsibilities.
CR_value	Resources brought into the venture by each firm were very valuable for the other firms.
Operational compatibility (Sarkar *et al.*, 2001)	
CB_technical	Technical capabilities of the two firms were compatible with each other.
CB_organizational	The organizational procedures of the two firms were compatible.
CB_employees	Employees of both firms had similar professional or trade skills.
Competitive relationship (Abell, 1980)	
	The goods and services provided by us and our partners relevant in the partnership …
CRS_functions	Serve similar functions.
CRS_technologies	Are created with the use of similar technology.
CRS_customer	Are used by similar users.
Trust (Deitz *et al.* (2010))	
	In our partnership, we have found our partner …
TR_credible	Can be counted on to do what is right.
TR_conscientious	Is always faithful.
TR_reliance	Is someone we have great confidence in.
TR_integrity	Has high integrity.
Opportunistic behavior (Parkhe, 1993)	
	As you know, cooperative relationships are sometimes subject to "opportunistic" behavior. That is, one firm may not abide by the terms of the agreement in order to exploit the other for short-term gain. Examples of opportunistic behavior are withholding or distorting information, shirking or failing to fulfill promises or obligations, appropriation of the partner firm's technology or key personnel, late payments, and delivery of substandard products. With respect to your partner firm in the present alliance:

(*Continued*)

Table 1. (*Continued*)

Construct	Item
OB_corporate image	They have always provided us a complete truthful picture of their business.
OB_honest	Complete honesty does not pay when dealing with my partner.
OB_facts	Sometimes my partner alters the facts slightly in order to get what they need.
OB_assignment completion	My partner carries out their duties even if we do not check up on them.
OB_promises	My partner has sometimes promised to do things without actually doing them later.
OB_pursuit of own interest	They seem to feel that it is OK to do anything within their means that will help their firm's interest.
Information exchange (Sarkar *et al.*, 2001)	
INFO_regular	There was frequent communication between the two firms (e.g., visits to each other's firms, meetings, written, and telephone communications).
INFO_informal	Exchange of information in this relationship took place frequently and informally.
INFO_easy	Making contact with people from other firms was hard for both firms.
Perceived success (Zollo *et al.*, 2002)	
PS_gain in knowledge	Satisfaction with the knowledge accumulated from participating in the collaborative agreement.
PS_possibility of business	Extent to which the alliance created new opportunities for the firm.
PR_expectations	Degree to which the alliance satisfied the partnering firm's initial objectives.
Partnership experience (Lambe *et al.*, 2002)	
CONT_exp_ partnership	We have a deep base of partnership experience.

- **Operationalization of the control variable:** The operationalization of the control variable "partnership experience" is done by means of a single-item measurement over a global indicator. The operationalization of the factor "partnership experience" is derived here directly from the definitional core of the factor. The global indicator asks about experience with partnerships that is similar to the partnership being rated in the questionnaire.

The analysis of the data set was performed using SPSS. First, the indicators collected and the constructs derived were tested for validity and reliability by factor analysis. Principal component factor analysis was applied with a varimax rotation, as an extraction method in each case. Then the correlation between the structural and dynamic factors on the one hand and the perceived success on the other hand were checked by means of multivariate linear regression. The assumptions applicable to the multivariate regression were checked and deemed to be met.

5. Results

The empirical results show that, out of the eight indicators of the resource-oriented approach, three factors, namely "complementary resources", "operational compatibility", and "competitive relationship" can be derived. From the 13 indicators of the relationship-oriented approach, the three dimensions of "trust", "bilateral exchange of information", and "opportunistic behavior" can be derived. The three items that measure the success of the partnership also yielded a single factor. Table 2 shows the separate factor analysis of the constructs used and the relevant quality criteria.

The results of the hypotheses tests conducted are shown in Figure 2. Accordingly, in the case of the structural factors, a significant influence by complementary resources and operational compatibility on perceived success can be confirmed. The competitive relationship of the partners, however, cannot be shown to have a significant influence. In the context of dynamic factors, a significant influence was shown both for the bilateral exchange of information as well as for opportunistic behavior.

Table 2. Results of the factor analysis.

		Structural factors			Dynamic factors			Success
		CR	CB	CRS	TR	INFO	OB	PS
		Factor loadings						
Complementary resources	CR_dependent	0.962						
	CR_value	0.962						
KMO = 0.500; α = 0.919; AVE = 92.6%								
Operational compatibility	CB_technical		0.918					
	CB_employees		0.910					
	CB_organizational		0.865					
KMO = 0.727; α = 0.879; AVE = 80.6%								
Competitive relationship	CRS_functions			0.944				
	CRS_technologies			0.911				
	CRS_customer			0.840				
KMO = 0.679; α = 0.875; AVE = 80.9%								
Trust	TR_integrity				0.944			
	TR_reliance				0.938			
	TR_conscientious				0.934			
	TR_credible				0.933			

(Continued)

Table 2. *(Continued)*

		Structural factors			Dynamic factors			Success
		CR	CB	CRS	TR	INFO	OB	PS
		Factor loadings						
KMO = 0.809; $\alpha = 0.953$; AVE = 87.8%								
Information exchange	INFO_informal					0.965		
	INFO_regular					0.960		
	INFO_easy					0.918		
KMO = 0.739; $\alpha = 0.940$; AVE = 89.8%								
Opportunistic behavior	OB_pursuit of own interest						0.935	
	OB_promises						0.933	
	OB_honest						0.894	
	OB_facts						0.883	
	OB_corporate image						0.878	
	OB_assignment completion						0.791	
KMO = 0.880; $\alpha = 0.944$; AVE = 78.7%								
Perceived success	PR_expectations							0.927
	PS_gain in knowledge							0.919
	PS_possibility of business							0.913
KMO = 0.755; $\alpha = 0.906$; AVE = 84.6%								

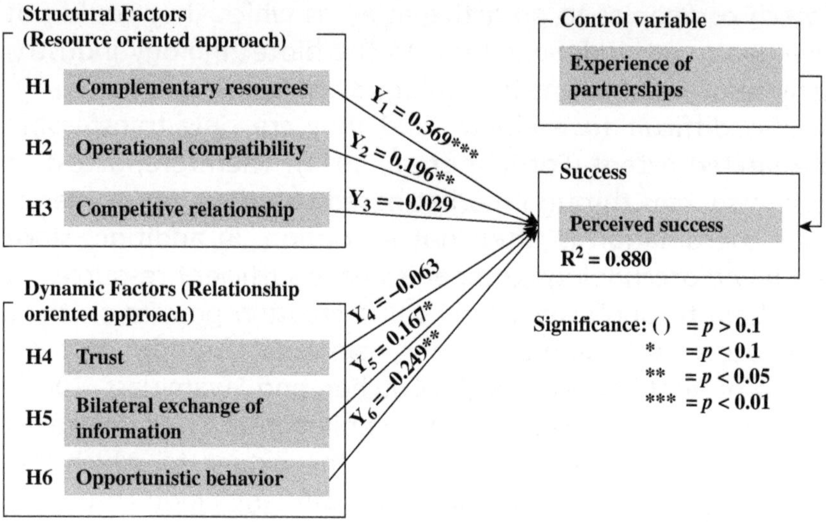

Figure 2. Results of the regression analysis.

Trust between the partners did not show a significant impact on perceived success, in this model. The two factors derived from the resource- and competence-based approach, thus, have a significant impact on the dependent variable. Thus, the postulated hypotheses can be confirmed in four cases. In two cases, a confirmation on the basis of the analyzed data set is not possible. In addition, partnership experience also plays a significant role as a control variable.

6. Discussion and Implications

The degree of complementarity of resources between the partners has a significantly positive effect on success in the partnership. The strongly positive correlation is striking, suggesting that the degree of complementarity of resources between partners is considered particularly important for the success of the partnership. The result also demonstrates that the complementary resources of the partner give great scope for biotech companies to be active in areas which they could not have dealt with independently. In the biotechnology industry, many resources, such as technological skills, are very company-specific, difficult to evaluate, and thus are only transferable to a limited extent (Fornahl *et al.*, 2011). Therefore, access to these resources through market-based coordination or hierarchical coordination is often not an option. In addition, since very few biotechnology companies have sufficient resources to take them through the whole value creation process on their own, access to complementary resources through partnerships is of vital importance (McCutchen and Swamidass, 2004). Consequently, the greater the complementarity of resources between the partners, the greater the extent to which the partnership promotes the individual company's own corporate objectives and creates new business opportunities and openings for the individual company (Deitz *et al.*, 2010). This in turn has a positive effect on the valuation of the partnership by the biotech company.

Apart from complementary resources, collaboration partners need a certain degree of operational compatibility at the same time. Companies must be able to assess which complementary skills of the partner are required and suitable, and, in addition, partners need to be capable of communicating with each other on a technical level and evaluate the results which are achieved in the context of the partnership. In this regard, operational compatibility creates the possibility of a high level of knowledge accumulation and has a positive effect on the potential for leveraging synergies.

The results further show, for the biotech industry, that a low competitiveness between companies leads to a higher stress level, a higher potential for conflict, as well as a counter-productive working atmosphere and consequently has a negative effect on the perceived success of the partnership.

The focus of the relationship-oriented approach — from which the dynamic success factors were derived — is on the long-term cooperation of the partner companies, as well as in the current operating configuration of the partnerships. The highly complex nature of the subject matter covered by the partnerships means that, in the biotech industry, it is all the more true that the benefits of a partnership can only be gained when there is effective communication between the partners. The challenging content of biotech partnerships increases the likelihood that, during the course of operations, *ad hoc* questions will arise that need to be quickly clarified with the partner company in the interest of an efficient workflow. Only if at this point the exchange of information with the partner is ensured can the benefits of the partnership be optimally utilized. The biotech companies questioned in the empirical analysis in which the bilateral exchange of information with their partner was at a high level therefore perceived the partnership as more successful than was the case for companies where there had been problems regarding this success factor.

The correlation between opportunistic behavior in the partnership and the perceived success of the partnership has been demonstrated to be significantly negative. The strong negative regression coefficient demonstrates, in this regard, that opportunism has a particularly critical impact on the perceived success of partnerships in the biotech industry. The business success of biotechnology companies depends to a great extent on the capabilities of all the companies in the partnership, as well as on the design of the partnerships in question. In other words, in comparison to other industries, the individual partnership has a particularly high priority for a biotech company. In the course of a partnership, the opportunity may arise of violating the mutual partnership agreement in order to realize short-term gains, to the detriment of the partner company. Although a more careful design of the partnership structures reduces the likelihood of opportunism, the risk remains that opportunistic behavior may have a negative influence on the perceived success of the partnership. This is particularly the case when there is a risk that "knowledge races" will develop between the partners in strategic partnerships, where the companies are trying to absorb as much knowledge as possible from their partner, while divulging as little knowledge as possible to their partner (Khanna *et al.*, 1998). Due to the importance of knowledge sharing in strategic partnerships in the biotech industry, the aspect of opportunistic behavior is therefore also of particular importance here (Baum *et al.*, 2000).

The extreme uncertainty in the R&D process also enhances the problem of inherently incomplete contracts. In the course of a partnership, because of the high degree of uncertainty in biotechnology, frequent changes in the exchange relationship in the partnership, which were not previously foreseen, may become necessary. These changes in the partnership thus ultimately increase the possibility of opportunistic behavior.

The structural success factors in this analysis refer to aspects of partnership design that must be considered *ex ante*. The dynamic success factors, however, relate to the ongoing design of the operational exchange relationship. The empirical results show that both groups influence the success of a strategic partnership in the biotech sector. It can be basically concluded that both the resource-oriented and the relationship-oriented approach are likely to explain the success of strategic partnerships in the biotech industry.

Specifically, it was found in terms of the structural factors that complementary resources increase the success of a cooperative venture. For this reason, before the formation of a strategic partnership, biotech companies should systematically evaluate the extent to which the partner company can actually bring in complementary resources to the partnership. So, in outbound partnerships with pharmaceutical companies, one should, on the one hand, pay attention to the extent of the partner's financial commitment. On the other hand, the extent to which the pharmaceutical company is able to bring additional research resources should also be taken into account when drafting the contracts. In inbound partnerships, the aspect of complementary resources should be taken just as seriously. It is recommended here that special attention should be paid to the quality aspects of the potential partner's research results and to ensure that the special abilities of the partner have little overlap with one's own abilities. In this way, one can increase the probability of improving one's own company's internal knowledge potential in the long term.

On the contrary, our results also show that prior to the formation of a strategic partnership, biotech companies should be concerned that collaboration partners are compatible enough — on a technological and organizational level — to increase the likelihood of a successful partnership. To this end, the implementation of technology management assessment and the use of instruments such as patent analysis are desirable. On this basis, the technological distance between partners measured based on their patent portfolio can be used as an indicator, where low technological distances correspond to technological closeness of the partners and high technological distances point toward very different technological skills (vom Stein *et al.*, 2014; vom Stein and Sick, 2014). The correlation between technological distance and collaboration success follows an inverted u-shape, indicating that partners need to be close enough to understand each other but on the contrary distant enough to innovate, creating new products, processes, or services. Bearing this in mind, we would recommend technological distance as a powerful and valuable tool to evaluate and chose collaboration partners in the biotech industry.

The benefits of a biotech partnership can be particularly availed of when a more intense bilateral exchange of information between the partners takes place. Biotech companies should continue to invest resources in the transfer of relevant knowledge during the course of a partnership. The biotech company can, for example, require that special contact persons are provided by the partner companies to be constantly available to supply their own research staff with the information they need about research results, publications, or patents. In addition, their own employees should work regularly at the partner company's site, so as to further increase the exchange of information between the two companies. Supplementary training may be needed to strengthen employees' communication skills and to overcome any reservations about open communication with the partner.

In the course of strategic partnerships in the biotech industry, there is a latent risk of opportunistic behavior on the part of the partner company. It was also shown that opportunistic behavior in a biotech partnership has a strong negative impact on the success of the partnership. It is therefore advisable, in strategic partnerships, to consistently apply measures that help to avoid opportunistic behavior. The design of appropriate incentive systems is one approach. As far as possible, these should be aligned with the common goal of the co-operative venture. One should also try to analyze the cooperation partner's incentive systems in as much detail as possible, with a view to check for factors that might support opportunistic behavior.

7. Conclusions, Limitations, and Future Work

Biotechnology companies are particularly dependent on partnerships with other companies throughout the value chain. This work shows that strategic partnerships have a particular relevance for businesses in research-intensive industries, such as the medical biotech industry. In addition, the work provides strong evidence that biotechnology companies can succeed in positively influencing the success of strategic partnerships by taking structural as well as dynamic factors into account.

Specifically, it can be shown that, prior to the formation of a partnership, paying attention to the complementary resources of the partner is very important for the success of the future strategic partnership. Despite the need for complementarity in the resources of the partner companies, the results of this work also show that biotech companies should be concerned, prior to the formation of a strategic partnership, that a certain overlap in technological and organizational issues is necessary in order to be able to understand each other and thus build a basis for creating new value. In addition, the consideration of two dynamic factors in the course of the partnership has a positive effect on success. Biotechnology companies should, on the one hand, continuously invest in the bilateral exchange of information during the course of a partnership. On the other hand, it can be shown that opportunistic behavior has a particularly negative effect in strategic partnerships in the biotech industry and should therefore be limited.

It can be concluded that the resource-oriented and relationship-oriented approaches are required to explain the success of strategic partnerships in the biotech industry. The two derived structural factors as well as the two dynamic factors explain the perceived success of a strategic partnership in the field of biotechnology. Therefore, the two basic theoretical concepts used here also provide a suitable basis for further research on cooperative exchange relationships in the biotech industry.

The limitations of this investigation suggest starting points for further research: One limitation of this work is the measurement of the factors in the model. Only the information from one company involved in the partnership was used, in every case, for the empirical data collection of the dependent and the independent variables. It would be logical to collect dyadic information from both partner companies, both in terms of the assessment of partnership success as well as in relation to individual independent variables. In assessing the success of a partnership, it is conceivable, for example, in this context that there has been a utility shift between the partners, so that one partner company views the partnership as successful whereas the other party has a negative assessment of the partnership (Balling, 1997). Regarding the assessment of individual independent variables, such as trust, a possible question might be whether a particularly high level of trust by one partner company towards its partner can compensate for a very low level of trust by the other partner.

Another limitation is based on the operationalization of individual factors. Despite the plausible empirical results for four of the six hypotheses, no significant relationship was observed for the two causal relationships between the independent variables "trust" and "competition" and perceived partnership success. One possible explanation for the lack of significant correlation between trust as measured and the perceived success of the partnership may lie in the operationalization of the factor of trust. Thus, different levels of trust can be distinguished in business relationships and business partnerships (Mouzas *et al.*, 2007). In addition to trust at the corporate level, trust between people, for example, can also be measured at the interpersonal level. A differentiated operationalization of the factor of trust could therefore lead to an improvement in the results as measured.

In conclusion, it can be stated, with respect to the limitations of this work that the latent variables that were operationalized here do not represent a complete listing of all possible factors influencing the success of strategic partnerships. External factors (such as the competitive environment) and partner-specific factors (e.g., how well the strategic orientations of the companies involved match each other) are also suitable topics for future studies to obtain further insight into the research question dealt with in this analysis.

References

Abell, D. F. (1980). *Defining the Business. The Starting Point of Strategic Planning*, Prentice-Hall, Englewood Cliffs, NJ.

Al-Laham, A., Amburgey, T. L. and Baden-Fuller, C. (2010). Who is my partner and how do we dance? Technological collaboration and patenting speed in US biotechnology, *British Journal of Management*, 21(3), 789–807.

Anderson, J. C. and Narus, J. A. (1990). A model of distributor firm and manufacturer firm working partnerships, *The Journal of Marketing*, 54(1), 42–58.

Baden-Fuller, C. and Morgan, M. S. (2010). Business models as models, *Long Range Planning*, 43(2–3), 156–171.

Baum, J. A. C., Calabrese, T. and Silverman, B. S. (2000). Don't go it alone. Alliance network composition and startups' performance in Canadian biotechnology, *Strategic Management Journal*, 21(3), 267–294.

Beuzekom, B. V. and Arundel, A. (2009). *OECD Biotechnology Statistics 2009*. OECD Paris, http,//www.oecd.org/sti/42833898.pdf.

Bianchi, M., *et al.* (2011). Organisational modes for open innovation in the bio-pharmaceutical industry. An exploratory analysis, *Technovation*, 31(1), 22–33.

Das, T. K. and Teng, B.-S. (1998). Resource and risk management in the strategic alliance making process, *Journal of Management,* 24(1), 21–42.

Das, T. K. and Teng, B.-S. (2000a). A resource-based theory of strategic alliances, *Journal of Management*, 26(1), 31–61.

Das, T. K. and Teng, B.-S. (2000b). Instabilities of strategic alliances. An internal tensions perspective, *Organization Science*, 11(1), 77–101.

Day, G. S. (1995). Advantageous alliances, *Journal of the Academy of Marketing Science*, 23(4), 297–300.

Deitz, G. D., *et al.* (2010). Joint venture stability and cooperation. Direct, indirect and contingent effects of resource complementarity and trust, *Industrial Marketing Management*, 39(5), 862–873.

Delerue, H. (2005). Relational risk perception and alliance management in French biotechnology SMEs, *European Business Review*, 17(6), 532–546.

DiMasi, J. A. and Grabowski, H. G. (2007). The cost of biopharmaceutical R&D. Is biotech different? *Managerial and Decision Economics*, 28(4–5), 469–479.

Douma, M. U., *et al.* (2000). Strategic alliances. Managing the dynamics of fit, *Long Range Planning*, 33(4), 579–598.

Duysters, G., Kok, G. and Vaandrager, M. (1999). Crafting successful strategic technology partnerships, *R&D Management*, 29(4), 343–351.

Fornahl, D., Broekel, T. and Boschma, R. (2011). What drives patent performance of German biotech firms? The impact of R&D subsidies, knowledge networks and their location, *Papers in Regional Science*, 90(2), 395–418.

Geringer, J. M. and Hebert, L. (1991). Measuring performance of international joint ventures, *Journal of International Business Studies*, 22(2), 249–263.

Gaister, K. W. and Buckley, P. J. (1996). Strategic motives for international alliance formation, *Journal of Management Studies*, 33(3), 301–332.

Glaister, K. W. and Buckley, P. J. (1999). Performance relationships in UK international alliances, *Management International Review*, 39(2), 123–147.

Gulati, R. (1998). Alliances and networks, *Strategic Management Journal*, 19(4), 293–317.

Hagedoorn, J. (1993). Understanding the rationale or strategic technology partnering. Interorganizational modes of cooperation and sectoral differences, *Strategic Management Journal*, 14(5), 371–385.

Hagedoorn, J. and Duysters, G. (2002). External sources of innovative capabilities. The preferences for strategic alliances or mergers and acquisitions, *Journal of Management Studies*, 39(2), 167–188.

Hagedoorn, J., Link A. N. and Vonortas, N. S. (2000). Research partnerships, *Research Policy*, 29(4–5), 567–586.

Havenaar, M. and Hiscocks, P. (2012). Strategic alliances and market risk, *Drug Discovery Today*, 17(15–16), 824–827.

Huang, Y.-A., Chung, H.-J. and Lin, C. (2009). R&D sourcing strategies. Determinants and consequences, *Technovation*, 29(3), 155–169.

Jiang, X., Li, Y. and Gao, S. (2008). The stability of strategic alliances. Characteristics, factors and stages, *Journal of International Management*, 14(2), 173–189.

Kale, P. and Singh, H. (2007). Building firm capabilities through learning. The role of the alliance learning process in alliance capability and firm-level alliance success, *Strategic Management Journal*, 28(10), 981–1000.

Khanna, T., Gulati, R. and Nohria, N. (1998). The dynamics of learning alliances. Competition, cooperation, and relative scope, *Strategic Management Journal*, 19(3), 93–210.

Lambe, C. J., Spekman, R. E. and Hunt, S. D. (2002). Alliance competence, resources, and alliance success. Conceptualization, measurement, and initial test, *Journal of the Academy of Marketing Science*, 30(2), 141–158.

Luo, Y. (2007). Are joint venture partners more opportunistic in a more volatile environment? *Strategic Management Journal*, 28(1), 39–60.

Madhok, A. and Tallman, S. B. (1998). Resources, transactions and rents. Managing value through interfirm collaborative relationships, *Organization Science*, 9(3), 326–339.

March-Chordà, I. and Yagüe-Perales, R. M. (2011). Biopharma business models in Canada, *Drug Discovery Today*, 16(15–16), 654–658.

McCutchen, W. W. and Swamidass, P. M. (2004). Motivations for strategic alliances in the pharmaceutical/biotech industry. Some new findings, *The Journal of High Technology Management Research*, 15(2), 197–214.

Mohr, J. and Spekman, R. (1994). Characteristics of partnership success. Partnership attributes, communication behavior, and conflict resolution techniques, *Strategic Management Journal*, 15(2), 135–152.

Morgan, R. M. and Hunt, S. D. (1994). The commitment-trust theory of relationship marketing, *The Journal of Marketing*, 58(3), 20–38.

Morgan, S., *et al.* (2011). The cost of drug development. A systematic review, *Health Policy*, 100(1), 4–17.

Mouzas, S., Henneberg, S. and Naudé, P. (2007). Trust and reliance in business relationships, *European Journal of Marketing*, 41(9–10), 1016–1032.

Mowery, D. C., Oxley, J. E. and Silverman, B. S. (1996). Strategic alliances and interfirm knowledge transfer, *Strategic Management Journal*, 17(1), 77–91.

Murphy, W. J. (1988). Interfirm cooperation in a competitive economic system, *American Business Law Journal*, 26(1), 29–45.

Nielsen, B. B. (2007). Determining international strategic alliance performance. A multidimensional approach, *International Business Review*, 16(3), 337–361.

Nienaber, A. and Schewe, G. (2014). Enhancing trust or reducing perceived risk, what matters more when launching a new product? *International Journal of Innovation Management*, 18(1), 1450005-1–1450005-24.

Ohmae, K. (1989). The global logic of strategic alliances, *Harvard Business Review*, 3–4, 143–154.

Park, S. H. and Russo, M. V. (1996). When competition eclipses cooperation. An Event history analysis of joint venture failure, *Management Science*, 42(6), 875–890.

Parkhe, A. (1993). Strategic alliance structuring. A game theoretic and transaction cost examination of interfirm cooperation, *The Academy of Management Journal*, 36(4), 794–829.

Pekar, P. and Allio, R. (1994). Making alliances work. Guidelines for success, *Long Range Planning*, 27(4), 54–65.

Rothaermel, F. T. and Deeds, D. L. (2004). Exploration and exploitation alliances in biotechnology. A system of new product development, *Strategic Management Journal*, 25(3), 201–221.

Sarkar, M. B., *et al.* (2001). The influence of complementarity, compatibility, and relationship capital on alliance performance, *Journal of the Academy of Marketing Science*, 29(4), 358–373.

Saxton, T. (1997). The effects of partner and relationship characteristics on alliance outcomes, *The Academy of Management Journal*, 40(2), 443–461.

Spekman, R., *et al.* (1996). Creating strategic alliances which endure, *Long Range Planning*, 29(3), 346–357.

Stuart, T. E. (2000). Interorganizational alliances and the performance of forms. A study of growth and innovation, *Strategic Management Journal*, 21(8), 791–812.

Suarez, M. V. and García-Canal, E. (2003). Complementarity and leverage as drivers of the stock market reaction to global alliance formation, *Long Range Planning*, 36(6), 565–578.

Taylor, A. (2005). An operations perspective on strategic alliance success factors. An exploratory study of alliance managers in the software industry, *International Journal of Operations & Production Management*, 25(5), 469–490.

Villiger, R. (2009). Licensing. Pro and cons for biotech, *Drug Discovery Today*, 14(5–6), 227–230.

vom Stein, N. and Sick, N. (2014). Technological distance in academic collaborations — Evidence from battery research, *International Journal of Innovation Management*, 18(6), 1440011-1–1440011-22.

vom Stein, N., Sick, N. and Leker J. (2014). How to measure technological distance in collaborations — The case of electric mobility, *Technological Forecasting and Social Change*, http://dx.doi.org/10.1016/j.techfore.2014.05.001.

Wittmann, C. M., Hunt, S. D. and Arnett, D. B. (2009). Explaining alliance success. Competences, resources, relational factors, and resource-advantage theory, *Industrial Marketing Management*, 38(7), 743–756.

Zollo, M., Reuer, J. and Singh, H. (2002). Interorganizational routines and performance in strategic alliances, *Organization Science*, 13(6), 701–713.

Part 3

Innovation Management Perspectives

Chapter 7

Open Innovation in the Medical Device Industry

Hua-Hsin Wan* and Xiaohong Quan†

Department of Organization and Management, San Jose State University, California, USA

**hwanh31@yahoo.com*

†*xiaohong.quan@sjsu.edu*

Abstract

Using a case study of Acclarent, a medical device company, this chapter attempts to propose a framework to further illustrate the process of open innovation in the medical device industry. We examined five elements in the mechanism of the open innovation process. This chapter shows how the success of Acclarent — a medical device start-up — depends on effective management of the flow of knowledge to satisfy unmet needs, while integrating in-depth knowledge of FDA regulations and third-party payers' reimbursement policies into the product innovation process.

Keywords: Open innovation, medical device company, Acclarent.

1. Introduction

The concept of open innovation manifests the importance of firms employing "external ideas as well as internal ideas, and internal and external paths to market" (Chesbrough, 2003a) as they progress with their technology development. The underlying assumption of open innovation is the "mobility of knowledge workers" and the availability of capital which enables the generation of innovative ideas outside of the "silos" of corporate research labs (Chesbrough, 2003b).

The power of open innovation lies in the fact that knowledge created through such an open mind-set and corporate policy can be reused and it can lead to increasing returns (Arthur, 1996). Moreover, both the breadth and depth of the collective knowledge can surpass the knowledge contribution of an individual provider (Chesbrough and Appleyard, 2007).

Although the idea of open innovation paves an alternative path to the advancement of technology, theoretical discussions are still insufficient to expound the mechanism of open innovation. Open innovation contributes to broadening the "realm" for knowledge creation by focusing on "different sources of external knowledge" and the balancing role of both external and internal sources of knowledge (van de Vrande *et al.*, 2010). Nevertheless, the theory does not provide us with a clear guidance on how new knowledge, the core of innovation, is constructed. In this chapter, using the case of Acclarent, we plan to contribute to existing theories through an in-depth examination on "how" knowledge is created or recreated through such a process.

2. Theoretical Background

West and Bogers (2011) conducted an extensive literature review on open innovation research and they developed a four-phase model for inbound open innovation to categorize prior studies in open innovation. These four phases include "obtaining, integrating and commercializing external innovation, as well as work on nonreciprocal innovation flows". For the purpose of this chapter, we only allude literature related to the first phase in their model.

In terms of obtaining external innovation, studies have examined external stakeholders (Ili *et al.*, 2010; Tether and Tajar, 2008), e.g., suppliers (Li and Vanhaverbeke, 2009; Schiele, 2010), competitors (Lim *et al.*, 2010), or universities (Cassiman *et al.*, 2010; Fabrizio, 2009), as well as market feedback (Dodgson *et al.*, 2006), networks (Vanhaverbeke, 2006; Zeng *et al.*, 2010), and communities (Stam, 2009; Janzik, 2010) as sources of external knowledge. In addition, Tortoriello and Krackhardt (2010) demonstrated that the nature of relationship between a firm and an external stakeholder may determine the effectiveness of the search for external innovation. Moreover, there is also an increasing amount of research scrutinizing the role of third-party actors in enabling external innovation (e.g., Jeppesen and Lakhani, 2010; Mortara *et al.*, 2010).

In addition to studies on obtaining external innovation, other research investigating different aspects in open innovation include: analyzing firms adopting an outside in (versus an inside out) approach of open innovation (e.g., Lichtenthaler and Ernst, 2007; Witzeman *et al.*, 2006), examining small and medium-sized enterprises (SMEs) rather than the traditionally large, multinational enterprises (e.g., De Jong and Marsili, 2006; Massa and Testa, 2008; Ndou *et al.*, 2011); exploring firms' cultural dimensions of implementing open innovation (Herzog and Leker, 2010), studying different types of alliance strategies to maximize start-up firms' innovation performance (Neyens *et al.*, 2010), and incorporating analysis of user innovation, customer interaction, online community, and alliance networks in the existing literature (e.g., Hienerth, 2006; Lettl, 2007; Spaeth *et al.*, 2010; Van Rijswijk *et al.*, 2008; Weber *et al.*, 2012).

While existing research on open innovation has certainly expanded the scope of the original concept and enlightened us on various open channels of sources of ideas, there is still a lack of attention on the process of knowledge (re)creation, which is the underpinning of innovation.

Our proposed model in investigating how innovative knowledge is generated through interaction of both external and internal sources is meant to establish a framework of linking macro and micro levels of analysis regarding knowledge exchange and flow, thereby enhancing the value of the open innovation paradigm.

Using a case study of Acclarent, a medical device company, this chapter attempts to illustrate how the process of open innovation is implemented in the medical device industry, which can shed some light to the mechanism of open innovation.

In our proposed framework, we focus on five essential elements to capture the mechanism of innovation in medical device businesses. These five elements include the following: sources of ideas, the interrelationship (quality of relationship) between innovators and the sources of ideas, types of knowledge, characteristics of knowledge, and path for knowledge acquisition. We first give a brief introduction of the case, then illustrate the five elements in the following sections. Data are obtained through both face-to-face interviews and secondary resources.

3. Research Method

Since previous studies examining open innovation in the medical device industry are scarce, we employed both primary and secondary research to obtain first-hand data as well as background information on medical device companies and the industry. The medical device companies we selected for interview are from the MDR website. We used locations, annual revenue, and patents as major criteria for determining medical companies in our sample. As a preliminary research, we employ a case study method in this chapter to have an in-depth understanding of the phenomena. Our literature review on the medical device industry indicated that many medical device companies were centered in the Silicon Valley area.

Acclarent was chosen because it was located in Menlo Park, a hub for many medical device companies in Silicon Valley. The company had 16 active patents in 2009. In our in-depth interview with Bill Facteau, CEO of the company, he provided us with ample data on the company's innovation procedures and practices, and challenges the company faced in developing new products. In addition, we were able to find valuable secondary information from the book related to the process of innovating medical technologies, co-authored by Joshua Makower, founder of Acclarent, which offered us insightful details on how the idea of the Acclarent's Balloon Sinuplasty devices was formed. The combined interviews, case studies, and archival research thus presented us a much more clear and affluent resource on the innovation of Acclarent's Balloon Sinuplasty product as well as key issues concerning innovation in the medical device industry. The rich information we collected rendered Acclarent worthy for a case study.

4. The Case of Acclarent

4.1. *Background*

Acclarent Inc., is a medical device company dedicated to the development of innovative technologies to meet the needs of ENT patients in a better manner. By 2010, the company acquired 16 patents and there were 120 patent applications pending. The company typically has 3–4 new products every year, and the Balloon Sinuplasty, an instrument designed to improve quality of life for sinusitis patients, is their major product line. Approximately 50% of the balloon sinus patents are related to their key products. Acclarent's revenue in 2009 was 95 million (Facteau) and it was acquired by Ethicon Inc., a Johnson & Johnson company, in the same year.

Joshua Makower, Acclarent's founder, is an entrepreneur in the medical device industry. He started a medical technology incubator named ExploraMed I in 1995, which spawned EndoMatrix and TransVascular. In 2003, Medtronic acquired TransVascular for a deal valued up to $90 million. The success sale of TransVascular left Makower in a position to decide on what was to be done next (Zenios *et al.*, 2010). After a thorough assessment of what he would like to accomplish in his career and his strengths and weaknesses, he started his next project acceptance criteria which he believed would have a reasonably high chance of success which included: (1) focus on real-world problems (no more science experiments), (2) work on problems that affected a large number of people, and (3) devote to projects that would not involve any patient deaths. In order to accomplish his goal, he restarted ExploraMed II, which served as a platform for launching two to three medical device businesses (Zenios *et al.*, 2010). After forming a trusted team and researching several clinical areas which met Makower's project criteria, a company that focuses on ear, nose, and throat (ENT), Acclarent, was established in 2004.

4.2. *Sources of innovative ideas*

Since innovation starts with idea generation and development, "understanding the sources of ideas is critical for innovation" (Desouza *et al.*, 2008). Three subjective groups may play an important role in being the sources for innovative ideas in the medical device sector: physicians (customer), patients (user), and insurance companies (buyer) (see Figure 1).

Physicians are the major customers for medical device manufacturers as they are usually the decision-makers for the adoption of medical devices in the treatment process. Patients are the users who physically experience the effect and quality of the medical devices. It is therefore essential for medical device manufacturers to improve physicians' and patients' satisfaction with their devices when they invent a new product.

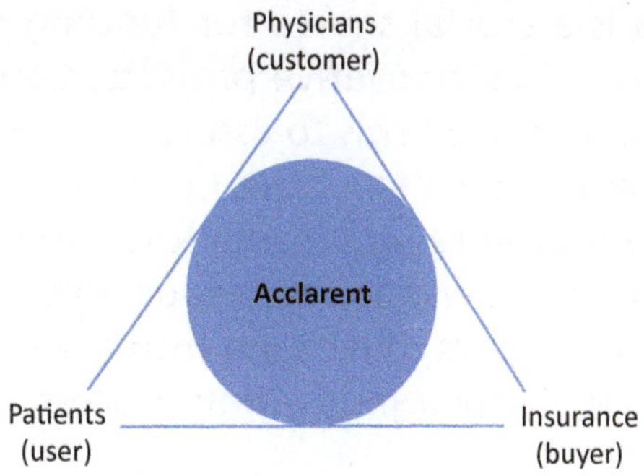

Figure 1. Sources of ideas.

As a medical device company, one of Acclarent's areas of innovation is in the ear, nose, and throat (ENT) field. To better understand the problems in the ENT field in order to propose innovative solutions, Acclarent adopted an open innovation strategy. The founder of Acclarent, Joshua Makower, asserts that, rather than starting with a solution, an existing invention, or ideas from academia, innovation of medical device starts with "focusing on a set process", which evidences a thorough examination and in-depth understanding of an area of medicine (Stommen, 2010). As a result, Makower, John Chang (Vice President of Acclarent), and engineers at the company collaborated closely with ENT physicians and their patients to identify clinical problems and uncover their unmet needs. That is where the invention starts. They observe life surgeries, identify clinical problems, find out physicians' unmet needs, and then propose solutions. In the process of developing new concepts, Acclarent has a Science Advisory Board where they obtain advices from physician consultants. The strong partnership with physicians allows Acclarent to develop thorough and profound knowledge of the medical problems which, in turn, drives the innovation.

In addition, insurance companies play an important role in the innovation process of the medical device industry. The reimbursement from insurance companies for employing certain medical devices is a crucial source for funding medical device corporations' on-going innovative projects. Consequently, it is critical for medical device firms to assure the acceptance of the insurance company of their inventive product in order to obtain compensation. Because reimbursement criteria determine the success or failure of a new medical product in the market, medical device manufacturers must take into consideration these criteria and policies in their innovation process.

4.3. *Relationship between innovators and sources*

The Acclarent's case also reveals that the relationships between innovators and the sources of ideas determine whether there is a flow of different knowledge for generating a new set of knowledge. In studying the relationship between an organization and its publics, Hon and Grunig (1999) mainly identified four indicators to measure the relationship outcomes: trust, control mutuality, relationship commitment, and relationship satisfaction. Since the relationship between innovators and the source of ideas is like that between an organization and its various publics, we adopt three of the four indicators to examine the quality of the relationship between innovators and their sources of ideas. Figure 2 provides an overview of the relationships between Acclarent and its external sources of ideas. Moreover, we attempt to investigate how such a quality of the relationship may affect different types of knowledge sharing in the innovation process.

Innovators must build up trust with physicians in order to acquire practical clinical knowledge and to gain access to first-hand information of surgical procedures. Trust, according to Hon and Grunig (1999), is "one party's level of confidence in and willingness to open oneself to the other party" (p.14). Gambetta (1988) also asserts that trust in an individual means "the probability that he (or she) will perform an action that is beneficial or at least not detrimental to us is high enough for us to consider engaging in some form of cooperation with him

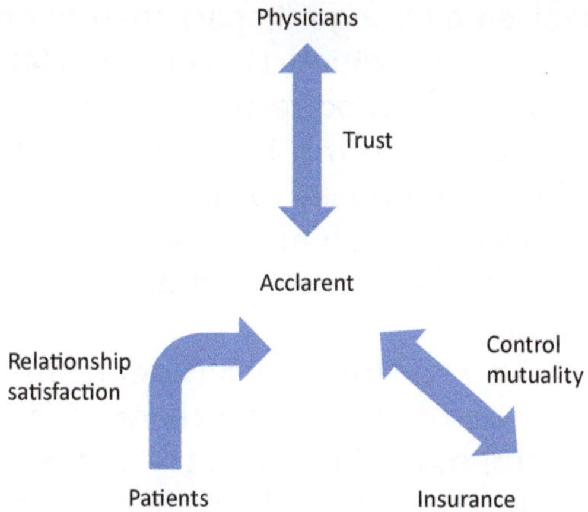

Figure 2. Relationship between Acclarent and its external sources of ideas.

(or her)" (p. 217). If there is no trust between innovators and physicians, it is unlikely for the innovators to attain experiential knowledge from physicians.

According to Rastogi (2000), effective sharing of complex knowledge cannot be accomplished without trust and cooperation. Therefore, mutual trust between individuals is key to promote interpersonal complex knowledge sharing (Chowdhury, 2005).

In addition, innovators should have relationship satisfaction with patients (user) in order to solicit their feedback on any type of medical treatment. Relationship satisfaction is defined as "the extent to which one party feels favorably toward the other because positive expectations about the relationships are reinforced" (Hon and Grunig, 1999, p. 14). Patients may not be willing to collaborate with innovators by sharing their feedback if they don't believe the purpose of investing in such a relationship is to benefit themselves ultimately. In a study examining the effect of the type of the mentor and the quality of the relationship on employees' work and career attitudes, Ragins *et al.* (2000) discovered that satisfaction with a mentoring relationship exerted a stronger impact than the presence of a mentor on attitudes. In addition, Liao *et al.* (2004) contend that when employees have a good relationship with the firm, they would like to share working knowledge with coworkers voluntarily and unconditionally (p. 33). It can thus be inferred that relationship satisfaction may serve as a crucial factor in influencing individuals' attitudes and/or behaviors such as knowledge sharing.

Moreover, the relationship between innovators and insurance companies (buyer) can be characterized as "control mutuality". Control mutuality refers to "the degree to which partners agree about which of them should decide relational goals and behavioral routines" (Stafford and Canary, 1991, p. 224). Since the criteria for reimbursement from insurance companies are essential guidelines for medical device firms to obtain compensation for their product usage, these criteria thus affect the product innovation process as innovators must consider how their invention fits with existing rules so that they can secure financial returns.

4.4. *Types of knowledge*

Idea generation is often derived from agitation of different types of knowledge. There are two types of knowledge: explicit knowledge and tacit knowledge (e.g., Nonaka and Takeuchi, 1995; Nonaka *et al.*, 2000).

- **Explicit knowledge:** This type of knowledge can be found in documented information or materials such as reports, articles, manuals, patents, pictures, images, video, sound, and software (Nonaka and Takeuchi, 1995; Nonaka *et al.*, 2000).
- **Tacit knowledge:** Tacit knowledge is personal knowledge derived from individual experience and is shared and exchanged through direct contact (Borghoff and Pareschi, 1997). In Acclarent's case, knowledge learned from the physician's personal clinical practice experience, for example,

is considered tacit knowledge because such knowledge is mainly obtained through the accumulation of physicians' personal know-how of medical operation.

4.5. *Characteristics of knowledge*

In addition to types of knowledge, knowledge can also be categorized in terms of its characteristics. Such categorization may provide a framework in steering innovators to search for needed or useful knowledge. Because various sources of ideas may possess different knowledge, in this study, the knowledge categorization is developed pertaining to Acclarent's circumstances. Based on its characteristics, knowledge can be classified into professional, process, operational, and discipline knowledge.

(1) **Professional knowledge:** This type of knowledge refers to specific knowledge related to a particular professional field of interest. Professional knowledge can be obtained from interaction with professionals or from documented information such as books, journals, reports, and manuals. Therefore, it can be both tacit and explicit knowledge.
(2) **Process knowledge:** The process knowledge in this study is different from the term used in process management, where process knowledge means "explicit, formalized knowledge about executing sequences of work activities" (Borghoff and Pareschi, 1997, p. 838). In Acclarent's case, process knowledge refers to information gathered by observing life surgeries, identifying clinical problems, discovering physicians' unmet needs, and researching possible solutions. Since process knowledge can be acquired through information sharing and through documented materials, it can be both tacit and explicit knowledge.
(3) **Operational knowledge:** Operational knowledge mainly includes knowledge of FDA regulations and the insurance company's reimbursement policies. Such type of knowledge

may not be the core for idea generation, but it is still vital as it may serve to validate the feasibility of innovative ideas. In this study, operational knowledge is mainly explicit knowledge. However, the interpretation of FDA regulations and the discretion of reimbursement policies can be tacit knowledge.

(4) **Discipline knowledge:** Discipline knowledge comes from the innovators' own educational background and training. Bright innovative ideas may be generated from integration of discipline knowledge in related fields or in totally different fields. Discipline knowledge is mostly documented information, and thus explicit knowledge.

4.6. *Path for knowledge acquisition*

The path for knowledge acquisition refers to "means" for obtaining different types of knowledge in the idea generation process. Such means can be broadly classified into one-way or two-way communication based on the nature of relationship between innovators and sources of ideas. In this study, knowledge acquisition from physicians is mainly through two-way communication in that innovators need to interact with physicians to attain their experiential knowledge. However, knowledge can also be acquired via one-way communication by observing life surgeries.

The knowledge on patients (end user) can be collected through feedback solicitation (two-way communication) or through examining existing literature (one-way communication) related to patients' response and recovery process pertaining to certain medical treatments.

For medical device manufacturers (innovators), comprehension of the insurance company's reimbursement policies primarily results from thorough investigation of their reimbursement criteria and the medical code system (one-way communication). Nevertheless, innovators can strive for maximizing their benefit in the classification of reimbursement criteria by seeking support from physician associations and by engaging in negotiation with insurance companies (two-way communication).

Table 1 summarizes the five components that we proposed as a framework to explain the mechanism of open innovation process in the medical device industry.

4.7. *How does knowledge contribute to innovation?*

The ability to generate new knowledge and to create value is important for innovation. According to Carneiro (2000), the success of an innovative product is connected to research activities and changing orientation, which are dependent on the development of knowledge levels and the innovative efforts of knowledge workers.

In analyzing intraorganizational knowledge transfer on business innovation, Tsai (2001) also asserts that knowledge transfer among organizational units stimulates the creation of new knowledge, thus contributing to organizational units' ability to innovate (Tsai, 2001; Kogut and Zander, 1992; Tsai and Ghoshal, 1998). In addition, Spencer (2003) contends that knowledge is viewed as a resource that accelerates technical progress (p. 218). By acquiring technological knowledge from the innovation system such as research institutes, universities, and innovative corporations for the use of their own researchers, firms can increase their innovative performance (p. 218). Therefore, knowledge sharing and exchanging can lead to the generation of new knowledge, which is an important driving force for innovation.

4.8. *Nature of the innovative product — Disruptive innovation*

Acclarent's main product may also be understood as disruptive innovation originating from the process of external knowledge transfer through interaction with other sources of innovation.

Table 1. Mechanism for the open innovation process in medical device industry.

Dimension				
Sources of idea	Innovator (Manufacturer)	Physicians (customer)	Patients (user)	Insurance (buyer)
Quality of relationship		Trust	Relationship satisfaction	Control mutuality
Types of knowledge	Mostly explicit	Tacit/explicit	Tacit/explicit	Explicit/tacit
Knowledge characteristics	Discipline knowledge	Professional knowledge	Process knowledge	Operational knowledge
Path for knowledge acquisition	1. One-way Communication (e.g., books) 2. Two-way communication (e.g., interactive learning)	1. Two-way communication (e.g., interaction) 2. One-way communication (e.g., observation)	1. Two-way communication (e.g., primary research) 2. One-way communication (e.g., secondary research)	1. One-way communication (e.g., secondary research) 2. Two-way communication (e.g., negotiation)

Disruptive innovation is not a breakthrough innovation, rather, it is a process by which complicated, expensive products and services are transformed into simple, affordable ones (Christensen, 2009, p. 3). The innovation, therefore, should focus on understanding the "jobs" people need to do to maintain their health and how to make these jobs easier, more convenient, and more pleasant for them (p.13).

The innovative idea of Acclarent's main product — Balloon Sinuplasty device — was derived from John Makower and his team's clinical observations of how patients with sinusitis underwent the standard form of sinus surgery called functional endoscopic sinus surgery (FESS) to treat severe cases of chronic sinusitis. FESS involves cutting and removing abnormal and obstructive tissues in an effort to open the sinus drainage pathways (Zenios *et al*., 2010, p. 55). The process is bloody "because a significant amount of bone and tissue was being removed in every procedure" (p. 55). Observing the whole practice of the FESS led Makower and his team to conclude that there is "a need for a minimally invasive approach to treating chronic sinusitis that had less bleeding, less pain, less bone and tissue removal, less risk of scarring, and that was faster, easier, and safer to perform" (p. 55). This is how the team went on to explore the feasibility of using a balloon catheter instrument instead of surgical incision in the sinus surgery procedure.

To be defined as disruptive innovation, an innovative technology or product is usually cost efficient, easier to perform, and reasonably effective compared to existing technologies or products. In contrast to using traditional FESS for sinus treatment, the Balloon Sinuplasty procedure costs less, requires no excising tissues and bones, and helps minimize postoperative trauma. The balloon technique involves using an inflated balloon to enlarge the sinus ostium by compressing mucosa and displacing local bony structures, rather than employing surgical excision of the mucosa and bones. Such a technique is less invasive than standard surgery and, therefore, it reduces postoperative scarring, thereby increasing the patients' satisfaction measure. The price for opting the Balloon Sinuplasty procedure is approximately $1,000–2,000 lower than that for the FESS.

Acclarent published the CLEAR study involving 6-month, 1-year, and 2-year follow-up clinical studies on the effectiveness of Balloon Sinuplasty System. The results revealed significant improvement among sinus patients who underwent the procedure. In the 6 months study, 115 patients (358 peripheral sinuses) were treated and there was an 80.5% overall sinus patency. In the 1-year study, 70 patients (217 peripheral sinuses) underwent the balloon catheter surgery and the overall functional sinus patency was 91.6%, with statistically and clinically significant improvement in the Sino-Nasal Outcomes Test (SNOT-20 scores). In the 2-year study, 65 patients (195 peripheral sinuses) were treated and there was an 85% improvement in postoperative changes in symptoms. Revision rate was 3.6% of sinuses involving six of 65 patients (9%). As a result, Acclarent concluded that these studies indicated that the use of *Balloon Sinuplasty* instruments in sinus surgery is safe and effective. In addition, patients' satisfaction with this minimally invasive technology is consistently positive over the 2 years after the surgery (Acclarent's Clear Study).

4.9. *Further look: The role of regulation and reimbursement in medical device innovation*

As an external factor influencing the innovation actors, the role of FDA regulation and reimbursement system has been unique in the process of open innovation in the medical device industry.

FDA regulations exert a major impact on medical firms' innovation. FDA regulations govern many activities that medical device companies conduct, or activities conducted on their behalf to ensure the safety and effectiveness of the medical devices distributed domestically or exported to other countries. FDA regulations play an important role in the economic success of small innovative firms due to the direct and indirect regulatory costs (especially delays in generating revenues) occurred during the commercialization in the innovative products stage. In medical device industry, if product innovation is derived from compliance to the regulations, you need to involve clinical trials in the innovation process, which could cost millions of dollars, according to William Facteau, Acclarent's CEO. Many venture capitals do not want to invest in medical device companies because it is too expensive and risky in terms of ROI, and because there is so much uncertainty involved due to the healthcare reform, stated Facteau. Such a trend may cause medical device companies to select a path where clinical trials are not required in inventing new products. Consequently, further investigations of how FDA's regulations facilitate or hinder innovation in the medical device industry (especially small firms) are called for.

For medical device companies, obtaining adequate coverage and reimbursement from third-party payers such as private health insurance companies, Medicare, and Medicaid for all or part of the costs and fees associated with using medical devices, is critical for the medical device product acceptance and the widespread adoption in the marketplace (Risk Factors). Reimbursement constitutes part of the revenue for medical device companies and may be a crucial source of funding for continuous innovation in these companies. Acclarent claimed that approximately 15 third-party payers did not currently cover or reimburse the sinus procedure performed with its Balloon Sinuplasty devices because they believe such devices are new and in the investigational stage (Risk Factors). These private payers have generally required using a separate billing code that is unique for Balloon Sinuplasty (Risk Factors). Nevertheless, the fact that the Balloon Sinuplasty instrument is considered a "tool" rather than a "procedure" allows Acclarent to get reimbursement from existing Category I Current Procedure Terminology, or CPT, codes relating to the various sinuses treated using FESS procedure. "These codes do not currently distinguish between FESS performed with Balloon Sinuplasty devices and traditional instruments" (Risk Factors). In addition to the reimbursement from third-party payers, Acclarent got 6% of its revenue from international sales of its Balloon Sinuplasty devices by 2008 (Risk Factors).

Acclarent's case suggests that the third-party reimbursement policies and the medical coding system may significantly impact the profits of medical device companies. As a result, the structure of the medical codes and payment guidelines can be vital affecting the medical device company's innovation process. To determine if the Balloon Sinuplasty team should proceed further with the invention, Acclarent hired a professional reimbursement consulting firm to evaluate whether the use of their Balloon Sinuplasty devices could fit within the existing FESS codes. The team's idea was able to be carried out due to the positive feedback they received from the consulting firm as well as a legal/reimbursement expert (Zenios *et al.*, 2010).

Acclarent's case also reveals that there is complex knowledge regarding how to "categorize" the nature of an innovative device since different a categorization could influence the pathway to innovation and the potential development of the end product. Future research should further investigate how reimbursement criteria, policies, and coding systems may have an effect on a medical device company's innovation process.

5. Discussion and Conclusion

Most of the existing literature in open innovation tends to focus on high-tech companies when investigating factors related to open innovation. This chapter adds to prior research in this field by extending the theory to the realm of medical industry. Acclarent's case indicates that open innovation is one of the essential elements for a medical device company to explore the unmet needs in the market, thereby sustaining its innovative capability in a highly competitive industry. We examined the five elements in the mechanism of the open innovation process.

"Fulfilling the unmet needs" is necessary but not sufficient for an innovative product to be successful in its commercialization. Since medical device companies are regulated by FDA, familiarity with FDA's regulations to obtain clearance for product premarket approval is critical in determining whether the innovative product can be commercialized. In addition, revenue for medical device companies depends, to a large degree, on third-party payers' reimbursement. Therefore, a thorough understanding of third-party payers' reimbursement criteria and medical codes system is essential for medical device firms to be profitable.

A more important contribution of our study to the open innovation literature is the development of a framework in examining the mechanism of the core of the innovation process — knowledge exchange and flow. As West and Bogers (2011) argue: "accessing internal and external knowledge bases are key to the innovation process". In fact, an innovation may be the result of fresh recombination of existing knowledge that creates new commercial value (Khilji *et al.*, 2006).

Previous literature on open innovation has investigated the role of different sources of ideas in facilitating innovation. However, a further investigation of how diverse knowledge is

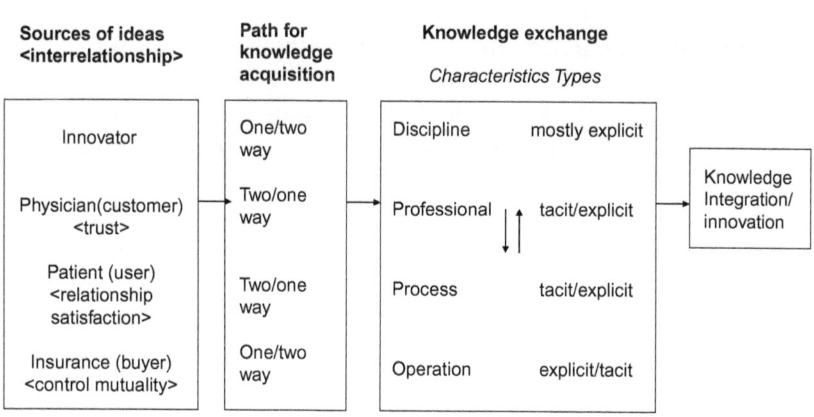

Figure 3. A model of knowledge exchange and flow in the process of open innovation.

exchanged and integrated among various sources thereby leading to bright innovative ideas is warranted. With the case study of a medical device company, integrating theories from both the field of open innovation and the field of communications, our model (see Figure 3) intends to close such a gap by linking macro and micro level of analysis in a hope to open a new path to expand and enrich the scope of open innovation research.

The lesson learned from Acclarent's case is that the success of a medical device start-up depends on how well the company can effectively manage the flow of knowledge to satisfy unmet needs, while integrating their in-depth knowledge of FDA regulations and third-party payers' reimbursement policies into the product innovation process. Future empirical research is needed to investigate the complex interplay among the various actors in the open innovation process.

References

Acclarent Inc. Clear Study, Retrieved July 28, 2011, from http://www.acclarent.com/clinical-education/clinical-data/clear-study.

Arthur, W. B. (1996). Increasing returns and the new world of business, *Harvard Business Review*, 74(4), 100–110.

Borghoff, U. M. and Pareschi, R. (1997). Information technology for knowledge management, *Journal of Universal Computer Science*, 3(8), 835–842.

Carneiro, A. (2000). How does knowledge management influence innovation and competitiveness? *Journal of Knowledge Management*, 4(2), 87–98.

Cassiman, B., Di Guardo, M. C. and Valentini, G. (2010). Organizing links with science: Cooperate or contract? A project-level analysis, *Research Policy*, 39(7), 882–892.

Chesbrough, H. W. (2003a). Open innovation: The new imperative for creating and profiting from technology, *Harvard Business School Press*, Boston, MA.

Chesbrough, H. W. (2003b). The era of open innovation, *MIT Sloan Management Review*, 35–41.

Chesbrough, H. W. and Appleyard, M. M. (2007). Open innovation and strategy, *California Management Review*, 50(1), 57–76.

Chowdhury, S. (2005). The role of affect- and cognition-based trust in complex knowledge sharing, *Journal of Managerial Issues*, 17(3), 310–326.

Christensen, C. M., Grossman, J. H. and Hwang, J. (2009). *The Innovator's Prescription: A Disruptive Solution for Health Care*, McGraw Hill, New York.

De Jong, J. P. J. and Marsili, O. (2006). The fruit flies of innovations: A taxonomy of innovative small firms, *Research Policy*, 35(2), 213–229.

Desouza, K. C. *et al.* (2008). Customer-driven innovation, *Research-Technology Management*, 51(3), 35–44.

Dodgson, M., Gann, D. and Salter, A. (2006). The role of technology in the shift towards open innovation: The case of Procter & Gamble, *R&D Management*, 36(3), 333–346.

Fabrizio, K. R. (2009). Absorptive capacity and the search for innovation, *Research Policy*, 38(2), 255–267.

Gambetta, D. (1988). Can we trust trust? in Gambetta, D. (ed.), *Trust: Making and Breaking Cooperative Relation*, Basil Blackwell, Oxford.

Herzog, P. and Lecker, J. (2010). Open and closed innovation — different innovation cultures for different strategies, *International Journal of Technology Management*, 52(3/4), 322–343.

Hienerth, C. (2006). The commercialization of user innovation: The development of the rodeo kayak industry, *R&D Management*, 36, 273–294.

Hon, L. C. and Grunig, J. (1999). *Guidelines for Measuring Relationships in Public Relations*, The Institute for Public Relations, Gainesville, FL.

Ili, S., Albers, A. and Miller, S. (2010). Open innovation in the automotive industry, *R&D Management*, 40(3), 246–255.

Janzik, L. (2010). Contribution and participation in innovation communities: A classification of incentives and motives, *International Journal of Innovation and Technology Management*, 7(3), 247–262.

Jeppesen, L. B. and Lakhani, K. R. (2010). Marginality and problem-solving effectiveness in broadcast search, *Organization Science*, 21(5), 1016–1033.

Khilji, S. E., Tomasz, M. and Bernstein, B. (2006). Developing an integrated innovation model for biotech firms, *Journal of Product Innovation Management*, 23(6), 528–540.

Kogut, B. and Zander, U. (1992). Knowledge of the firm, combinative capacities and the replication of technology, *Organization Science*, 3, 383–397.

Lettl, C. (2007). User involvement competence for radical innovation, *Journal of Engineering and Technology Management,* 24(1/2), 53–75.

Li, Y. and Vanhaverbeke, W. (2009). The effects of inter-industry and country difference in supplier relationships on pioneering innovations, *Technovation*, 29(12), 843–858.

Liao, S. H., Chang, J. C., Cheng, S. C. and Kuo, C. M. (2004). Employee relationship and knowledge sharing: A case study of a Taiwanese finance and securities firm, *Knowledge Management Research & Practice*, 2, 24–34.

Lichtenthaler, U. and Ernst, H. (2007). External technology commercialization in large firms: Results of a quantitative benchmarking study, *R&D Management,* 37, 383–397.

Lim, K., Chesbrough, H. and Ruan, Y. (2010). Open innovation and patterns of R&D Competition, *International Journal of Technology Management*, 52(3/4), 295–321.

Massa, S. and Testa, S. (2008). Innovation and SMEs: Misaligned perspectives and goals among entrepreneurs, academics, and policy makers, *Technovation,* 28, 393–407.

Mortara, L. *et al*. (2010). Developing a technology intelligence strategy at Kodak European research: Scan & target, *Research-Technology Management*, 53(4), 25–38.

Ndou, V., Del Vecchio, P. and Schina, L. (2011). Open innovation networks: The role of innovative marketplaces for small and medium enterprises' value creation, *International Journal of Innovation and Technology Management,* 8(3), 437–453.

Neyens, I., Faems, D. and Sels, L. (2010). The impact of continuous and discontinuous alliance strategies on startup innovation performance, *International Journal of Technology Management*, 52(3/4), 392–410.

Nonaka, I. and Takeuchi, H. (1995). *The Knowledge-Creating Company,* Oxford University Press, New York, Oxford.

Nonaka, I., Toyama, R. and Konno, N. (2000). SECI, Ba, and leadership: A unified model of dynamic knowledge creation, *Long Range Planning,* 33, 5–34.

Ragins, B. R., Cotton, J. L. and Miller, J. S. (2000). Marginal mentoring: The effects of type of mentor, quality of relationship, and program design on work and career attitudes, *Academy of Management Journal*, 43, 1177–1194.

Rastogi, P. N. (2000). Knowledge management and intellectual capital — The new virtuous reality of competitiveness, *Human Systems Management,* 19(1), 39–48.

Risk Factors. Retrieved June 6, 2008, from http://google.brand.edgar-online.com/EFX_dll/EDGARpro.dll?FetchFilingHtmlSection1?SectionID=5983684-49637-142405&SessionID=ElDvWjaYAmKf5X7.

Schiele, H. (2010). Early supplier integration: The dual role of purchasing in new product development, *R&D Management*, 40(2), 138–153.

Spaeth, S., Stuermer, M. and Krogh, G. (2010). Enabling knowledge creation through outsiders: Toward a push model of open innovation, *International Journal of Technology Management*, 52(3/4), 411–431.

Spencer, J. W. (2003). Firms' knowledge-sharing strategies in the global innovation system: Empirical evidence from the flat panel display industry, *Strategic Management Journal,* 24, 217–233.

Stafford, L. and Canary, D. J. (1991). Maintenance strategies and romantic relationship types, gender and relational characteristics, *Journal of Social and Personal Relationships*, 8, 217–242.

Stam, W. (2009). When does community participation enhance the performance of open source software companies? *Research Policy,* 38(8), 1288–1299.

Stommen, J. (2010). Medical innovator and entrepreneur, *The Healthcare Syndicate*, Retrieved July 18, 2010, from http://www.thehealthcaresyndicate.com/.

Tether, B. S. and Tajar, A. (2008). Beyond industry-university links: Sourcing knowledge for innovation from consultants, private research organizations and the public science-base, *Research Policy*, 37(6/7), 1079–1095.

Tortoriello, M. and Krackhardt, D. (2010). Activating cross-boundary knowledge: The role of Simmelian ties in the generation of innovations, *Academy of Management Journal,* 53(1), 167–181.

Tsai, W. (2001). Knowledge transfer in intraorganizational networks: Effects of network position and absorptive capacity on business unit innovation and performance, *The Academy of Management Journal*, 44(5), 996–1004.

Tsai, W. and Ghoshal, S. (1998). Social capital and value creation: The role of intrafirm Networks, *Academy of Management Journal*, 41, 464–476.

Van de Vrande, V., Vanhaverbeke, W. and Gassmann, O. (2010). Broadening the scope of open innovation: Past research, current state, and future directions, *International Journal of Technology Management*, 52(3/4), 221–235.

Vanhaverbeke, W. (2006). The inter-organizational context of open innovation, in Chesbrough, H., Vanhaverbeke, W. and West, J. (eds.), *Open Innovation: Researching a New Paradigm, Oxford University Press*, Oxford, pp. 205–219.

Van Rijswijk, M. *et al.* (2008). The process and experiences with creating user-driven innovation programs in the Netherlands, *Technology Analysis & Strategic Management*, 20, 309–320.

Weber, M., Weggeman, M. and Van Aken, J. (2012). Developing what customers really need: Involving customers in innovations, *International Journal of Innovation and Technology Management*, 9(3), 1–15.

West, J. and Bogers, M. (2011). Profiting from external innovation: A review of research on open innovation, in Paper presented at *the 9th International Open and User Innovation Workshop*, Vienna, Austria.

Witzeman, S. G. *et al.* (2006). Harnessing external technology for innovation, *Research Technology Management*, 49(3), 19–27.

Zeng, S. X., Xie, X. M. and Tam, C. M. (2010). Relationship between cooperation networks and innovation performance of SMEs, *Technovation*, 30(3), 181–194.

Zenios, S. J. *et al.* (2010). *Biodesign: The Process of Innovating Medical Technologies*, Cambridge University Press, New York, Cambridge.

Chapter 8

Exploring Technological Complexity in the Pharmaceutical Industry

Hao Hu[*,‡] and Liming Zhang[†,§]

[*]*State Key Laboratory of Quality Research in Chinese Medicine, Institute of Chinese Medical Sciences, University of Macau, Macao*

[†]*Business School, Sichuan University, Chengdu, China*

[‡]*haohu@um.edu.mo*

[§]*zhang@chem.ucsb.edu*

Abstract

Technological complexity is an inevitable challenge for latecomer firms aiming to upgrade themselves. Applying a perspective of firms within a sectoral system of innovation, this chapter studies the catch-up efforts of the leading Chinese pharmaceutical firms in the past few decades. The findings show that technological complexity tends to lengthen the catch-up process, raises capability requirement, requires more networking, and demands complicated institution design, which asks for a more evolutionary catch-up strategy with self-investment into system capability and network competence. The findings of this chapter provide references for catch-up efforts in other industries with technological complexity.

Keywords: Latecomer firm, technological complexity, pharmaceutical industry, China.

1. Introduction

Industrial catch-up of latecomer firms has become a more and more attractive subject in literature. In theory, catch-up is mostly regarded as a sustainable process that reduces the gap between the forerunners and the latecomers (Kim, 2011; Lee *et al.*, 2009). Researchers have paid much attention to not only how emerging giants achieved successful catch-up but also how small economies could catch-up with new industrial powers (Leseure *et al.*, 2009). Acknowledging the progress of industrial catch-up from developing countries, researchers also critically indicate that these newly emerged economies are still holding a weak position in the global industrial value chain (Steinfeld, 2004). The intense competition among domestic firms, low-profit work, and rapid improvement of foreign firms are eroding the catch-up efforts of new entrants, especially the rapid technical change that is complicating the whole catch-up process (Brandt and Thun, 2011).

Jung and Lee (2010) found that efficient catch-up by Korean firms was more likely to occur in industries where technologies were more explicit, predictable, and easily embodied in imported products or equipment. On the contrary, the catch-up in the industries with technological complexity often faces more challenges and experiences more setbacks and even failures. While it is more possible to comprehend successful catch-up by utilizing cost advantages in some industries, technological complexity will constrain the utilization of cost advantage in industrial catch-up (Zeng and Williamson, 2007). Therefore, how to realize catch-up in industries characterized with technological complexity becomes an important but unsatisfactorily answered question. Moreover, the changing global value is bringing more uncertainties for industrial upgradation, especially by causing shifts in the global market (Fold and Larsen, 2011). All of these require new understanding of catch-up in industries with technological complexity within the context of changing global value chain.

To address this concern, we study how latecomer firms realize catch-up in the industries with technological complexity in this chapter. We especially focus on the strategies chosen by firms and the development of technological capabilities during the process of catch-up. By applying firm-level analysis within the sectoral system of innovation in the Chinese pharmaceutical companies, we make contributions in several ways. First, we contribute to the field of catch-up by highlighting the distinguished catch-up difficulties due to technological complexity. Second, we propose strategic actions that latecomers could choose to meet the technological complexity. Third, we indicate the special effect of the big domestic market and institutional design following the logic of sectoral system of innovation.

The rest of this chapter is organized as follows. We briefly review the literature about catch-up, technological regimes, and firms within sectoral system of innovation in Section 2. Section 3 provides a background of the global pharmaceutical industry and the Chinese pharmaceutical industry. Sections 4 and 5 present methodology and findings from case firms. Section 6 discusses our case findings. Finally, we will summarize and conclude implications for future research and practice.

2. Literature Review

2.1. *Catch-up and technological complexity*

For the latecomer industries, catch-up not only requires careful design of maximizing value of domestic resources, such as labor, land, and raw materials, but also means facing the tough challenges of technological barriers. How to construct and apply technological capability is an important and difficult question in catch-up. In particular, whether latecomer industries could achieve success through technological leapfrogging is the most debatable topic (Child and Rodrigues, 2005), which is highly related to the features of technological complexity.

Technology as a knowledge base usually defines the emergence and evolution of an industry. Particularly, the nature of technology's influence in the choice of the path in industrial catch-up is where the technological complexity plays a significant role. The more system complexity a technology has, the slower the catch-up will be (Zeng and Williamson, 2007). Technology not only includes explicit knowledge but also embeds a lot of tacit knowledge. The more tacit knowledge embedded in technology, the more difficult it is for an industry to catch-up (Lee *et al.*, 2009; Guo *et al.*, 2013).

The technological complexity is also related to technological predictability. Lee and Lim (2001) indicate that technological predictability is the key in determining whether technological leapfrogging is feasible. For example, the main reason why the telecom equipment industry could leapfrog directly from analogue technology to digital technology was that the development path of telecommunication technology was obvious and digital technology was predictable for the inevitable development in technology (Mu and Lee, 2005). Always, the change of technology will bring new possibilities for latecomer industries to surpass forerunners in industrial catch-up (Rasiah *et al.*, 2010). For example, paradigm shifts of technology could provide latecomers with an opportunity to penetrate the market and universal standards (Wu and Zhang, 2010). But it also tests the latecomers' ability to predict the technology's future.

Leapfrogging is often associated with two risks: choosing the right technology or standards, and creating initial markets. To overcome these two risks, common actions of catch-up include entering new market segments quickly, manufacturing with high levels of engineering excellence, and to be the first-to-market by means of the best integrative designs (Lee, 2005). But these actions are usually more effective in industries with less technological complexity and this is why latecomer countries have better performance in the technological sectors with shorter cycle time, easier access to knowledge, and higher approachability (Park and Lee, 2006). In one word, problems of technological complexity in catch-up remain unsolved (Park, 2013).

2.2. *Latecomer firms within the sectoral system of innovation*

When latecomer firms are constrained by technological complexity, their own action scale is also limited, which emphasizes the necessity for considering catch-up in a broader view. Chaturvedi (2007) argues that a perspective of the sectoral system of innovation is more appropriate to study the catch-up of a specific industry, which necessitates a combinatory analysis of sectoral- and firm-level factors in catch-up. Therefore, a perspective of firms within the sectoral system of innovation is very appropriate for investigating catch-up in technological complexity (Kim and Lee, 2008).

In a catch-up process, firms have many options, such as niche market proposition, service innovation, collaborative research and development (R&D), and leveraging complementary technologies (Wu and Zhang, 2010). On the one hand, catch-up firms require technological catch-up before the catch-up in terms of firm value or brand values (Joo and Lee, 2010). On the other hand, catch-up firms needs to emphasize a resource-based catch-up strategy (Mathews, 2002) and carry out a series of activities on management processes and products (Forbes and Wield, 2008). Essentially, the catch-up not only means technological development but also requires a systematic restructuring of the whole organization (Nolan and Yeung, 2001).

As the main industrial actors, firms and their related interactions with the other industrial actors decide industrial catch-up greatly. For domestic firms, they must deal with the complicated relationship with multinational corporations, which can benefit the catch-up of domestic firms through their technology transfer and business interaction, thus, improving management and technological capabilities of the domestic firms (Mu and Lee, 2005;

Fan, 2010). However, multinational corporations are usually the biggest competitors for domestic latecomer firms, and their reverse effect on local catch-up is often unpredictable. Besides, it could also trap firms into low-profit work resulting in missing an industrial chance in some cases, though competition among domestic firms could promote industrial upgradation to some extent (Xie and Wu, 2003). The internationalization effort is another important determinant for industrial catch-up. For example, the practices of Samsung (South Korea) and Acer (Taiwan) approve the importance of the firm's internationalization efforts (Hobday, 1998). Moreover, firms could accelerate their catch-up through frequent interaction with universities (institutes). Based on the experience of Chinese firms, secondary innovation emphasizing internal development and self-development through integrating external capability is regarded as an effective catch-up choice (Fan *et al.*, 2007; Wu *et al.*, 2009).

According to the framework of the sectoral system of innovation, catch-up firms can't ignore the effect of becoming an institution. In a comparative study of Japan and South Korea, researchers have found that different institutional systems led firms choose different innovation managements, which eventually resulted in a varied innovation output (Hemmert, 2008). Specifically, the government could intervene according to the domestic firms' development stage to ensure they could catch-up with MNCs (Fan, 2006). A typical example is that in 1970, the Indian government denied compound patents in drugs to promote domestic firms to accumulate manufacturing capabilities but reestablished patent policy in 1995 to support the innovative drug efforts of domestic firms (Athreye *et al.*, 2009), which provided enough time and market space for the catch-up of local pharmaceutical firms. In addition to institutional framework from the government, domestic demand plays a significant role in directing industrial catch-up. Whether domestic demand could provide large enough market space is thought to be important for domestic firms to bring up technological capability and earn valuable time to compete with multinational firms.

In general, although past literature has generated meaningful knowledge and understanding about the catch-up analysis of a firm, catch-up within the perspective of the sectoral system of innovation could provide insightful instructions specific to technological complexity.

3. Global Transfer of Pharmaceutical Industry: A Background

Modern pharmaceutical industry is also a typical representative of technological complexity. The core R&D of innovative drugs involves a long chain of events, starting from the selection of the appropriate drug to the final clinical trials and marketing activities. Simultaneously, it crosses multiple academic disciplines, including chemistry, biology, medical science, material science, and computer science. The major drawback of the pharmaceutical industry is discontinuous invention of innovative drugs (Athreye and Godley, 2009). Theoretically, every innovative drug is a revolutionary breakthrough compared to the past drugs and comprises completely new technological elements or ingredients.

Traditionally, the global pharmaceutical industry is controlled by pharmaceutical companies in the USA and Europe. Before the 1990s, more than 90% of the market was centered in advanced economies such as North America, West Europe, and Japan (Chandler, 2005). However, in the past three decades certain significant changes have happened. Now, more and more pharmaceutical consumption is happening in the emerging economies, which is expected to occupy 30% of the global market by 2020 (Grabowski, 2011). Especially, the transfer of the global pharmaceutical industry not only brings new industrial uncertainties but also provides opportunities for latecomers, such as India and China.

As a model of a latecomer industry in the global pharmaceutical industry, India made great progress in the modernization of its pharmaceutical industry and realized industrial catch-up, partially (Kale and Little, 2007; Athreye and Godley, 2009). But India still faces a lot of challenges in discovering innovative branded drugs (Chaturvedi, 2007). The experience of India can't generate a complete and convincing answer for catch-up in the global pharmaceutical industry (Chittoor *et al.*, 2009).

On the contrary, China has different experiences in pharmaceutical catch-up. With its rising economy and huge population, the Chinese pharmaceutical market has been enlarging rapidly in the past decade and has become the third largest pharmaceutical market in the world. But domestic pharmaceutical firms' lack of innovative drug products has to wildly compete on generic drug pricing while innovative drugs from global pharmaceutical companies are enjoy pricing advantages and doctors' preferences (Wang, 2006). Although there are more than 5,000 domestic pharmaceutical firms, most of them have no R&D facilities and are not strategically located, which makes them difficult to benefit from global R&D offshoring (Hamdouch and He, 2009). Recognizing its own weakness in the global pharmaceutical sector, Chinese government wants to reach a balance between the developing domestic pharmaceutical industry and controlling drug expenditure to guarantee even access of drug for poor and uninsured patients (Chan and Daim, 2011). Up until now, the joint efforts of the government, industry, and academia to improve industrial capacity are currently at a very early stage (Mao and Zheng, 2009; Qiu *et al.*, 2014), which calls for rigorous inquiry on the current catch-up activities of the leading pharmaceutical firms in China.

4. Methodology

4.1. *Case study*

In order to track the catch-up process and to obtain deep insights, we choose the case study method to analyze and present the strategy and technological capability choices that have been

Table 1. Background information of case firms.

Firm	Founding year	Year of public listing	Ownership	Employee number	Main business areas
Hengrui Co.	1970	2000	Private	4,500	Anti-neoplastic, anesthetic, role in electrolytic infusion
Huadong Co.	1952	1999	State-controlled	4,300	Immunosuppressant, treatment of diabetes mellitus
Humanwell Co.	1988	1997	Private	4,627	Anesthetic, birth control pills
Xiansheng Co.	1995	2007	Private	4,000	Anti-neoplastic, anti-infection drugs, cardiovascular drug

made in the Chinese pharmaceutical sector. Since multiple cases are more appropriate to derive at conclusions and ensure externality (Eisenhardt and Graebner, 2007), we use the multiple case method in this study. Considering that the Chinese pharmaceutical industry is mostly composed by generic drug producers, drug innovation rather than sales should be chosen as a criterion for case selection. Although few New Chemical Entities have been created by the Chinese pharmaceutical firms, we choose case companies by considering whether they had innovative outputs in me-too drugs or Abbreviated New Drug Applications (ANDA) approvals. Besides, to ensure that the data satisfy the criteria for triangle review, the case company should be publically listed in the stock exchange market. According to these criteria, under the instruction of industrial experts, we selected four companies as our final cases. The background information for the four case companies is summarized in Table 1.

4.2. *Data collection*

The analysis of case companies needs data covering strategy, product, and technological capability, etc., in different development stages. The primary data for the case companies were collected through multiple sources: (1) archival documents, including annual reports, newspaper articles, industrial magazine reports, and analysts' reports; (2) interviews with senior managers, R&D scientists, and salespersons; (3) technological presentations (seminars), including listening to the speeches of the case company representatives at technology and industry conferences (seminars); (4) a collection of industrial opinions, including communication with financial analysts and university (research institute) professors who are connected with the case firms. The whole data collection process lasted from January 2009 to November 2011.

4.3. *Data analysis*

After data collection, all the data are analyzed by a combined approach of process and theme (Edmondson and McManus, 2007). We track the main business and management events during the whole developmental process of the case companies. All the data are also categorized into three themes: market, product, and technological capability. Market theme concerns about overseas vs. domestic market target, therapeutic segment, and prescription vs. over-the-counter (OTC) drugs; product theme is about the innovative nature of drugs; and technological capability theme is about technology acquisition, technology cooperation, and cultivation of own technological capability. We summarize all the information in a more cohesive way. Then we present the catch-up of the case companies based on these three themes.

5. Findings

5.1. *Huadong Co.*

Huadong Co. was started as state-owned Zhejiang Pharmaceutical Factory. In 1993, it founded its marketing department and began academic promotion activities. So far, the market positioning of Huadong Co. is mainly focused on the domestic market. Its main clients are hospitals above the county level and its product portfolio is mainly composed of prescription drugs. In 2005, the company announced the expansion of its business to the international market by exporting bulk drugs. The company has received a series of international certifications.

Huadong Co. chooses immunosuppressive drugs and diabetes medication as its key business and is strengthening its research on anti-infective, anti-hepatitis B, and anti-cancer drugs, as well as involved in modernizing Traditional Chinese Medicine. Earlier, the company's focus was on the fields of Traditional Chinese Medicine. In 1991, they developed a national first-class new drug which was made from fermented Cordyceps powder. In 1999, it developed *Fen injection,* which is the third industrialized leukocyte colony-stimulating factor in the world. In 2002, it developed the me-too drug *Cyclosporine* first in China to compete with Novartis, who is the original developer of this innovative drug. In the field of diabetes, Huadong Co. acquired the patent of *Acarbose* in 2002 to obtain the market share of *Acarbose*'s original producer Bayer. In 2006, Huadong Co. launched *Sai Keping*, another me-too drug first marketed in China in order to compete with Roche, who originally launched the product in China. In 2008, it introduced the first me-too drug *Tacrolimus* capsules of Astellas. In the field of peptic ulcer drugs, Huadong Co.'s *Pantoprazole* is also a me-too drug.

These star products above reflect the "either the first or the only" philosophy of Huadong Co., which lead the company's market segmenting strategy. The common feature of these key products is that there is a multinational pharmaceutical enterprise in every corresponding therapy. Huadong Co. follows and benefits from foreign pharmaceutical companies' doctors and by patient education. Once the market gradually matures, the company gets the market share from the original products by first introducing its me-too products at lower prices.

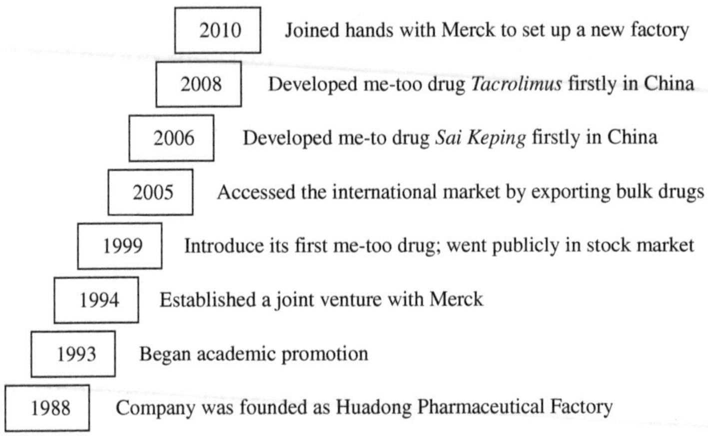

Figure 1. Catch-up process of Huadong Co.

Consequently, the company becomes an influential player in the therapeutic segment by relatively lowering the price and improving the reputation of the first me-too drugs.

Huadong Co. emphasizes the development of an appropriate internal and external balance in R&D. On the one hand, Huadong Co. insists on the long-term cooperation with pharmaceutical companies such as Merck. On the other hand, Huadong Co. continues to strengthen its own R&D capacity. The whole development process of Huadong Co. could be summarized as shown in Figure 1.

5.2. *Hengrui Co.*

Founded in 1991, Hengrui Co. started from generic drugs and has become China's leading R&D-oriented and academic marketing pharmaceutical company. Now the company's main drugs include anti-neoplastic drugs, anesthetic drugs, and anti-infective drugs. Especially in the field of anti-neoplastic drugs, Hengrui Co. ranked No. 1 in terms of sales in China. Hengrui Co. has China's largest research and production bases of anti-neoplastic and anesthetic drugs. Hengrui Co. has taken the domestic prescription drug market as its key target market and has adopted academic promotion as its main marketing model.

The company's catch-up began in 1994 when it set up a research center. Until 1996, Hengrui Co. successfully developed over 20 new products and was involved in the market of anti-tumor and anesthetic drugs among which five species were national key new products. Its bulk pharmaceutical chemicals have also infiltrated the US market. In order to achieve the upgrade from just producing generic drugs to innovative generic drugs, Hengrui Co. set up the Shanghai Research Center in 2000. This research center is primarily engaged in the discovery of innovative drug research and established anti-neoplastic agents, cardiovascular drugs, endocrine drugs, and surgery medication. In 2001, drugs such as *Etoposide*, *Cyclophosphamide*, *Mesnaum*, and *Thiotepa* obtained the Food and Drug Administration of USA (FDA) certification. In the year 2005, Hengri Co. established its subordinate company in USA and set up two laboratories in New Jersey and North Carolina.

In 2006, Hengrui Co. decided to transform itself into a branded generics company after increasing the investment in R&D capabilities. It has marketed about 10 new medicines with independent intellectual property rights into the domestic market. Hengrui Co. is also actively involved in R&D outsourcing for the purpose of entering the high-end market through innovative product development. It chose to cooperate with multinational pharmaceutical companies such as Chiron and Medicir. In 2009, Hengrui Co. submitted *Retagliptin*'s ANDA application to FDA. Approval for the first me-better drugs *Erin PuBu* and *Irinotecan* was obtained 2011. In general, Hengrui Co. has successfully completed the transition from a generic to a branded generic company, and has started production of me-better drugs.

Hengrui Co. attaches great importance to the construction of its own R&D facilities. In recent years, Hengrui Co. has attracted a number of Chinese scientists who have extensive experience in developing innovative drugs in multinational

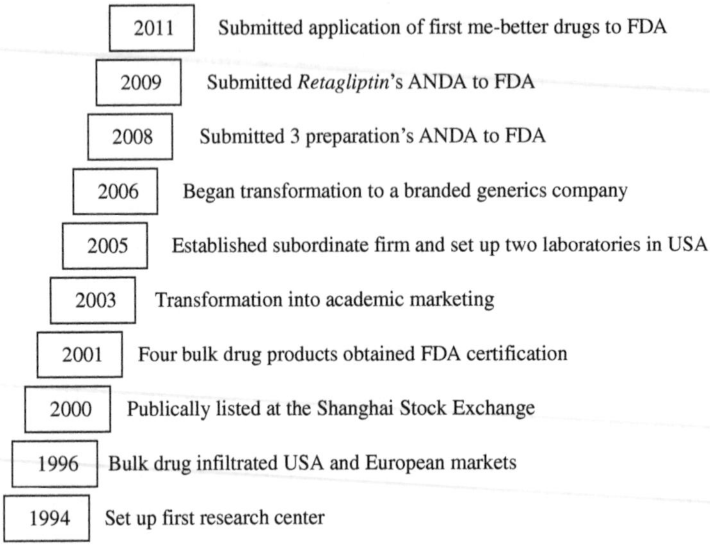

Figure 2. Catch-up process of Hengrui Co.

pharmaceutical companies. These scientists brought advanced experience from overseas projects to Hengrui Co. to help the company reach a high-level R&D capability. Now, it has the capability of covering the entire innovation chain of drug development and carrying out R&D work independently. It also allows Hengrui Co. to enjoy a dominant position, making Hengrui Co. more selective in deciding its partners. The whole development process of Hengrui Co. could be summarized as shown in Figure 2.

5.3. *Humanwell Co.*

Humanwell Co. was set up in 1988 by a few pharmaceutical experts and was listed publicly in the stock market in 1997. Its core market is narcotic drugs, which are strictly regulated by the government. Its first key product was *Fentanyl citrate*, which was introduced to the market in 2001 and enjoys exclusive market rights in China. In 2003, Humanwell Co. successfully cooperated with local universities and institutes to develop the national second-class drug *Remifentanil*. It divided the whole R&D project into several parts and subcontracted them to several universities and institutes to accelerate the process. In the meantime, this firm also quickly started to construct production lines. With such kind of parallel project management, it shortened the originally planned 6 years to 3 years, bringing about rapid science and technology transformation. In 2005, it introduced a national third-class new drug *Sufentanil*, which is the first me-too version in China. In 2006, it successfully imitated *Midazolam*, which is classified as a national second-class new drug. In 2009, its *Phosphorus propofol* (a national first-class new drug) and *Isoflurane* (a national second-class new drug) obtained clinical trial approval from the State Food and Drug Administration of China.

Other than contributions to the narcotics field, Humanwell Co. also began to get itself involved in the business of reproductive health drugs and steroid hormones. Furthermore, Humanwell Co. utilized acquisition and joint ventures to enter into the frontier of biopharmaceutical business. The company also plans to explore the advanced markets by exporting narcotic drugs in bulk. Now it is trying to obtain several certifications from FDA. Moreover, Humanwell Co. has also tried to enter into the African market by establishing subsidiaries there.

In recent years, Humanwell Co. tried to build its own technological capabilities, transitioning from being completely dependent on external universities to a more balanced R&D structure. It initiated a "research institute without barrier" program, which aims to build research platforms with local famous universities to conduct advanced research on development, manufacturing technology, and the clinical study of narcotic drugs. It plans to invest in the R&D of 21 analgesic drugs in the near future. In general, the whole development process of Humanwell Co. could be summarized as shown in Figure 3.

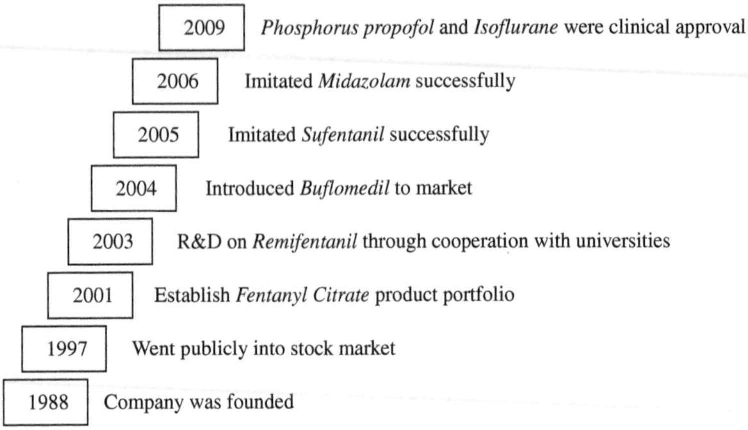

Figure 3. Catch-up process of Humanwell Co.

5.4. *Xiansheng Co.*

Founded in 1995, Xiansheng Co. was first famous agent for marketing children's oral cold medicines. Nevertheless, Xiansheng Co. was aware of the drawbacks of being a pure sales company and began to build up its own manufacturing facility. In 2000, Xiansheng Co. set up its drug research center to enter into the area of therapeutic drugs for the nervous system by pioneering the research and development work of *Bicun* (Edaravone injection), in collaboration with the China Pharmaceutical University. As an emergency medicine, *Bicun* is the only oxygen free-radical scavenger in the world that has the clear mechanism to target and treat cerebral infarction. Xiansheng Co. is the first company in China and the second company in the world that successfully developed this kind of drug.

In 2003, Xiansheng Co. formally set up its drug research institute. And in 2006, the firm acquired *Endu* (a new anti-tumor drug) to foray into the field of cancer treatment. *Endu* is the first anti-tumor drug that underwent Phase IV clinical studies in China. Besides development in product, Xiansheng Co. rapidly leapfrogged into the finance market. With the investment and financial assistance from the Lenovo Group, Xiansheng Co. got publically listed in the New York Stock Exchange (NYSE) in 2007, becoming the first Chinese pharmaceutical firm that was listed in NYSE, which brought much reputation and more opportunities in the international market.

Since 2009, Xiansheng Co. has ventured into the fields of antibodies and vaccines, reaching an agreement with some world-renowned companies to jointly develop a number of internationally innovative drugs. In 2009, Xiansheng Co. developed the world's first anti-VEGF rabbit monoclonal antibody drug together with a USA company. Xiansheng Co. also made an agreement with the OSI Biotechnology Company to jointly develop a new anti-tumor drug (OSI930). In late November of 2010, Xiansheng Co. announced that it had reached a strategic partnership agreement with Bristol-Myers Squibb (BMS) for the research and development of an anticancer drug (BMS-817378), through which Xiansheng Co. enjoyed the exclusive right to market BMS-817378 in China. Besides, its bulk drug (*Montmorillonite*) passed the EU GMP certification in 2010.

The company tries to improve its technological capabilities in two ways. On the one hand, Xiansheng Co. keeps strengthening its own R&D abilities. In addition to establishing its drug research institute, it established Beijing Laboratory in 2007, aiming to form a strategic R&D layout. Its general strategy is to rank first in me-too drug producers in China by studying and improving pharmaceutical production. On the other hand, Xiansheng Co. continues to positively cooperate with foreign pharmaceutical companies, particularly by purchasing relatively advanced research projects and taking over the rest of the R&D work. Through acquisition of advanced pharmaceutical projects, it could reduce the R&D risk and enhance its own R&D capabilities. The whole development process of Xiansheng Co. could be summarized as shown in Figure 4.

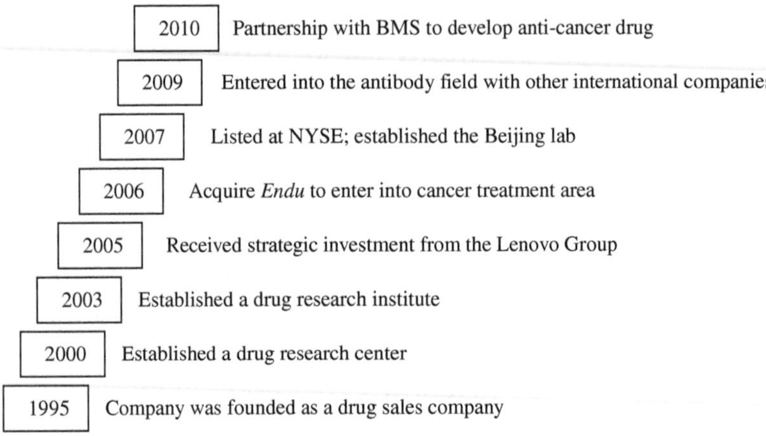

Figure 4. Catch-up process of Xiansheng Co.

6. Discussion

Within the changing context of the global pharmaceutical sector, the leading Chinese pharmaceutical firms take active actions to seek breakthrough in the technological complexity of drug innovation. During this process, they demonstrated characteristic features of their catch-up strategies and technological capabilities. Through a detailed case study, we can summarize the key features of such case companies as shown in Table 2.

Different organizations have varied strategies and strengths in different technological regimes (Park and Lee, 2006), and we can find that these case firms have showed some similarities in terms of market positioning, product choice, and technological capability planning, which reflects the impact of the technological complexity in the pharmaceutical industry. Using the framework of firms within the sectoral system of innovation, we can provide a detailed analysis here.

First, firms fixed the domestic market as their core target market. Most of their revenues and operations are based on the domestic market. Although they have some business overseas such as bulk drugs, those businesses do not contribute

Table 2. Catch-up features of case firms.

Firm	Target market (Overseas vs. Domestic)	Therapeutic segment (Popular vs. Niche)	Prescription vs. OTC	Drug product	Technology acquisition	Technology cooperation	Cultivation of technological capabilities
Hengrui Co.	Mainly domestic	Popular	Prescription	Me-too drugs and some me-better drug	Few	Cooperation with overseas pharmaceutical firms	High
Huadong Co.	Mainly domestic and some overseas	Niche	Prescription	Me-too drugs	Few	Stable cooperation with key pharmaceutical companies	Middle
Humanwell Co.	Domestic	Niche	Prescription	Me-too drugs	Few	Cooperation with local universities and institutes	Middle
Xiansheng Co.	Mainly domestic	Popular	Prescription	Me-too drugs	Many	Cooperation with overseas pharmaceutical firms	Middle

significantly to firm growth. Although catch-up is more likely to occur in sectors with more monopolistic market structures (Jung and Lee, 2010), our study finds that the market space also plays a great role in supporting catch-up. The big market space provides support to catch-up firms at their early stages. When they are unable to enter the advanced market and are also facing competition pressure from multinational pharmaceutical companies in the domestic market, the big domestic market gives them time and a chance to generate revenues to solve the problems of technological complexity.

Second, "improvement innovation" of prescription drugs in the large consumer market has been the main product choice. Most of the products in case companies are prescription drugs, which means higher profitability compared to OTC products. They also choose therapeutic segments that have a large number of patients, such as anti-tumor and anti-infection. In particular, Humanwell Co. has concentrated its business on the anesthetic area. While it is highly regulated by the government, the rapid increase in the number of surgeries in China guarantees anesthetic drugs as an attractive business area. Most of the products are me-too drugs that have a similar chemical structure as the original innovative drugs but have some "improvement innovation" in some aspects, such as dosage or molecular structure. Case firms carry out differentiated market segmenting, price discounting, and closer marketing to compete with the innovative drugs of multinational pharmaceutical companies. They aim to obtain remarkable market shares but do not expect to control the specific therapeutic market. As previously found, catch-up firms may choose emulation to develop flexible routines rather than blind imitation (Li and Kozhikode, 2008). These case companies demonstrated a more stable and evolutionary strategy choice to apply incrementalism to respond to the technological complexity of pharmaceutical innovation.

Third, different technological capability paths have been chosen in response to technological complexity. During the process, the leading firm may have varied choices (Forbes and

Wield, 2008), which is exactly reflected on the technological capability paths of case companies. In the process of constructing its own R&D capability, four case companies have all paid enough attention by investing in establishing R&D facilities, buying experimental equipment, and hiring qualified R&D experts. Among them, Hengrui Co. shows a higher level of capability consequential to its imitation of the R&D organizing structure of multinational pharmaceutical companies, staffing experts from overseas, and recruiting domestic outstanding Ph.D. degree holders.

Nevertheless they have a distinguished choice about technology cooperation: Huadong Co. and Xiansheng Co. cooperated mainly with key pharmaceutical companies that have close business links with them; Humanwell Co. decided to cooperate with domestic universities (institutes); whereas Hengrui Co. cooperated with target foreign firms that could make up for its specific technological shortage. None of them get technological capability through cooperation with domestic firms. And in terms of technology acquisition, Xiansheng Co. is the only case company that emphasizes purchasing premature drug projects.

Literature has highlighted the importance of international cooperation (Mathews, 2006), international trade (Mendoza, 2010), and other "interactive learning" with international collaborators (Kristinsson and Rao, 2008) in catch-up. Our case firms also demonstrated to some extent that interactions with international or multinational pharmaceutical companies are important to strengthen latecomers' technological capability. But such kind of interaction is limited in many aspects, implying that overseas pharmaceutical firms and multinational pharmaceutical companies do not have too much motivation to exchange or transfer their technological capability to domestic Chinese pharmaceutical firms. Besides, the isolation of technological cooperation among domestic pharmaceutical firms sharply indicates difficulties in integrating industrial strength in overcoming technological complexity. On the contrary, domestic universities and public institutes provide some help to the industry by coordinating the work of these case firms, which supports the argument of the public research institutions' crucial role for industrial catch-up (Mazzoleni and Nelson, 2007).

Compared with the catch-up process of Indian pharmaceutical firms, our study has also identified some differences. First, the emergence of biotechnology has increased the technology complexity for Chinese pharmaceutical firms. While Indian pharmaceutical firms mainly began their catch-up process through chemical bulk drugs, Chinese pharmaceutical firms today have to learn cutting-edge technologies in biotechnology for pharmaceutical innovation. Second, Chinese pharmaceutical firms have to compete with global pharmaceutical companies in the domestic market today. At the beginning of catch-up, Indian pharmaceutical firms accumulated technological and financial resources by exporting generic drugs to advanced economies. On the contrary, many global pharmaceutical companies entered into the growing Chinese pharmaceutical market directly. Local Chinese pharmaceutical firms have to deal with foreign market competition and own technological accumulation at the same time. Third, Chinese pharmaceutical firms have to meet the diverse requirements from the government. While the Chinese government has introduced a series of policies to encourage pharmaceutical innovation in recent years (Huang, 2012), the central government strongly emphasizes drug price control and safe supply, which generates conflicting institutional pressures for Chinese pharmaceutical firms.

Thus, based on the case study of catch-up by the leading Chinese pharmaceutical companies, we could identify risks in technological complexity and firm's catch-up in a sectoral system of innovation, which could be summarized as a proposed framework as shown in Figure 5.

From Figure 5, we can see that technological complexity will generate much tougher challenges. First, technological complexity will lengthen the catch-up process, forcing latecomer firms to spend more time and effort to realize catch-up. Second,

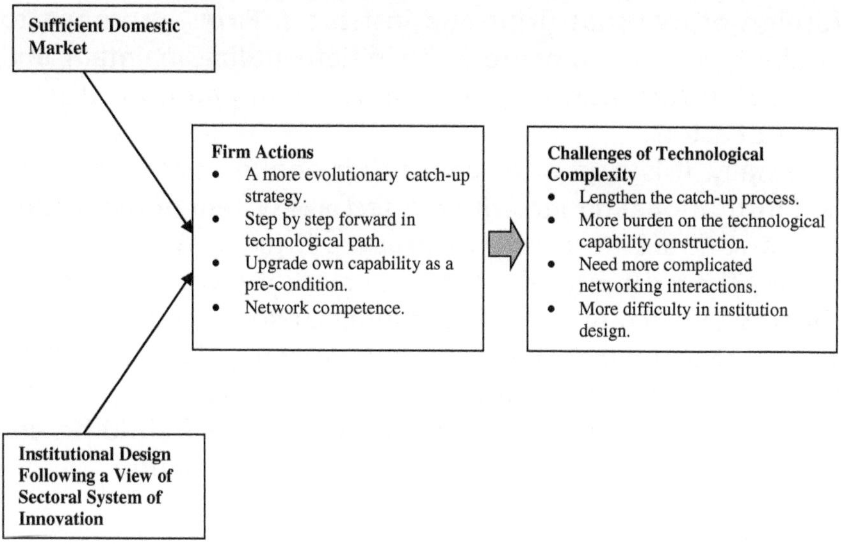

Figure 5. Framework of catch-up in technological complexity.

technological complexity will burden technological capability construction even more. Each firm has to enrich and improve its interdisciplinary capabilities. Third, technological complexity needs more complicated networking interaction among the industrial actors. Fourth, institutions will become more crucial and difficult to be designed. As the move into the more advanced capability requires a redesign of the related institutions (Figueiredo, 2008), technological complexity makes it hard for institutions to meet the complex and sometimes conflicting system requirements.

To overcome these risks, catch-up firms could implement a series of interrelated actions. Facing more system problems than ever, firms have to choose a more evolutionary rather than radical catch-up strategy. An ideal option would be selecting and sticking to specific market segments, combined with a step-by-step forward strategy in the technological path. Firms have to upgrade their capability as a precondition before beginning external cooperation, especially cooperation with foreign or overseas firms and institutes. Firms also need to establish network competence to initiate, utilize, maintain, and manage interorganizational cooperation among different types of actors.

Finally, it is crucial to realize that enough domestic space and institutional design within a sectoral system of innovation framework are necessary to support firms' action discussed above. The existence of a big local market gives firms decent chances to catch-up with frontrunners, experiment with their work, and accumulate resources and capability. Besides, only by following a view of sectoral system of innovation could the work of institutional design integrate opinions from different parties and reflect the systematic complexity demand.

7. Concluding Remarks

As highlighted by the sectoral system of innovation, technology as a representative of knowledge base will considerably affect the development of an industry (Malerba, 2005). Our study shows that technological complexity poses more challenges for firms that are striving for industrial catch-up. Thus, our study not only provides empirical findings about Chinese pharmaceutical firms but also contributes to the literature in two main aspects. First, our study enriches the field of catch-up by clarifying the impact of technological complexity on catch-up process. Second, applying the firms' perspective in a sectoral innovation system, our study contributes to the literature on sectoral innovation system by highlighting the roles and specific strategies of catch-up firms in reshaping the sectoral innovation system.

Our study has valuable implications for both managers and policy-makers. Ambitious leaders from catch-up firms need to apply a long-term strategy view to complete system construction. It is crucial for latecomers to systematically balance every aspect of technological innovation's capability to establish their own system capability (Yam *et al.*, 2004). Moreover, when considering the key impact of absorptive and transformation capability in industrial catch-up (Guan *et al.*, 2006), managers should invest enough energy to improve firms' internal capability of technology innovation and management innovation. With its management innovation and network competence, latecomers may experience great acceleration in catch-up.

Our study also has implications for policy-designers. To meet the challenges of technological complexity, the design of institutions must reflect the requirements of the sectoral system of innovation. Particularly, policy-makers should think clearly on how to make use of the domestic market as a driver for catch-up firms. For example, although the government has the responsibility to control drug price to ensure medical equity, it also needs careful arrangements for innovative drugs both from multinational pharmaceutical companies and me-too drugs from domestic latecomers to provide appropriate possibility and motivation for local R&D. Government should also play an important role in initiating network integration of firms and universities (institutes) at different positions of the value chain. In addition, another role for the government to play is to transition from being an institutional initiator to an institutional supporter and to leave space for industrial actors to manage their complex relationships in a situation of technological complexity.

As the main catch-up activities in Chinese pharmaceutical firms have just begun in the past decade, it is still too early to reach a complete understanding about catch-up in situations with technological complexity. This research should be advanced through longitudinal observation on the future evolution of pharmaceutical industry in China. While our study focuses on the pharmaceutical sector, other industries in which technological complexity is significant still need to be further understood, such as medical devices (Zhang *et al.*, 2013). Technological complexity will be more and more popular in the current industries that are crossing traditional technological boundaries to provide more innovative products (Kiamehr *et al.*, 2014).

Then, continuous investigation on efforts with respect to the technological complexity will enrich our knowledge and provide more guidance for industrial practice.

Acknowledgment

This work was supported by the research fund of the University of Macau (MYRG160(Y1-L2)-ICMS11-HH).

References

Athreye, S. and Godley, A. (2009). Internationalization and technological leapfrogging in the pharmaceutical industry, *Industrial and Corporate Change*, 18(2), 295–323.

Athreye, S., Kale, D. and Ramani, S. V. (2009). Experimentation with strategy and the evolution of dynamic capability in the Indian pharmaceutical sector, *Industrial and Corporate Change*, 18(4), 729–759.

Brandt, L. and Thun, E. (2011). Going mobile in China: Shifting value chains and upgrading in the mobile telecom sector, *International Journal of Technological Learning, Innovation and Development*, 4(1/2/3), 148–180.

Chan, L. and Daim, T. U. (2011). Multi-perspective analysis of the Chinese pharmaceutical sector: Policy, enterprise and technology, *Journal of Technology Management in China*, 6(2), 171–190.

Chandler, A. D. J. (2005). *Shaping the Industrial Century: The Remarkable Story of the Modern Chemical and Pharmaceutical Industries*, Harvard University Press, Cambridge, MA.

Chaturvedi, S. (2007). Exploring interlinkages between national and sectoral innovation systems for rapid technological catch-up: Case of Indian biopharmaceutical industry, *Technology Analysis & Strategic Management*, 19(5), 643–657.

Child, J. and Rodrigues, S. B. (2005). The internationalization of Chinese firms: A case for theoretical extension? *Management and Organization Review*, 1(3), 381–410.

Chittoor, R. *et al.* (2009). Third-world copycats to emerging multinationals: Institutional changes and organizational transformation in the Indian pharmaceutical industry, *Organization Science*, 20(1), 187–205.

Edmondson, A. C. and McManus, S. E. (2007). Methodological fit in management field research, *Academy of Management Review*, 32(4), 1155–1179.

Eisenhardt, K. M. and Graebner, M. E. (2007). Theory building from cases: Opportunities and challenges. *Academy of Management Journal*, 50 (1), pp. 25–32.

Fan, P. (2006). Promoting indigenous capability: The Chinese government and domestic telecom-equipment firms, *China Review*, 6(1), 9–35.

Fan, P. (2010). Catch-up through staged development and innovation: The case of Chinese telecom companies, *Journal of Science and Technology Policy in China*, 1(1), 64–91.

Fan, P., Gao, X. and Watanabe, K. N. (2007). Technology strategies of innovative Chinese domestic companies, *International Journal of Technology and Globalisation*, 3(4), 344–363.

Figueiredo, P. N. (2008). Government policies and sources of latecomer firms' capability building: A learning story from Brazil, *Oxford Development Studies*, 36(1), 59–88.

Fold, N. and Larsen, M. N. (2011). Upgrading of smallholder agro-food production in Africa: The role of lead firm strategies and new markets, *International Journal of Technological Learning, Innovation and Development*, 4(1/2/3), 39–66.

Forbes, N. and Wield, D. (2008). Innovation dynamics in catch-up firms: Process, product and proprietary capabilities for development, *Industry and Innovation*, 15(1), 69–92.

Grabowski, H. (2011). The evolution of the pharmaceutical industry over the past 50 years: A personal reflection, *International Journal of the Economics of Business*, 18(2), 161–176.

Guan, J. C. *et al.* (2006). Technology transfer and innovation performance: Evidence from Chinese firms, *Technological Forecasting & Social Change*, 73(6), 666–678.

Guo, B., Gao, J. and Chen, X. L. (2013). Technology strategy, technological context and technological catch-up in emerging economies: Industry-level findings from Chinese manufacturing, *Technology Analysis & Strategic Management*, 25(2), 219–234.

Hamdouch, A. and He, F. (2009). R&D offshoring and clustering dynamics in pharmaceuticals and biotechnology: Key features and insights from the Chinese case: *Journal of Innovation Economics*, 2(4), 95–117.

Hemmert, M. (2008). Innovation management of Japanese and Korean firms: A comparative analysis, *Asia Pacific Business Review*, 14(3), 293–314.

Hobday, M. (1998). Latecomer catch-up strategies in electronics: Samsung of Korea and ACER of Taiwan, *Asia Pacific Business Review*, 4(2), 48–83.

Huang, S. F. (2012). How can innovation create the future in a catching-up economy?: Focusing on China's pharmaceutical industry, *Journal of Knowledge-based Innovation in China*, 4(2), 118–131.

Joo, S. H. and Lee, K. (2010). Samsung's catch-up with Sony: An analysis using US patent data, *Journal of the Asia Pacific Economy*, 15(3), 271–287.

Jung, M. and Lee, K. (2010). Sectoral systems of innovation and productivity catch-up: Determinants of the productivity gap between Korean and Japanese firms, *Industrial and Corporate Change*, 19(4), 1037–1069.

Kale, D. and Little, S. (2007). From imitation to innovation: The evolution of R&D capabilities and learning processes in the Indian pharmaceutical industry, *Technology Analysis & Strategic Management*, 19(5), 589–609.

Kiamehr, M., Hobday, M. and Kermanshah, A. (2014). Latecomer systems integration capability in complex capital goods: The case of Iran's electricity generation systems, *Industrial and Corporate Change*, 23(3), 689–716.

Kim, Y. (2011). From catch-up to overtaking: Competition and innovation in the semiconductor industries of Korea and Japan, *Asian Journal of Technology Innovation*, 19(2), 297–311.

Kim, Y.-Z. and Lee, K. (2008). Sectoral innovation system and a technological catch-up: The case of the capital goods industry in Korea, *Global Economic Review*, 37(2), 135–155.

Kristinsson, K. and Rao, R. (2008). Interactive learning or technology transfer as a way to catch-up? Analysing the wind energy industry in Denmark and India, *Industry and Innovation*, 15(3), 297–320.

Lee, K. (2005). Making a technological catch-up: Barriers and opportunities, *Asian Journal of Technology Innovation*, 13(2), 97–131.

Lee, K. and Lim, C. (2001). Technological regimes, catching-up and leapfrogging: Findings from the Korean industries, *Research Policy*, 30 (3), pp. 459–483.

Lee, K., Cho, S.-J. and Jin, J. (2009). Dynamics of catch-up in mobile phones and automobiles in China: Sectoral systems of innovation perspective, *China Economic Review*, 2(1), 25–53.

Leseure, M., Hurreeram, D. and Bennett, D. (2009). Playing catch-up with China: Challenges and strategies for smaller developing countries, *Technology Analysis & Strategic Management*, 21(5), 617–637.

Li, J. and Kozhikode, R. K. (2008). Knowledge management and innovation strategy: The challenge for latecomers in emerging economies, *Asia Pacific Journal of Management*, 25(3), 429–450.

Malerba, F. (2005). Sectoral systems of innovation: A framework for linking innovation to the knowledge base, *Economics of Innovation and New Technology*, 14(1–2), 63–82.

Mao, D. and Zheng, Q. (2009). Encouraging an environment for pharmaceutical R&D in China, *Journal of Pharmaceutical Innovation*, 4(3), 152–154.

Mathews, J. A. (2002). Competitive advantages of the latecomer firm: A resource-based account of industrial catch-up strategies, *Asia Pacific Journal of Management*, 19(4), 467–488.

Mathews, J. A. (2006). Catch-up strategies and the latecomer effect in industrial development, *New Political Economy*, 11(3), 313–335.

Mazzoleni, R. and Nelson, R. R. (2007). Public research institutions and economic catch-up, *Research Policy*, 36(10), 1512–1528.

Mendoza, R. U. (2010). Trade-induced learning and industrial catch-up, *Economic Journal*, 120(546), 313–350.

Mu, Q. and Lee, K. (2005). Knowledge diffusion, market segmentation and technological catch-up: The case of the telecommunication industry in China, *Research Policy*, 34(6), 759–783.

Nolan, P. and Yeung, G. (2001). Large firms and catch-up in a transitional economy: The case of Shougang Group in China, *Economics of Planning*, 34(1–2), 159–178.

Park, K.-H. and Lee, K. (2006). Linking the technological regime to the technological catch-up: Analyzing Korea and Taiwan using the US patent data, *Industrial and Corporate Change*, 15(4), 715–753.

Park, T.-Y. (2013). How a latecomer succeeded in a complex product system industry: Three case studies in the Korean telecommunication systems, *Industrial and Corporate Change*, 22(2), 363–396.

Rasiah, R., Lin, Y. and Sadoi, Y. (2010). Explaining technological catch-up in Asia, *Journal of the Asia Pacific Economy*, 15(3), 221–224.

Steinfeld, E. S. (2004). China's shallow integration: Networked production and the new challenges for late industrialization, *World Development*, 32(11), 1971–1987.

Wang, Y. R. (2006). Price competition in the Chinese pharmaceutical market, *International Journal of Health Care Finance & Economics*, 6(2), 119–129.

Wu, X. and Zhang, W. (2010). Seizing the opportunity of paradigm shifts: Catch of Chinese ICT firms, *International Journal of Innovation Management*, 14(1), 57–91.

Wu, X. *et al.* (2009). Secondary innovation: The path of catch-up with 'Made in China', *China Economic Review*, 2(1), 93–104.

Xie, W. and Wu, G. (2003). Differences between learning processes in small tigers and large dragons: Learning processes of two color TV (CTV) firms within China, *Research Policy*, 32(6), 1463–1479.

Yam, R. C. M. *et al.* (2004). An audit of technological innovation capabilities in Chinese firms: Some empirical findings in Beijing, China, *Research Policy*, 33(8), 1123–1140.

Zeng, M. and Williamson, P. J. (2007). *Dragons At Your Door: How Chinese Cost Innovation Is Disrupting Global Competition*, Harvard Business School Press, Boston.

Zhang, L. M., Lam, W. O. and Hu, H. (2013). Complex product and system, catch-up, and sectoral system of innovation: A case study of leading medical device companies in China, *International Journal of Technological Learning, Innovation and Development*, 6(3), 283–302.

Chapter 9

Biotechnology Innovation

Mark J. Ahn[*,¶], Anne S. York[†], So Young Sohn[‡,||]
and Payam Benyamini[§]

[*]*Portland State University, Portland, Oregon, USA*

[†]*College of Business, Creighton University, Omaha, Nebraska, USA*

[‡]*Yonsei University, Seoul, Korea*

[§]*University of California, Los Angeles, California, USA*

[¶]*mark@pukanapartners.com*

[||]*sohns@yonsei.ac.kr*

Abstract

Disruptive technology platforms from emerging companies hold great promise for exploiting innovation, but often face legitimacy hurdles due to their liability of newness. Nascent firms must learn new roles with limited precedent and establish ties with an environment that may not fully understand or value their existence. Using a legitimacy-based lens in the context of the biotechnology industry, we posit a sequential construct — cognitive, regulative, and normative legitimacy — to evaluate emergent technology platforms. Our model of biotechnology platform emergence may provide insights for understanding how breakthroughs achieve legitimacy in the scientific community, mobilize resources and talent, and attain commercial success.

Keywords: Biotechnology, legitimacy, disruptive innovation.

1. Introduction

Disruptive technology platforms from emerging companies hold great promise to exploit innovation, accelerate growth, and create value (Laurie *et al.*, 2006). However, disruptive technology platforms often face significant legitimacy hurdles due to their small size and liability of newness, as well as the relative lack of power over multiple stakeholder claims, control over resource flows, and strong exchange relationships (Stinchcombe, 1965; Singh *et al.*, 1986; Hannan and Carroll, 1992; Aldrich and Fiol, 1994; Ruef and Scott, 1998).

While the liability of newness is a factor for all new ventures, it is exacerbated for firms in emerging industries (Aldrich and Fiol, 1994; Rao *et al.*, 2008) created around new technologies (Deeds *et al.*, 2004). Within the emerging industry context, organizations lack the "familiarity" (cognitive legitimacy) and "credibility" (regulative and normative legitimacy) that constitute the fundamental basis of "interaction" (Aldrich and Fiol, 1994, p. 647). In this regard, population ecologists (Freeman *et al.*, 1983; Hannan *et al.*, 1995) have provided evidence of lower founding and higher disbanding rates when industries are small and have drawn on the institutional theory (Meyer and Rowan, 1977; DiMaggio and Powell, 1983) to explain this phenomenon in terms of firms initially lacking legitimacy due to low density (Aldrich and Fiol, 1994).

Organizational ecologists, on the contrary, have stipulated that as they become better understood, new industries become "taken-for-granted" (resulting in a decrease in organizational failure) as the number of organizations in an industry asymptotically increases, until a point at which increased competition negates any further legitimacy gains (Hannan and Freeman, 1984; Baum and Oliver, 1992; Hannan and Carroll, 1992; Rao, 2002). As such, organizations in emerging industries at the frontiers of technology development have to learn new roles with limited precedent for their actions, and they must educate the broader community to establish ties with an environment that may not fully understand or value their existence.

Understanding the process by which disruptive technology platforms become legitimized and reach increasing returns to scale is critical in high-technology industries generally (Christensen and Overdorf, 2000; Brekke and Sandlie, 2003; Pera and Trounson, 2004; Stylios *et al.*, 2005) and in biotechnology specifically (Zimmerman and Deeds, 1987; George *et al.*, 2008; Ahn *et al.*, 2009). In its relatively short history, for example, recombinant DNA technology has transitioned from being a research laboratory technique to becoming a dominant biotechnology platform underlying the commercial development of multibillion dollar blockbuster therapeutics (Cohen *et al.*, 1973; Colowick and Kapian, 1980; Brower, 1998; Brekke and Sandlie, 2003). Thus, exploring how "platforms" evolve within an industry, as well as how industry players manage this process, is an important area for researchers, practitioners, and policymakers.

This chapter asks: How does an emerging technology platform gain legitimacy within an industry, such as biotechnology, with an already embedded, dominant technology? To use a biological analogy, we posit that biotechnology platforms evolve much like the blueprint of life, DNA. That is, a hallmark of natural selection is the beneficial acceleration of mutations in an organism's genome that result in permanent changes that enable organisms to adapt, survive, reproduce, and pass on heritable information. In legitimacy terms, small changes in knowledge — in the face of continuous selection pressure (e.g., scientific publications, patents, financing, performance results) — accumulate into increasing rates of returns leading to technology breakthroughs and commercial success. In this case, we assess the sequence of changes in dominant biotechnology platforms — from an initial focus on manufacturing recombinant therapeutic proteins to engineered monoclonal antibodies (mAbs) — and how small changes eventually led to a transformative technology shift which resulted in significant clinical and commercial breakthroughs (e.g., Herceptin, for the treatment of breast cancer).

As such, this chapter extends current legitimacy research by measuring its impact on underlying technology shifts within the nascent biotechnology industry. The majority of population-level studies of legitimacy have focused on measuring "density" (Hannan *et al.*, 1995; Kuilman and Li, 2009). We complement these approaches, based primarily on population ecology, by looking at the inter-relationship between more specific measures (e.g., scientific publications, patents, strategic alliances) relevant to our foci population. In addition, we provide a sequential perspective on the legitimization process (e.g., cognitive, regulative, normative) in gaining acceptance, accumulating resources and talent, and achieving commercial success.

2. Defining Organizational Legitimacy

Rather than developing as one contingent theory, organizational legitimacy has drawn from different conceptual histories (Suchman, 1995; Barkemeyer, 2007), specifically: institutional, resource dependence, and population ecology theories. Legitimacy can be traced back to sociologist Parsons (1960) who noted that, as organizations are dependent on scarce resources from some larger social system, the value systems of an organization must be congruent with that superordinate system (Dowling and Pfeer, 1975; Pfeer and Salancik, 1978). A number of integrative definitions were developed in the 1990s (Aldrich and Fiol, 1994; Scott, 1995; Suchman, 1995; Ruef and Scott, 1998) and extend to shaping organizational reputation (Deephouse and Carter, 2005). In particular, Suchman's (1995, p. 574) definition of legitimacy as "... a generalized perception or assumption that the actions of an entity are desirable, proper, or appropriate" is adopted here. This definition allows for a multidimensional understanding of legitimacy typology including cognitive, regulative, and normative legitimacy.

Cognitive legitimacy is measured by assessing public "knowledge" about an entity or activity — namely understandability and, in a more developed form, "taken-for-grantedness" (Aldrich and Fiol, 1994; Scott, 1995; Suchman, 1995; Ruef and Scott, 1998). Berger and Luckmann (1966, p. 86) provided a foundation for cognitive understanding by noting that "... legitimation is not just a matter of 'values.' It always implies 'knowledge' as well". For instance, Mezias and Miller (2008, p. 2) outline that "legitimacy issues arise for new ventures when a lack of knowledge renders them difficult to classify and comprehend". Of all technologies, biotechnology is one of the newest, least studied, and arguably most complex in arriving at the ultimate end-point of legitimation, "taken-for-grantedness" (Fiol and O'Connor, 2005). The biotechnology industry is unique in that the process of product development is concurrent with the discovery of fundamental scientific knowledge (Pisano, 2006).

Regulative legitimacy is the adherence to explicit rules and regulations. For example, Rao (2002, p. 308) outlined regulative legitimacy as "laws authorizing the use of a product and stipulating the conditions of its use". In biotechnology, for example, new biopharmaceutical products generally sequentially progress through the following steps: (1) Conduct *in vitro* and *in vivo* pre-clinical testing to establish biological activity against the targeted disease and preliminary toxicology, (2) File an Investigational New Drug (IND) application to allow human clinical trials, (3) Conduct Phase I, II, and III clinical trials to establish statistically significant safety and efficacy in humans, and (4) File a New Drug Application (NDA) for approval for a specific type and stage of disease (Wierenga and Eaton, 2006).

Normative legitimacy is the adherence to norms of behavior and standards of practice (Suchman, 1995). In the biotechnology industry, for example, the pre vailing norm for the treatment of indolent non-Hodgkin's lymphoma (NHL) was to "watch and wait" for the slow-growing cancer to spread and then episodically treat patients with chemotherapy.

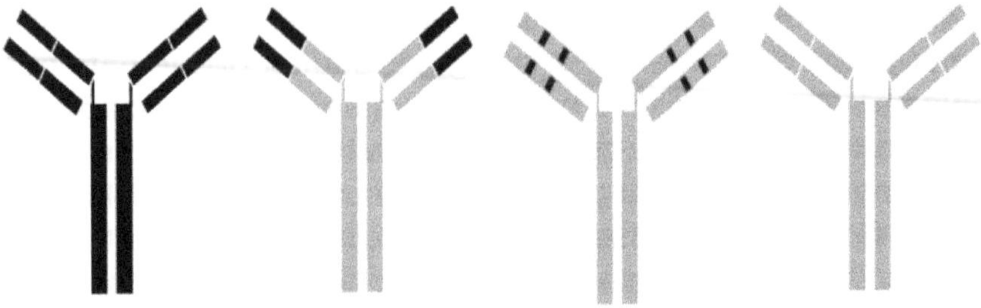

Figure 1. Evolution of monoclonal antibody platform technology. Mouse mAbs are generated using mouse hybridoma technology. Recombinant DNA technology is used to advance the development of chimeric, humanized, and fully human antibodies. Chimeric antibodies are generated by cloning mouse variable genes into human constant region genes. The introduction of mouse complementarity-determining regions (CDR) onto human constant and variable domains produces humanized antibodies. *In vitro* screening of phage-display libraries and human hybridoma technology is employed for the development of fully human antibodies.

To overcome the limitations associated with murine mAbs, new strategies were employed to make mAbs more "human-like", by utilizing recombinant DNA technology to generate chimeric variants, that is, antibodies possessing human protein sequences (Boulianne *et al.*, 1984; Morrison *et al.*, 1984) (Figure 1).

Although chimeric mAbs have been shown to be less immunogenic than their murine counterparts, significant immunogenicity has nonetheless been observed, resulting in their rapid clearance from circulation and limited efficacy (Bell and Kamm, 2000). As the legitimacy of antibody-based therapeutics evolved, subsequent efforts focused on an alternative to mouse hybridomas by producing humanized or fully human antibodies through generating heterohybridomas (human lymphocytes fused with mouse myeloma cells) carrying human immunoglobulin genes, developing *Escherichia coli*-based antibody expression systems,[2] or screening combinatorial phase-display libraries containing a large collection of variant antibody-like molecules (Thomson *et al.*, 1986; Skerra and Plückthun, 1988; McCarerty *et al.*, 1990).

The production of fully human mAbs has been possible since the early 1990s, but patent disputes for the technologies hindered their commercial development, until being resolved in 1997. Compared to their murine counterparts, fewer humanized mAbs entered clinical trials between the late 1980s and early 1990s; however, this class of mAbs has been the primary source of antibody-based products since 1997 (Reichert, 2001).

2.2. *Building legitimacy and monoclonal antibody platforms*

The history of mAb technology illustrates the importance of sequentially building legitimacy — from cognitive to regulative to normative — in the biotechnology industry. The development and dissemination of reproducible scientific knowledge through peer-reviewed publications is a critical antecedent of cognitive legitimacy (i.e., understandability in the first instance) for biotechnology platforms (Chubin, 1994; Spier, 2002). Further, the growth of scientific understanding and awareness attracts increasing interest and resources (e.g., competitive research grants) in advancing and extending knowledge (Azoulay *et al.*, 2007).

[2] *Escherichia coli* is a gram-negative bacterium that is commonly found in the lower intestine of warm-blooded organisms. Because of its long history of laboratory culture and ease of manipulation, *E. coli* also plays an important role in modern biological engineering and industrial microbiology. Due to the work of Cohen and Boyer with *E. coli*, the use of plasmids and restriction enzymes to create recombinant DNA became a foundation for biotechnology. Plasmids are small accessory DNA molecules that enable researchers to introduce new genes into microbes, allowing for the mass production of useful proteins in industrial fermentation processes. In this way, *E. coli* has been used to produce hormones such as insulin, vaccines, and a variety of enzymes.

Based on the required foundation of cognitive legitimacy, the next step is the establishment of regulative legitimacy for biotechnology platforms. In this case, as the body of scientific knowledge and interest grows in emergent biotechnologies, universities and research institutes begin to establish intellectual property (IP) rights in order to attract investor interest in licensing or forming new spin-off companies due to the large capital requirements for product development (e.g., average drug development is 12 years and over $1 billion to approval) (DiMasi *et al.*, 2003; Adams and Brantner, 2006). Specifically, once there is a broad scientific understanding or acceptance (which can be reproduced and extended), then the field becomes more competitive for mobilizing resources (e.g., research grants), which allows for IP rights to be claimed on the basis of demonstrating innovative utility and obtaining financing (e.g., venture capital). For example, medical research grant recipients with larger numbers of grants are far more likely to obtain patents than other researchers, indicating that advances in IP formation are accelerated by competitive grant awards (Azoulay *et al.*, 2007).

Even with patents, early clinical development with therapeutic mAbs faced significant hurdles due to limited efficacy (e.g., short half-life or circulating time, inadequate penetration into diseased tissue) and side effects (e.g., allergic reactions, adverse reactions which limited repeat dosing) (Oldham, 1983; Waldman, 1991; Oldham and Dillman, 2008). During the 1980s, a review article in *Journal of Clinical Oncology* bleakly concluded: "... there has been little evidence to support the use of monoclonal antibody alone with clinically apparent tumor burdens" (Oldham, 1983, p. 583). Indeed, despite a substantial increase in the number of products and over 40 clinical trials in the 1980s, only one product based on murine antibodies — Orthoclone OKT3, used for transplant rejection — was approved (Reichert, 2001; Waldman, 1991). Consequently, mAbs were predominantly viewed as a high-risk, esoteric approach to drug development. As a result, mAbs fell in and out of favor with venture capital firms, and large multinational pharmaceutical companies largely ignored them.

However, from these difficult early beginnings, mAb technology has progressed to overcome early technical difficulties to, arguably, become the dominant platform in the biotechnology industry in the last decade. Consequently, broad adoption of a new technology paradigm — specifically, a change in the norms around treatment (reflecting normative legitimacy) — is required. This can be measured through the amount of revenues generated which reflects clinical standards of care and use by physicians, payers, and patients.

As an example of the dramatically expanded efficacy of mAbs, consider Rituxan, based on the seminal work of Miller *et al.* (1982). Rituxan is a breakthrough innovation for treating NHL, a disease that went over 25 years without a change in the standard of care and survival (Cofier, 2002). Due to the innovative nature of Rituxan, the FDA approved the treatment in less than 7 years after it was discovered versus the industry average of 12 years (Grillo-López, 2000). Five years after Rituxan was approved, a clinical review of NHL therapies concluded: "because of its activity, coupled with a favorable toxicity profile, Rituxan has become almost ubiquitous in the treatment of most B-cell malignancies" (Cheson, 2003, p. 391). Rituxan's commercial success reflects its clinical efficacy in improving survival — sales went from $5 million in 1997 to $2.9 billion in 2008, which represented 30% of Genentech's product sales in that year.

In turn, venture capital investors and large multinational pharmaceutical firms have shown significant interest in this technology segment through direct investment, strategic alliances (Kumar and Das, 2007; Gopalakrishnan *et al.*, 2008), and organizational learning (Morgan and Berthon, 2008). This can be explained as a dynamic of legitimacy spillover, where greater legitimacy for one organization leads to an increase in the legitimacy of similar organizations (McKendrick *et al.*, 2003; Kuilman and Li, 2009). Today, mAbs represent the most dominant platform in terms of commercial interest and success in the biopharmaceutical industry. Currently, 21 mAb products are approved for marketing in the US (three murine, five chimeric, 11 humanized, and two fully human) including eight multibillion dollar blockbusters such as Avastin, Rituxan, Enbrel, and Erbitux (Table 1) — with more than 200 potential products in clinical development.

In addition, mAbs have experienced significant pricing power reflecting their breakthrough clinical value. For example, mAbs indicated for cancer treatments have a 94% premium compared to all other cancer treatments during the 1992–2008 period (Bach, 2009). Further, there are more than 200 mAbs in clinical trials (63% cancer, 16% immunology, 11% anti-infective, 5% cardiovascular, and 5% others). Another indicator of increased legitimacy for mAbs is attracting increasingly higher valuations, even at the earlier stages of development (Nelson and Reichert, 2009). Consider, for example, multinational pharmaceutical Merck's license of a Phase II (development stage) monoclonal antibody product candidate from Medarex. Merck paid $60 million up front and will pay up to $165 million in development and regulatory milestones, plus sales milestones and double-digit royalties (BioCentury, 2009).

Due to the unique biotechnology industry architecture characterized by long product development cycle times, large capital costs, and high amounts of regulatory burden (Pisano, 2006), the monoclonal antibody technology platform segment provides a robust way of exploring legitimization dynamics associated with emerging biotechnologies. The mAb platform exhibited most of the characteristics of an emerging industry (i.e., a technology platform which dramatically departed from the then dominant recombinant DNA product development paradigm), while being situated within a developing industry in its own right. Such an analysis is of interest because the emergence of new technologies within a broader industry is more frequent than the creation of a totally new industry which has been the focus of the majority of legitimacy theory and

Table 1. Monoclonal antibody product approvals by the US FDA 1986–2008.

Antibody	Brand name	Approval date	Type	Approved treatment(s)	Target
Muromonab-CD3	Orthoclone OKT3	1986	Murine	Transplant rejection	T cell CD3 Receptor
Abciximab	ReoPro	1994	Chimeric	Cardiovascular disease	Inhibition of glycoprotein IIb/IIIa
Daclizumab	Zenapax	1997	Humanized	Transplant rejection	IL-2Ra receptor (CD25)
Rituximab	Rituxan, Mabthera	1997	Chimeric	Non-Hodgkin lymphoma	CD20
Basiliximab	Simulect	1998	Chimeric	Transplant rejection	IL-2Ra receptor (CD25)
Infliximab	Remicade	1998	Chimeric	Several autoimmune disorders	Inhibition of TNF-a signaling
Palivizumab	Synagis	1998	Humanized	Respiratory Syncytial Virus	An epitope of the RSV F protein
Trastuzumab	Herceptin	1998	Humanized	Breast cancer	ErbB2
Gemtuzumab	Mylotarg	2000	Humanized	Acute myelogenous leukemia (with calicheamicin)	CD33
Alemtuzumab	Campath	2001	Humanized	Chronic lymphocytic leukemia	CD52
Adalimumab	Humira	2002	Human	Several autoimmune disorders	Inhibition of TNF-a signaling
Efalizumab	Raptiva	2002	Humanized	Psoriasis	CD11a

(*Continued*)

Table 1. (*Continued*)

Antibody	Brand name	Approval date	Type	Approved treatment(s)	Target
Ibritumomab tiuxetan	Zevalin	2002	Murine	Non-Hodgkin lymphoma (with yttrium-90 or indium-111)	CD20
Tositumomab	Bexxar	2003	Murine	Non-Hodgkin lymphoma	CD20
Bevacizumab	Avastin	2004	Humanized	Colorectal cancer	Vascular endothelial growth factor (VEGF)
Cetuximab	Erbitux	2004	Chimeric	Colorectal cancer, head and neck cancer	Epidermal growth factor receptor
Omalizumab	Xolair	2004	Humanized	Mainly allergy-related asthma	Immunoglobulin E (IgE)
Natalizumab	Tysabri	2006	Humanized	Multiple sclerosis and Crohn's disease	Alpha-4 (a4) integrin
Panitumumab	Vectibix	2006	Human	Colorectal cancer	Epidermal growth factor receptor
Ranibizumab	Lucentis	2006	Humanized	Macular degeneration	Vascular endothelial growth factor A (VEGF-A)
Eculizumab	Soliris	2007	Humanized	Paroxysmal nocturnal hemoglobinuria	Complement system protein (C5)

Source: US FDA.

empirical studies (e.g., automobile, film, banking). In this way, we can describe the monoclonal antibody segment as a "sub-population" defined as "a subset of a general population by combining all the membership-defining features of the general population with some more specific features idiosyncratic to the sub-population" (Kuilman and Li, 2009, p. 231). In sum, we posit that legitimacy in the context of emergent biotechnology platforms follows a sequential construct — cognitive, regulative, and normative legitimacy — which impacts the timing and acceleration of platform acceptance summarized in the following propositions (P):

P_1: *In emerging biotechnology platforms, cognitive legitimacy is required in order to achieve regulatory, and then normative, legitimacy.*

P_2: *The time period required to develop cognitive legitimacy is longer than that required to achieve regulatory and normative legitimacy.*

P_3: *Once the first technology in an emerging platform has achieved all three types of legitimacy, new products that follow in the same platform face a significantly increased acceleration in their progression across the three types of legitimacy.*

3. Methodology

To explore the evolution of legitimacy in the biotechnology industry, our data describe the second technology wave in biotechnology — hybridomas which produce monoclonal antibody-based therapeutics. Life histories have been collected for many populations (e.g., as part of population ecology), but have mostly focused on such generic events as "foundings and disbandings" (Aldrich and Fiol, 1994, p. 665; Rao, 2002), and there remains much scope toward expanding on this project by collecting more complex and direct data (Baum and

Oliver, 1991, 1992). As a perception held by an audience external to an organization, legitimacy is an unobservable construct. Consequently, legitimacy has usually been inferred indirectly through the actions of external audiences (e.g., population density, media articles). For instance, Terreberry (1968) argued that legitimacy can be assessed by the existence of an economic transaction between entities (Tornikoski and Newbert, 2007). Our measures of legitimacy are outlined in Table 2. Broadly, these measures relate to Aldrich and Fiol (1994), who argue that cognitive legitimacy can be measured by the level of public knowledge about a new activity (e.g., number of scientific publications) and that sociopolitical legitimacy (subsuming the regulative and normative dimensions) can be measured by public acceptance of a new activity. In the culmination, they can be seen to move from a picture of understandability (measures in journal publications) to the broader cognitive legitimacy dimension of "taken-for-grantedness" (e.g., generally accepted standards of treatment).

Table 2. Legitimacy dimensions and metrics.

Legitimacy dimension	Metric
Cognitive legitimacy (understandability)	Peer-reviewed scientific publications on mAbs.
Regulative legitimacy	Issued patents for mAbs demonstrating novelty, function, and exclusivity; Strategic alliances with larger partners demonstrate validation.
Normative legitimacy	Standards of patient care (i.e., adoption of new clinical practices) measured through revenues.
Cognitive legitimacy (taken-for-grantedness)	The sequential accumulation of the above legitimacy dimensions with increasing rates of return (e.g., knowledge, revenues).

- **Dependent variable:** Our dependent variable is post-FDA approval revenues from mAbs representing normative legitimacy. Zimmerman and Zeitz (2002) suggest using growth in revenues as a dependent variable, stating that while legitimacy can have many performance dimensions, growth in sales is particularly important for new ventures. We used global monoclonal antibody revenues from the Datamonitor (www.datamonitor.com) database that uses transparent, traceable, and auditable research methods to ensure quality and reliable information.
- **Independent variables:** Next, our independent variables — scientific publications, patents, and strategic alliances — represent cognitive and regulative legitimacy (Kumar and Das, 2007). Peer-reviewed scientific publications are the gold standard of the scientific method (Ingelfinger, 1974; Relman and Angell, 1989). The data source for patents and publications comes from Scopus (www.scopus.com), which is an abstract and citation database of research literature, which contains over 16,000 peer-reviewed journals from more than 4,000 publishers. The database covers scientific, technical, medical, and social sciences literature.

Further, novel scientific publications are often filed as patents and conferred by regulatory bodies such as the US PTO (Patent and Trademark Office), which provides a period of exclusivity in exchange for public disclosure of an invention. Patents also confer an external affirmation of potential value for investors by establishing non-obviousness, novelty, and utility; and typically cover product, method, or use. An example of an important biotechnology patent is PDL Bio pharma's family of patents for the humanization of mAbs. PDL received royalties of $276 million or 94% of revenues from nine approved products including multi billion dollar blockbusters such as Genentech's Avastin and Herceptin in 2008 (PDL Biopharma, 2009).

Our final independent variable relates again to normative legitimacy in strategic alliances that can span a broad array of structures including co-promotions, co-marketing, co-development, in-licensing, and mergers and acquisitions (Ahn *et al.*, 2009). Whatever the strategic alliance structure, higher milestone and royalty payments generally accrue to technologies that are more advanced in terms of the stage of development (Burrill & Co, 2009). The data source for strategic alliances was Biocentury (www.biocentury.com), which chronicles alliances in the biopharmaceutical industry worldwide.

Finally, we established a control variable to ensure we are measuring the monoclonal antibody segment, rather than simply spillover from the increased legitimacy of the biotechnology industry more generally. For example, Kuilman and Li (2009, p. 231) noted that: "increased population-level legitimacy (in biopharmaceuticals for example) should, however, also legitimate entry into any population sub-category (e.g., mAbs)". In this case, the general investment climate in the biotechnology industry may be an important variable in assessing the pace and intensity that a new technology is being pursued. The American Stock Exchange Biotech Index (BTK) was chosen as the benchmark index for the biotechnology industry. The BTK comprises 17 firms that are chosen to broadly represent the biotech sector. The index is rebalanced four times a year to maintain continuity and to keep any stock from dominating the index's value.

4. Results

Rather than relating all independent variables to the dependent variable directly, we conducted a two-step analysis: (1) relate the number of patents at time t to those of previous publications and patents and (2) then relate revenue (or sales) at time t to the number of previously obtained patents, as well as the current average strategic alliance deal size and the BTK as shown in Table 3. Using the proposed two-step approach, we sought to identify the relationship between publications (cognitive) and patents (regulative) first, and then explored the relationship between patents and revenues (normative) — in addition

Table 3. Legitimacy variables.

Type	No.	Variables	1	2	3	4	5	Mean	Standard deviation
Dependent	1	Revenues	—	0.32	0.76	0.59	0.84	2,657,188	6,842,937
Independent	2	Scientific Publications	0.32	—	0.59	0.40	0.45	5,444	4,678
	3	Patents	0.76	0.59	—	0.75	0.88	3,966	5,800
	4	Average Alliance Deal Size	0.59	0.40	0.75	—	0.88	9	19
		Biotech Industry Share							
Control	5	Prince Index (BTK)	0.84	0.45	0.88	0.88	—	124	222

to other variables such as strategic alliances and the overall biotechnology industry activity level represented by the BTK. This was done to avoid confounding effects of both publications and patents on the revenues.

First, we assembled the time series data consisting of mAb revenues, scientific publications, patents, strategic alliances, and the BTK. The starting point for mAb-related scientific publications was 1964 that reached two-digit numbers annually in 1970. In comparison, the first mAb patent appeared in 1976 and two-digit increases were observed beginning in 1980 — thus illustrating the considerable time gap between mAb publications and patents.

In order to predict the number of patents at time *t*, Pat_t, we used various time-lagged variables for the number of publications (e.g., Pub_{t-12}, Pub_{t-11}, Pub_{t-10}), along with time-lagged patents (Pat_{t-1}, Pat_{t-2}, Pat_{t-3}). When various variable selection algorithms were applied, they consistently displayed Markov-type properties from which the following model was selected at $R^2 = 95.37$:

$$\text{Pat}_t = 346.82 + 0.47 \times \text{Pub}_{t-12} + 0.63 \times \text{Pat}_{t-1}. \qquad (1)$$

That is, the number of publications 12 years prior and patents 1-year prior are good indicators for current patents in the mAb sector.

Next, we fitted mAb revenues against the number of related previous patents, the average strategic alliance deal size, and BTK. The mAb time series data show that mAb revenues began in 1995, 19 years after the first patent in 1976; and 16 years after significant increases in mAb-related patents. Thus, we used various time-lagged variables such as Pat_{t-19}; Pat_{t-18}; ... ; Pat_{t-13}, to fit the revenue at time *t*. Additionally, we included two additional independent variables — strategic alliances and the BTK. Several variable selection schemes were explored and the selected model with an $R^2 = 0.9788$ was selected as follows:

$$\text{Rev}_t = 170491 + 14656 \times \text{Pat}_{t-16} + 7231.5 \times \text{Pat}_{t-15} - 10082 \times \text{Pat}_{t-14}. \quad (2)$$

Of note, the data suggest that strategic alliances and the BTK are insignificant in predicting revenues (Figure 2).

We can observe that there are increasing returns to legitimacy. For example, the time between the seminal discovery by Koehler and Milstein in 1975 to the first drug approval was 21 years, the time from first to second monoclonal antibody drug approval was 8 years, and the average time from the third to the 21st mAb approved was 0.6 years.

An illustrative example previously noted is Rituxan, the first cancer mAb approved and revenue leader to date. Repeating the same two-step analysis for Rituxan, we can observe a

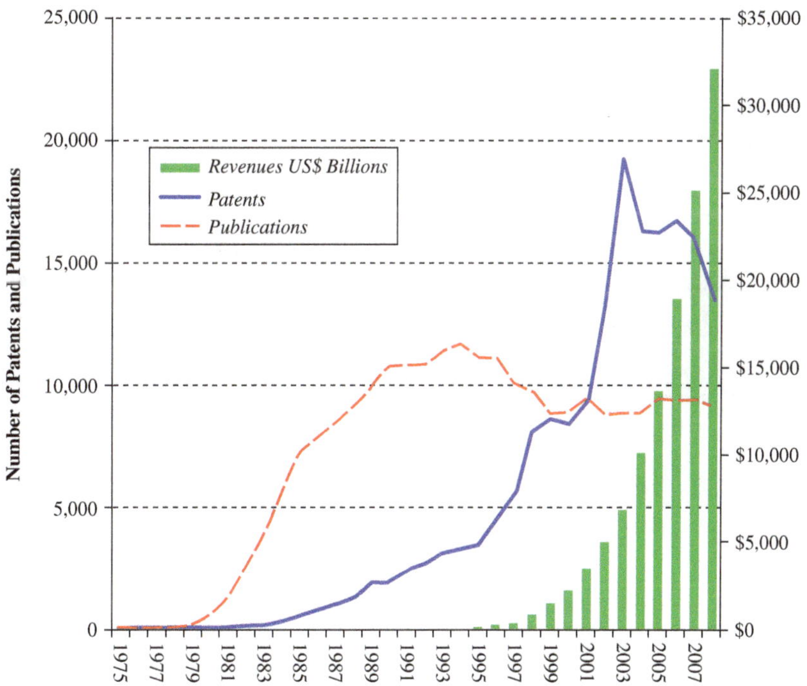

Figure 2. Monoclonal antibodies — scientific publications and patents versus revenues (US$ millions).

significantly shorter time gap between the first publication in 1987 and patent in 1988, as well as between the first patent in 1988 and revenues in 1998 — versus the corresponding data for all mAbs. Relative to the entire mAb field, Rituxan's accelerated development and commercialization illustrate the path-dependent and temporal typology of legitimacy paved by pioneering technologies and products. As the fourth mAb approved in the US, increasing rates of legitimacy due to prior antecedents conferred significant benefits to Rituxan on several levels — from the time between laboratory discovery at Stanford in 1991 to out-licensing and initial human clinical trials with start-up IDEC Pharmaceuticals in 1993, to a

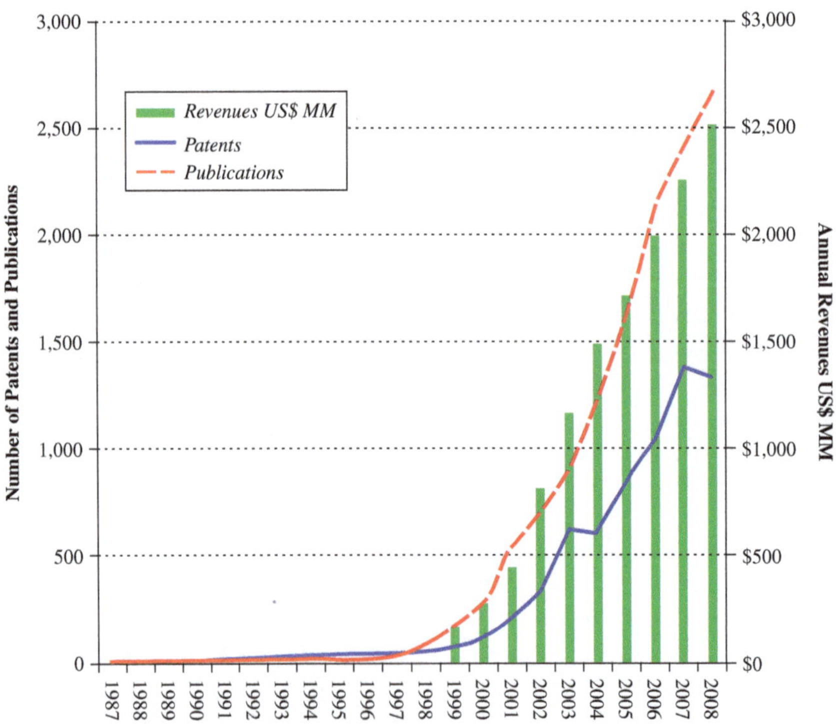

Figure 3. Rituxan (rituximab) scientific publications and patents versus revenues (US$ millions).

development alliance with Genentech and subsequent US commercial approval in 1997, to full commercial globalization and product extension with Roche (which eventually purchased Genentech in 2009). As such, the case of Rituxan illustrates the cumulative effect of increasing legitimacy in the mAb field generally (Figure 3).

5. Conclusion

As an industry characterized by its academic foundations, as well as continued reliance on emerging insights, the biotechnology industry provides a rich context to explore the progression of emergent technology platforms within a nascent industry. In this case, the mAb platform development dramatically illustrates the arc of achieving biotechnology legitimacy within an already existing industry. From its beginnings in the laboratory where its two inventors did not even seek patent protection on their breakthrough technology, through encountering a wide range of problems during its early years, mAb technology has grown into a highly legitimated platform worth billions and is fully integrated into the scientific (i.e., number of publications), clinical (i.e., number of patents), and commercial (i.e., revenues) environments.

In exploring how an emerging technology platform gains legitimacy within an industry with an already embedded, dominant technology paradigm, this chapter has utilized a temporal understanding of legitimacy to assess the development of biotechnology platforms. We measured cognitive legitimacy in relation to biotechnology platforms through the development and dissemination of reproducible scientific knowledge through peer-reviewed publications (i.e., understandability). Reproducibility creates a virtuous cycle of knowledge creation and extension, which enables the opportunities for resource mobilization (e.g., grants, graduate research) which, in turn, exponentially grows legitimacy.

With the foundation of cognitive legitimacy marked by significant academic progress, regulative legitimacy for biotechnology platforms may be represented by the issuance of patents that provide IP. Patents also confer an external affirmation of potential value for investors by establishing non-obviousness, novelty, and utility. In biotechnology, regulative legitimacy can also further occur as the regulatory authority (e.g., US FDA) confers approval to commence clinical trials through to marketing approval for specific diseases for which firms must prove statistically significant superiority versus the prevailing standard of treatment.

Gaining product approval, however, does not ensure changes to the norms of the customer and the user behavior that establish value and sustainability (e.g., six out of 10 approved products are unprofitable (PhRMA (2008)). In this context, normative legitimacy of biotechnology platforms is rejected in changing the clinical norms of behavior or standards of care as evidenced by revenues (e.g., typically measured as a continuum from pre-marketing intent-to-treat surveys to new and follow-on prescription rates post-approval, and, ultimately, to revenues and market share). Finally, our findings also suggest that legitimacy in this context is sequential and path dependent (i.e., scientific publications to patents to revenues) and is viral — legitimacy tends to spur increasing returns.

These results concerning the development of emergent biotechnology platforms have several implications for practitioners, policymakers, and researchers. For practitioners, the exponential growth of legitimacy has implications for managing and investing in emerging technologies. Essentially, a broader range of bets (e.g., portfolio of investments in small firms) and contingencies (e.g., options to license after proof of principle is reached) to tap into emerging technologies may be more efficient than waiting until a technology is established and legitimated. Large biotechnology and pharmaceutical companies must add to their pipelines through establishing networks; however, a company's cost structure may become prohibitive if they wait to target already legitimated technologies. This is clearly shown in the mAb case, one example being the difference between Genentech's license of Rituxan for $30 million at Phase II clinical trials in 1986 versus Amgen purchasing Vectibix from Abgenix in Phase III for $2.2 billion in 2005. Instead, Amgen could have boldly made earlier bets (i.e., established many weak ties through research alliances or minority equity stakes) on promising, albeit unproven, nascent technologies. Such lessons are relevant for current emerging platforms such as regenerative medicine (i.e., stem cells), gene silencing (i.e., RNAi), nanotechnology, and gene therapy.

While strategic alliances with larger multinational pharmaceutical companies are clearly a validating event for smaller firms, we did not find alliances to be a significant factor in our model. This lack of significance may be due to the observation that alliances tend to be a lagging variable after scientific research is established and reproduced by academic scientists and smaller companies (i.e., patent claims are already established which creates the need for alliances by larger companies seeking access to new technologies). In addition, alliances occur along the entire continuum of the biotechnology life cycle, which may make the variable "too noisy", although a more fine-grained investigation of the role that alliances play would be a helpful next step in the empirical development and understanding of the legitimacy process.

In addition, long product development cycle times and a highly regulated industry architecture make resilience a key aspect of sustainability, particularly since the vast majority of biotechnology firms have no revenues and require continuous rounds of financing based on research and development progress. As Joshua Berger, CEO, Vertex advised: *Follow your own business plan. Don't follow the winds that blow back and forth. You can't be successful by following the trends of the moment, especially if your business has a relatively long product cycle, as ours does. It sounds simple, but it's very hard to do* (Thomas, 2009).

For policymakers, these findings reinforce the critical role of public funding of basic science in academia and research institutes to establish new technology platforms and spur economic competitiveness. Further, our results also suggest that in order to maximize efficiency, investment and commitment from a policy perspective must match the long R&D cycle time required to move an industry from nascent to established and legitimated.

In summary, from a legitimacy-based perspective, this research has extended theory by providing a specific construct — cognitive, regulative, normative, and sequential — to evaluate nascent technology platforms. Our model of biotechnology platform emergence can be used to better understand how breakthrough insights achieve legitimacy in the scientific community, mobilize resources from public and private funding, and attain commercial success. As such, it may be a useful framework for biotechnology industry managers, charged with accelerating technology platforms, building product pipelines, and developing commercial products for addressing unmet medical needs.

References

Adams, C. P. and Brantner, V. V. (2006). Estimating the cost of new drug development: Is it really 802 million dollars? *Health Affairs*, 25, 420–428.

Ahn, M. and Meeks, M. (2007). Building a conductive environment for life science based entrepreneurship and industry clusters, *Journal of Commercial Biotechnology*, 14, 20–30.

Ahn, M., Davenport, S., Meeks, M. and Bednarek, R. (2009). Exploring technology agglomeration patterns for multinational pharmaceutical and biotechnology firms, *Journal of Commercial Biotechnology*, 16, 17–32.

Aldrich, H. E. and Fiol, C. M. (1994). Fools rush in? The institutional context of industry creation, *Academy of Management Review*, 19, 645–670.

Alkan, S. S. (2004). Landmark: Monoclonal antibodies: The story of a discovery that revolutionized science and medicine. *Nature Reviews Immunology*, 4, 153–156.

Azoulay, P., Michigan, R. and Sampat, B. (2007). The anatomy of medical school patenting, *New England Journal of Medicine*, 357, 2049–2056.

Bach, P. B. (2009). Limits on medicare's ability to control rising spending on cancer drugs, *New England Journal of Medicine*, 360, 626–633.

Barkemeyer, R. (2007). Legitimacy as a key driver and determinant of CSR in developing countries. Paper presented at Marie Curie Summer School on Earth System Governance.

Baum, J. A. C. and Oliver, C. (1991). Institutional linkages and organizational mortality, *Administrative Science Quarterly*, 36, 187–218.

Baum, J. A. C. and Oliver, C. (1992). Institutional embeddedness and the dynamics of organizational populations, *American Sociological Review*, 57, 540–559.

Bell, S. and Kamm, M. A. (2000). Antibodies to tumour necrosis factor as a treatment of Crohn's disease, *Lancet*, 355, 58–860.

Berger, P. L. and Luckmann, T. (1966). *The Social Construction of Reality: A Treatise in the Sociology of Knowledge*. Doubleday and Company Inc, New York.

BIO (Biotechnology Industry Organization) (2007). *BIO 2005–2006: Guide to Biotechnology*. BIO, Washington DC.

BioCentury (2009). Available at: www.biocentury.com [Accessed on 17 September 2009].

Boulianne, G. L., Hozumi, N. and Shulman, M. J. (1984). Production of functional chimaeric mouse/human antibody, *Nature*, 312, 643–646.

Brekke, O. H. and Sandlie, I. (2003). Therapeutic antibodies for human diseases at the dawn of the twenty-first century, *Nature Review of Drug Discovery*, 2, 52–62.

Brower, V. (1998). Naked DNA vaccines come of age, *Nature Biotechnology*, 16, 1304–1305.

Burrill & Co. (2007). *Biotech 2007 Life Sciences: A Global Transformation*. Burrill Life Sciences Media Group, San Francisco.

Cheson, B. (2003). Radioimmunotherapy of non-Hodgkins lymphomas, *Blood*, 1010, 391–398.

Christensen, C. and Overdorf, M. (2000). Meeting the challenge of disruptive change, *Harvard Business Review*, 78, 66–76.

Chubin, D. E. (1994). Grants peer review in theory and practice, *Evaluation Review*, 18, 20–30.

Cohen, S. N., Chang, A. C., Boyer, H. W. and Helling, R. B. (1973). Construction of bio logically functional bacterial plasmids *in vitro*, *Proceedings of National Academy of Sciences*, 70, 3240–3244.

Colowick, S. P. and Kapian, O. N. (1980). Recombinant DNA, *Methods in Enzymology*, Vol. 68, Academic Press, New York, ISBN 012181968X.

Deeds, D. L., Mang, P. Y. and Frandsen, M. L. (2004). The influence of firms' and industries legitimacy on the flow of capital into high-technology ventures, *Strategic Organization*, 2, 9–34.

Deephouse, D. L. and Carter, S. M. (2005). An examination of differences between organizational legitimacy and organizational reputation, *Journal of Management Studies*, 42, 329–360.

DiMaggio, P. J. and Powell, W. W. (1983). The iron cage revisited: Institutional isomorphism and collective rationality in organizational fields, *American Sociological Review*, 48, 147–160.

DiMasi, J. A., Hansen, R. W. and Grabowski, H. G. (2003). The price of innovation: New estimates of drug development costs, *Journal of Health Economics*, 22, 151–185.

Dowling, J. and Pfefer, J. (1975). Organizational legitimacy: Social values and organizational behavior, *The Pacific Sociological Review*, 18, 122–136.

Fiol, C. M. and O'Connor, E. J. (2005). Stuff matters: Artifacts, identity, and legitimacy in the U.S. medical profession, in Rafaeli, A. and Pratt, M. G. (eds.), *Artifacts and Organizations: Beyond Mere Symbolism*, Routledge, London and New York.

Freeman, J., Carroll, G. R. and Hannan, M. T. (1983). The liability of newness: Age dependence in organizational death rates, *American Sociological Review*, 48, 692–710.

George, G., Kotha, R. and Zheng, Y. (2008). Entry into insular domains: A longitudinal study of knowledge structuration and innovation in biotechnology firms, *Journal of Management Studies*, 45, 1448–1474.

Gopalakrishnan, S., Scillitoe, J. L. and Santoro, M. D. (2008). Tapping deep pockets: The role of resources and social capital on financial capital acquisition by biotechnology firms in biotech-pharma alliances, *Journal of Management Studies*, 45, doi:10.1111/j.1467- 6486.2008.00777.x.

Hannan, M. T. and Carroll, G. R. (1992). *Dynamics of Organizational Populations: Density, Legitimation, and Competition*, Oxford University Press, New York and Oxford.

Hannan, M. T. and Freeman, J. (1984). Inertia and organizational change, *American Sociological Review*, 49, 149–164.

Hannan, M. T., Carroll, G. R., Dundon, E. A. and Torres, J. C. (1995). Organizational evolution in a multinational context: Entries of automobile manufacturers in Belgium, Britain, France, Germany, and Italy, *American Sociological Review*, 60, 509–528.

Ingelfinger, F. J. (1974). Peer review in biomedical publication, *American Journal of Medicine*, 56, 686–692.

Khazaeli, M. B., Conry, R. M. and LoBuglio, A. F. (1994). Human immune response to monoclonal antibodies, *Journal of Immunotherapy*, 15, 42–52.

Kohler, G. and Milstein, C. (1975). Continuous cultures of fused cells secreting antibody of predefined specificity, *Nature*, 256, 495–497.

Kuilman, J. and Li, J. T. (2009). Grades of membership and legitimacy spillovers: Foreign banks in Shanghai, 1847–1935, *Academy of Management Journal*, 52, 229–245.

Kumar, R. and Das, T. K. (2007). Interpartner legitimacy in the alliance development process, *Journal of Management Studies*, 44, doi:10.1111/j.1467-6486.2007.00709.x.

Laurie, D., Doz, Y. and Sheer, C. (2006). Creating new growth platforms, *Harvard Business Review*, 84, 80–90.

McCafferty, J., Griffiths, A. D., Winter, G. and Chiswell, D. J. (1990). Phage antibodies: Filamentous phage displaying antibody variable domains, *Nature*, 348, 552–554.

McKendrick, D. G., Jaree, J., Carroll, G. R. and Khessina, O. M. (2003). In the bud? Disk array producers as a (possibly) emergent organizational form, *Administrative Science Quarterly*, 48, 60–93.

Meyer, J. W. and Rowan, B. (1977). Institutionalized organizations: Formal structure as myth and ceremony, *The American Journal of Sociology*, 83, 340–363.

Mezias, S. J. and Miller, J. I. (2008). Storming legitimacy barriers: Attention and favourability during emergence of the American film industry, *Academy of Management Proceedings*, pp. 1–6.

Miller, R. A., Maloney, D. G., Warnke, R. and Levy, R. (1982). Treatment of B-cell lymphoma with monoclonal anti-idiotype antibody, *New England Journal of Medicine*, 306, 517–822.

Morgan, R. E. and Berthon, P. (2008). Market orientation, generative learning, innovation strategy and business performance inter-relationships in bioscience firms, *Journal of Management Studies*, 45, doi:10.1111/j.1467-6486.2008.00778.x.

Morrison, S. L., Johnson, M. J., Herzenberg, L. A. and Oi, V. T. (1984). Chimeric human antibody molecules: Mouse antigen-binding domains with human constant region domains, *Proceedings of the National Academy of Sciences USA*, 81, 6851–6855.

Nelson, A. L. and Reichert, J. M. (2009). Development trends for therapeutic antibody fragments, *Nature Biotechnology*, 27, 331–337.

OECD (2012). Biotechnology policies, Available at: www.oecd.org {Accessed 17 September 2009}.

Oldham, R. K. (1983). Monoclonal antibodies in cancer therapy, *Journal of Clinical Oncology*, 1, 582–590.

Oldham, R. K. and Dillman, R. O. (2008). Monoclonal antibodies in cancer therapy: 25 years of progress, *Journal of Clinical Oncology*, 26, 1774–1777.

Parsons, T. (1960). *Structure and Process in Modern Societies*, Free Press, Glencoe.

Pera, M. F. and Trounson, A. O. (2004). Human embryonic stem cells: Prospects for development, *Development*, 131, 5515–5525.

PhRMA (Pharmaceutical Research and Manufacturers of America) (2008). *Pharmaceutical Industry Profile 2006,* PhRMA, Washington DC.

Pisano, G. (2006). *Science Business: The Promise, the Reality, and the Future of Biotech,* Harvard Business School Press, Boston.

Rao, H. (2002). 'Tests tell': Constitutive legitimacy and consumer acceptance of the auto- mobile: 1895–1912, *Advances in Strategic Management*, 19, 307–335.

Rao, R. S., Chandy, R. K. and Prabhu, J. C. (2008). The fruits of legitimacy: Why some new ventures gain more from innovation than others, *Journal of Marketing*, 72, 58–75.

Reichert, J. M. (2001). Monoclonal antibodies in the clinic, *Nature Biotechnology*, 19, 819–822.

Relman, A. S. and Angell, M. (1989). How good is peer review? *New England Journal of Medicine*, 321, 827–829.

Ruef, M. and Scott, W. R. (1998). A multidimensional model of organizational legitimacy: Hospital survival in changing institutional environments, *Administrative Science Quarterly*, 43(4), 877–904.

Scott, W. R. (1995). *Institutions and Organizations*, Sage, Thousand Oaks, CA.

Singh, J., Tucker, D. and House, R. (1986). Organizational legitimacy and the liability of newness, *Administrative Science Quarterly*, 31, 171–193.

Skerra, A. and Plückthun, A. (1988). Assembly of a functional immunoglobulin Fv fragment in *Escherichia coli*, *Science*, 1240, 1038–1041.

Spier, R. (2002). The history of the peer-review process, *Trends in Biotechnology*, 20, 357–358.

Stinchcombe, A. L. (1965). Organizations and social structure, in March, J. G. (ed.), *Handbook of Organizations*, Rand-McNally, Chicago.

Stylios, G. K., Giannoudis, P. V. and Wan, T. (2005). Applications of nanotechnologies in medical practice, *Injury*, 36, S6–S13.

Suchman, M. C. (1995). Managing legitimacy: Strategic and institutional approaches, *Academy of Management Review*, 20, 571–610.

Terreberry, S. (1968). The evolution of organizational environments, *Administrative Science Quarterly*, 12, 590–613.

Thomas, J. (2009). Biotech CEO: Firms that adapt to recession will thrive, *Charlotte Business Journal*. Available at: www.charlotte.bizjournals.com [Accessed 2 June 2009].

Thomson, K. M., Hough, D. W., Maddison, P. J., Melamed, M. D. and Hughes-Jones, N. (1986). The efficient production of stable, human monoclonal antibody-secreting hybridomas from EBV-transformed lymphocytes using the mouse myeloma X63-Ag8.653 as a fusion partner, *Journal of Immunological Methods*, 94, 7–12.

Waldman, T. A. (1991). Monoclonal antibodies in diagnosis and therapy, *Science*, 252, 1657–1662.

Wierenga, D. and Eaton, C. (2006). Office of research and development, *Pharmaceutical Manufacturers Association*. Available at: www.pharma.org [Accessed 17 December 2009].

Zimmerman, M. A. and Deeds, D. L. (1987). Legitimacy and the initial public offerings of biotechnology firms, *Frontiers for*

Entrepreneurship Research. Available at: www.babson. edu/entrep/fer/papers97 [Accessed 17 December 2009].

Zimmerman, M. A. and Zeitz, G. J. (2002). Beyond survival: Achieving new venture growth by building legitimacy, *Academy of Management Review*, 27, 414–431.

Part 4

New Product Development Perspectives

Chapter 10

Ambidexterity and Ambiguity

Eric Christian Brun

Department of Industrial Economics, Risk Management and Planning, University of Stavanger, Norway

eric.brun@uis.no

Abstract

The research goal of this chapter is to explore and explain the relation between ambiguity management and contextual ambidexterity in innovation. Based on qualitative analysis of case data, a model is presented showing how managing ambiguity is an underlying process of contextual ambidexterity. Requisite variety, perspective-taking, and interpretive skills help generate ambiguity to achieve exploration, while analytic skills help reduce ambiguity to achieve exploitation. Contextual ambidexterity is achieved through a process of alternating between generation, sustention, and reduction of ambiguity. High ambiguity tolerance (AT) emphasizes exploration, while low AT emphasizes exploitation. The findings contribute to a more detailed theoretical understanding of the contextual ambidexterity concept and can help practitioners to achieve contextual ambidexterity in their innovation projects.

Keywords: Ambidexterity, ambiguity tolerance, innovation, new product development.

1. Introduction

Recent reviews (Raisch and Birkinshaw, 2008; Simsek, 2009) point to the need for more research to understand the phenomenon of ambidexterity and its underlying processes. This chapter responds to that call.

Gibson and Birkinshaw (2004) draw a distinction between *structural ambidexterity*, which involves structurally separating business units for exploration and exploitation, and *contextual ambidexterity*, which they define as "the behavioral capacity to simultaneously demonstrate alignment and adaptability across an entire business unit" (p. 209). Contextual ambidexterity is however not well understood, and Raisch and Birkinshaw (2008) have accordingly called for more research to help substantiate our understanding of this phenomenon.

Gibson and Birkinshaw (2004) suggest that contextual ambidexterity is best achieved "not by structural, task or temporal separation, but by building a business-unit context that encourages individuals to make their own judgements…" (p. 211). Making a judgment is associated with how one perceives a situation and interprets it. A variety of individuals may interpret the same situations differently, giving rise to ambiguity. Also, "encouraging individuals to make their own judgments" can be seen as alluding to a notion of *tolerance*. The approach taken in this chapter is therefore that contextual ambidexterity — as advocated by Gibson and Birkinshaw (2004) — may be associated with a tolerance for ambiguity and managing ambiguity.

Brun and his colleagues (Brun and Sætre, 2008, 2009; Brun *et al.*, 2008, 2009) have studied the ambiguity element of "fuzziness" in innovation and argue that a new product development (NPD) project needs to meet two conflicting needs. One need is to come up with an innovative product concept; the other need is to execute the project in a cost- and time-efficient manner. The first need calls for generation and sustention of ambiguity to create ideas and achieve flexibility, while the second need calls for reduction of ambiguity to obtain the clarification and agreement necessary to achieve operational efficiency. Managing ambiguity in NPD, they therefore contend, requires a balancing act of generating or sustaining ambiguity to achieve flexibility and innovation and reducing ambiguity to achieve operational efficiency. The article by Brun and Sætre (2009) in *Creativity and Innovation Management* describes the link between all the foregoing articles by Brun and his colleagues. However, their currently published research has not related ambiguity management to concepts of ambidexterity.

The motivation for the research reported in this chapter has therefore been to contribute to the research agenda on ambidexterity, by exploring the possible relation between contextual ambidexterity and management of ambiguity. The study has been done in the context of technological innovation — in particular, NPD in established companies — with the NPD project as the unit of analysis.

The research objective of this chapter is to present a model by which the relation between ambiguity management and contextual ambidexterity in innovation can be understood.

2. Literature Review

2.1. *Ambidexterity in innovation*

NPD has a dual purpose both within incremental and radical innovation. One purpose is to develop new and innovative product concepts. The other purpose is to develop these product concepts into manufactured products that are launched in the market. Early in the NPD process the first purpose will have high priority, as the NPD project team searches for new product concepts and market opportunities. During this part of the process, emphasis will be on flexibility, exploration, and creation of new knowledge. An overall requirement of an NPD project is that it must be run in a time- and cost-efficient manner, and this concern is present already in the early, creative phase of the

NPD project. As the project progresses toward preparing for manufacturing and market launch, the concern for operational efficiency will gain importance, and emphasis will be laid on exploiting the knowledge developed in the early phases. NPD as an innovation process therefore implies a tension between exploration and exploitation.

The challenge of resolving the tension between exploration and exploitation has been subject to extensive research. Early contributions saw the challenge as one of trade-offs (Burns and Stalker, 1961; March, 1991; Thompson, 1967), claiming that exploration and exploitation are incompatible, implying that an organization can only be good at one of the two. Later research demonstrated that depending on the situational uncertainty, some companies did indeed succeed in tailoring their organizations and process methods to shift between exploration and exploitation. Tushman and O'Reilly (1996) launched the concept of organizational ambidexterity (OA), i.e., the ability of organizations to perform well in both exploration and exploitation.

Later, research has advanced the discussion of OA. Raisch and Birkinshaw (2008) claim that the most common approach to OA has been to establish structurally separate units for exploration and exploitation. Sutcliffe and colleagues (2000) have called this a *binary* approach, whereas Gibson and Birkinshaw (2004) have used the term *structural ambidexterity* to describe such an approach. As an alternative, they promote the term *contextual ambidexterity*, which they define as "the behavioral capacity to simultaneously demonstrate alignment and adaptability across an entire business unit" (p. 209). In accordance with their view, researchers within the innovation literature have argued that some companies have demonstrated the ability to combine exploration and exploitation simultaneously and that further research should investigate how they manage to do so (e.g., Magnusson and Martini, 2008; Magnusson *et al.*, 2009).

Interest in the concept of OA has increased during the recent years, but approaches and units of analysis have varied widely among researchers. Simsek (2009) has provided a classification where he distinguishes between three main approaches: *behavioral*, *structural*, and *realized*. *Behavioral* approaches (e.g., Cegarra-Navarro and Dewhurst, 2007; Gibson and Birkinshaw, 2004) may study OA at the single business unit level and hold a view of OA that aligns with contextual ambidexterity. *Structural* approaches, on the contrary (e.g., Benner and Tushman, 2003; Tushman and O'Reilly, 1996), study OA at higher organizational levels and a hold view of OA in alignment with structural ambidexterity. Both behavioral and structural approaches focus on the processes and mechanisms used by organizations or organizational subunits to achieve ambidexterity. By contrast, the attention of the *realized* approaches is on the *state* of organizations that have managed to achieve high levels of ambidexterity. Realized approaches, hence, typically see an organization's achieved OA in terms of performance measures related to exploration and exploitation (e.g., He and Wong, 2004; Lubatkin *et al.*, 2006).

The research reported in this chapter falls within the behavioral approach. An earlier study of particular relevance within this approach is one of Rosing, Frese and Bausch (2011), where they link ambidexterity to what they call *opening* and *closing* leader behaviors. They define opening leader behaviors as "a set of leader behaviors that includes encouraging doing things differently and experimenting, giving room for independent thinking and acting, and supporting attempts to challenge existing approaches" (p. 967). Correspondingly, they define closing leader behaviors as "a set of leader behaviors that includes taking corrective action, setting specific guidelines, and monitoring goal achievement" (p. 967). Their conceptions of opening and closing behaviors are based on earlier research's notions that the core of exploration is the increase of variance, while the core of exploitation is the reduction of variance (Gupta *et al.*, 2006; March, 1991). Rosing and colleagues (2011) argue that "... ambidextrous leadership consists of three elements: (1) opening leader behaviors to foster exploration,

(2) closing leader behaviors to foster exploitation, (3) and the temporal flexibility to switch between both as the situation requires" (p. 966). Examples they give of opening behaviors include "allowing different ways of accomplishing a task", "encouraging experimentation with different ideas", and "giving room for own ideas". All of these implicitly suggest a link to ambiguity tolerance (AT), in that different ideas will emerge if a leader allows or encourages project team members to come up with a variety of interpretations of the project's challenges and opportunities.

Earlier research on top management teams (TMTs) also suggest a link between ambidexterity and ambiguity management. Tushman and O'Reilly (1997) argue that ambidexterity to a large extent is driven by TMTs' "internal processes that enable them to handle large amounts of information and decision alternatives and deal with conflict and ambiguity" (p. 172). Carmeli and Halevi (2009) argue that OA is enabled by "behavioral complexity" — an umbrella term previously suggested by Satish (1997) to cover multiple avenues of complexity research. Satish, in turn, indicates a link between behavioral complexity and AT arguing that "Higher complexity levels imply more abstract reasoning (Neuliep and Hazelton, 1986), more comfort with ambiguity, and greater breadth of focus towards multiple goals" (Harvey *et al.*, 1961; Satish, 1997, p. 2054).

2.2. *Ambiguity in innovation processes*

A well-known characteristic of innovation processes is their high level of uncertainty and ambiguity, especially in the early phases (e.g., Brown and Eisenhardt, 1995; Khurana and Rosenthal, 1997, 1998; Moenaert *et al.*, 1995; Reid and de Brentani, 2004).

However, it is important to address ambiguity as different from uncertainty. The latter can be understood as lack of information (Galbraith, 1974); in other words, it may be reduced or eliminated by providing more information. Ambiguity may be defined as different interpretations of the same cue. The cue can be a piece of text, a spoken statement, an image, etc., in short, a signal to perception. These different interpretations are formed because the actors interpreting the cue may draw on different cognitive bases to ascribe meaning to the cue. Terms that have been used in organizational literature to denote these cognitive bases are *paradigms* (Weick, 1995), *thought worlds* (Dougherty, 1992), and *frames of reference* (Daft and Lengel, 1986).

A common, implicit assumption in mainstream management literature is that ambiguity is undesirable and should consistently be reduced to provide precise information as a basis for rational decision-making. And certainly in NPD processes, an innovating company will eventually need to eliminate undesirable ambiguity before launching a product. There are however a number of contributions suggesting the opposite — that generating and sustaining ambiguity can be useful at certain stages in many organizational processes. Eric Eisenberg (1984) has argued that ambiguity is useful to retain strategic flexibility, and flexibility in turn has been highlighted by many authors as key to successfully managing innovation processes (Eisenhardt and Tabrizi, 1995; MacCormack and Verganti, 2003; Verganti, 1999). Other authors have argued for the usefulness of exploiting multiple interpretations to generate new alternatives for action in innovation processes (Lane and Maxfield, 1996; Sarasvathy and Dew, 2005). Leonard and Sensiper (1998) argue that groups that are intellectually homogenous will be less innovative than heterogeneous groups, because they will be more susceptible to engage in *groupthink* (Janis, 1982), hence, failing to produce the variety of viewpoints needed to feed innovation. Their argument implicitly suggests that the ambiguity resulting from the variety of reference frames within a heterogeneous group may play a role in stimulating innovation. Multiplicity of alternatives also takes an essential role in evolutionary approaches seeing innovation as occurring through processes of variation and selection (Aldrich, 1999; Burgelman, 1983). The notion of innovation as processes of variation and selection accords well with the claim by Leonard and Sensiper (1998) that ideas develop through a series of divergence and convergence. They see divergence as the creation of a variety of ideas and convergence as the selection of an idea to be processed, thus, closely resembling concepts of opening and closing leader behaviors put forth by Rosing and colleagues (2011). The illustration of idea development through divergence and convergence, also used by creativity researchers (e.g., Basadur *et al.*, 2000), may imply that ambiguity can fluctuate throughout an innovation process.

Brun and Sætre (2008) have shown that ambiguity in innovation projects can be effectively reduced through a hypothetical-deductive approach, by identifying the competing interpretations of a cue, treating each interpretation as a hypothesis, and subsequently testing each hypothesis as well as the assumptions underlying those hypotheses.

However, Brun *et al.* (2008) have also shown that NPD projects may benefit from sustaining ambiguity to retain fallback options and creative ideas. During the process of reducing ambiguity, the selection process is based on assumptions held by the involved actors, and these assumptions may or may not be valid. If they later prove invalid, and if all other interpretations have been eliminated, the company will have no options for further progress in its NPD project. By not fully reducing ambiguity, however, and instead leaving certain interpretations open, the project will retain these as fallback options and ideas, should the assumptions underlying the selected interpretation fail. The process model developed by Brun *et al.* (2008) is illustrated in Figure 1.

Following their conceptual model in Figure 1 from left to right, the process starts with a cue, which for example can be a product idea. This cue can have multiple interpretations, shown as A, B, C, and D, representing different interpretations of the product idea. If we first consider a process of ambiguity reduction, this will imply selecting one of these interpretations to be used as a basis for further progress. In Figure 1, interpretation

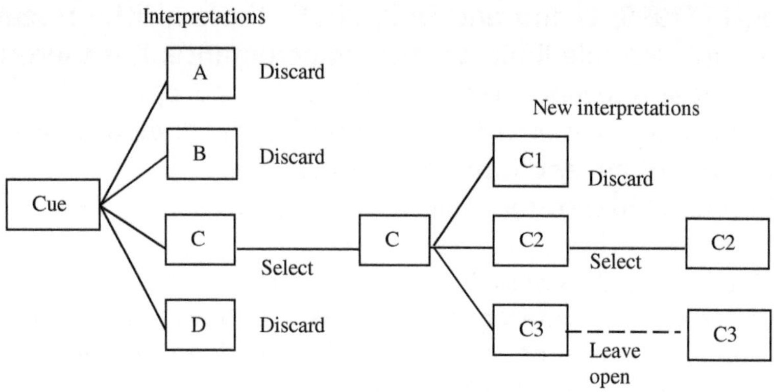

Figure 1. Development of ambiguity throughout innovation process.
Source: Adapted from Brun *et al.* (2008).

C is selected, and if the process were one of pure ambiguity reduction, A, B, and D would all be discarded. In the next step, interpretation C will become a new cue and be interpreted in light of how it can be developed further. The actors participating in the NPD process will again interpret the cue differently, for example as different product concept interpretations (C1, C2, and C3) at a more detailed level. Following the same logic as in the previous step, one might select C2 as a commonly agreed-on interpretation and discard C1, but one might choose to leave C3 open. If later in the process the assumptions underlying the selection of C2 (for example an assumed customer preference) prove invalid, then the project can revert to alternative C3. Similarly, one might have chosen to leave an alternative interpretation open in the first step, for example interpretation A, as a fallback option, in case the entire path resulting from interpretation C proved unsuccessful.

2.3. *Ambiguity tolerance*

Although many other authors have argued for the need to accept the presence of ambiguity as an ingredient of innovation processes (e.g., Ahmed, 1998; Griffin *et al.*, 2007; Nonaka and

Takeuchi, 1995; Zhang and Doll, 2001), there is little research suggesting sensible limits to such an acceptance. It is therefore of particular relevance here to address the concept of AT, which has been studied as an attribute of both individuals and organizations (Furnham and Ribchester, 1995).

Budner (1962) stated that:

> "Intolerance of ambiguity may be defined as 'the tendency to perceive (i.e., interpret) ambiguous situations as sources of threat', tolerance of ambiguity as 'the tendency to perceive ambiguous situations as desirable'" (p. 29).

He claimed that ambiguous situations were characterized by novelty, complexity, or insolubility and developed a scale for AT along these three dimensions. In 1982, Schere (1982) used Budner's scale in a study comparing entrepreneurs (defined as individuals who had started their own firms) with top executives and middle managers (who had not started firms). He found that entrepreneurs have higher AT levels than top executives and managers, and it was particularly along the Novelty dimension on the Budner scale that the difference in AT scores was most striking. Schere (1982) concluded that entrepreneurs have a higher tolerance than top executives and middle managers for the ambiguity they face in situations characterized by novelty and argued that tolerance for ambiguity is a distinguishing characteristic separating entrepreneurs from managers.

In another study, Begley and Boyd (1987) compared entrepreneurs (i.e., company founders) with managers (non-founders) of small businesses, on a number of psychological attributes. They also studied whether the subjects' scores on these attributes were related to the company's performance. Similar to Schere (1982), they found that entrepreneurs have significantly higher AT than non-founding managers. Interestingly though, they found a curvilinear (inverse U-shape) relation between AT in the manager group and company growth rate. Up to a certain level, increasing AT was associated with increasing company growth rate. Beyond this level though, growth declined with further increase in AT. Begley and Boyd (1987), hence, suggested that an optimum level for AT might exist and that beyond this level, excessive tolerance for ambiguity might impair a manager's ability to decisively respond to environmental change.

The implicit view largely held within management literature (with Eisenberg (1984) representing an exception) is that ambiguity has a negative influence and therefore one should consistently strive at reducing it. Innovation and entrepreneurship literature, though, commonly advocates high tolerance for ambiguity (although Begley and Boyd (1987) have issued a word of caution in that respect). These widely differing views of ambiguity found in the two bodies of literature demonstrate two stances toward AT. On one side is the *managerial* stance with a preference for low AT, and on the other side is the *entrepreneurial* stance with a preference for high AT, as reflected in Schere's (1982) research. In an NPD project in an established company, though, functional line managers as well as team members with entrepreneurial characteristics will be involved, causing the two stances toward AT to confront each other throughout the project. There is a lack of research addressing the management challenge of resolving this dilemma.

So far, we have discussed research addressing AT at an individual level. AT has however also been studied as an attribute of organizational units, mainly related to human resource issues such as job-related stress, job satisfaction, and promotions (Furnham and Ribchester, 1995). In the context of NPD, Ahmed (1998) claims that companies that want to build a culture of innovation need to accept and deal with ambiguity. However, little work has been done to investigate how variance in AT affects innovation processes. This chapter addresses the concept of AT as an attribute of the NPD team, resting on Budner's (1962) definition of AT as the tendency to perceive ambiguous situations as desirable.

3. Method

The research reported in this chapter builds on the work of Brun and colleagues (Brun and Sætre, 2008, 2009; Brun *et al.*, 2008, 2009). Their research was based on qualitative analysis of four case studies using the Grounded Theory (GT) method. Each case was an NPD project in an established Scandinavian company manufacturing medical devices. For the purpose of this research, cases from that industry were considered appropriate due to a number of characteristics. First, its business, engineering, and clinical environments represent widely different knowledge domains, so there was a high potential for encountering differences of interpretation, i.e., ambiguity. Second, it is characterized by a high degree of structured and disciplined NPD methodology (mainly due to regulatory requirements), hence, we could expect that ambiguity occurrences experienced in the cases were a natural part of the NPD process rather than aberrances due to an absence of disciplined approaches. Third, it has a high rate of NPD that is typically R&D intensive, i.e., requiring a high degree of exploration activities. And finally, the studied companies were small and medium-sized enterprises, and due to the limited size of SMEs one can expect their exploration and exploitation activities to be intertwined, rather than being organizationally separated in exploration and exploitation units. Hence one could expect that they had to rely more on contextual rather than structural ambidexterity to balance exploration and exploitation.

The interviewees included managers at top and middle level as well as project members without management responsibility. The data set consisted of 46 semi-structured interviews, 7 hours of meeting observations, 913 pages of document data, and 17 video files. Table 1 provides an overview of the cases.

The research reported in this chapter uses the same data set, but takes the analysis further. This research sought to *understand* a phenomenon rather than to achieve prediction and

Table 1. Overview of cases.

Cases	Company	Purpose of new product to be developed
Case 1	Alpha	Improve efficiency of both treatment and training of a specific first aid procedure.
Case 2	Beta	Improve "patient compliance"; i.e., the degree to which chronic patients adhere to their drug treatment schemes.
Case 3	Gamma	Improve quality control of coronary bypass surgery and vessel surgery.
Case 4	Delta	Improve patient safety during laparoscopic surgery.

control, hence the scientific stance taken here can be described as *interpretive* (Burrell and Morgan, 1979), more specifically, *descriptive interpretive* since the analysis has rested on the actual interpretations of the informants, rather than looking for hidden interpretations behind their words as one might in a critical/normative interpretive stance (Putnam, 1983). The research approach taken was to see if the relation between AT and contextual ambidexterity could be understood through a set of concepts and relations between them. This called for some method that utilized coding and category-building as a technique (Miles and Huberman, 1994). Of the ones thus far developed, GT approaches have become widely used and offer specific procedures for coding. Among the various GT approaches, the one described by Strauss and Corbin (1998) was considered to be consistent with the descriptive interpretive perspective taken. The choice was therefore made to build on the GT analysis done earlier by Brun and colleagues and perform additional analysis as follows:

- **Storyline write-up:** Writing up condensed storylines to identify when ambiguity was generated and when it was reduced throughout the project in each case. The purpose of this analysis step was to identify how ambiguity developed (i.e., was generated, sustained, or reduced) over time.

- **Content analysis:** Analyzing these storylines by classical content analysis. In this step, the storyline contents were analyzed to identify occurrences of "opening behaviors" and "closing behaviors" as defined by Rosing, Frese and Bausch (2011, p. 967).
- **Selective coding:** An additional process of *selective coding* — as described in Strauss and Corbin's (1998) approach to GT method — in which the data and the results from Brun and colleagues' research were compared to AT as a central concept, relying on Budner's (1962) definition of the term.
- **Identifying variety in NPD team:** A tabular display (Miles and Huberman, 1984) showing the teams' diversity compared to their generation of ambiguity.

4. Findings

4.1. *Storylines*

Each storyline is a summary of how ambiguity developed throughout the project in each case. For each storyline, a brief background to the project is given, followed by bullet points summarizing how ambiguity developed. Each bullet point starts by indicating the cue that was interpreted, followed by a description of the ambiguity development related to that cue. The bullet points are presented in the order they occurred — as far as possible — since some of them occurred somewhat overlapping.

4.1.1. *Alpha storyline*

Research had shown that when giving first aid to patients suffering from serious injury, even trained rescuers commonly made the mistake of performing a specific compression maneuver with insufficient quality. Alpha interpreted this problem as an opportunity to develop a product solution. Throughout the project, ambiguity developed as follows:

- **Cue: A product to improve first aid compressions**

Ambiguity was generated as there was a variety of interpretations as to what the appropriate product concept would be.

The first interpretation was that the device (called "the Snapper") would be a purely therapeutic product. It would be a small, palm-sized device to be placed on the patient's chest, producing an audible feedback when a compression was performed satisfactorily. It would be bundled with a pocket mask (an emergency breathing mask routinely carried by emergency medical personnel) in a package called "Pocket CPR".

The second interpretation was that "the Snapper" would be a *combined* therapeutic and training device. It could be used in a first aid training class, placing it on a training manikin, and subsequently carried with the user in a pocket mask kit, thus enabling the user to efficiently transfer a learned skill into a clinical situation.

The third interpretation was a training concept called "First Aid 1–2–3" where the audible feedback from compressions would be implemented as a built-in sound device in a training manikin. This interpretation arose from those participants who believed that a stand-alone Snapper would be too expensive if it was developed as a therapy product, whereas a less costly, built-in sound device would be sufficient to cover training needs.

Initially, the company chose to pursue all product concepts in parallel to keep options open. Ambiguity was thus sustained temporarily.

- **Cue: The Snapper as a therapeutic device**

Ambiguity arose as Alpha and the Food and Drug Administration (FDA) in the US had differing interpretations as to what an acceptable compression measurement principle would be. Furthermore, Alpha and FDA had differing interpretations as to whether the so-called "predicate devices" (i.e., devices operating by the same principle) existed on the market, which — if true — would greatly simplify the procedure to be granted market access in the US. FDA's interpretation was that predicate devices did not exist in this case. However. Alpha having an interest in the opposite interpretation, argued that predicate devices did indeed exist and thus generated ambiguity. After a process of correspondence with the FDA, Alpha chose to abandon their interpretation of the product concept for therapeutic use, at least for the US market. Ambiguity thus was reduced. However, some ambiguity was sustained as Alpha still wanted to hold open the option of targeting the therapy market outside the US. After a further process of development, testing and focus group discussions, the interpretation of the Snapper as a therapeutic device was fully rejected, i.e., ambiguity was reduced.

- **Cue: The global market for a therapeutic device**

Ambiguity was generated as there were interpretations of potential markets. One group of interpretations were related to geography — mainly dividing between the US and the rest of the world. Another group of interpretations were related to the type of use for the device — the therapy market or the training market. For both of these main markets, there was further differing interpretations as to who the main users would be: professional rescuers, instructors, or the lay public. Initially all options were held open, i.e., ambiguity was sustained. Ambiguity was gradually reduced as described in the previous bullet point, and the all interpretations of the therapeutic market niches were gradually abandoned.

- **Cue: A product concept to improve *training* of correct first aid compressions**

Ambiguity had previously been generated as a result of two product concept interpretations; the Snapper as a stand-alone device or as a built-in sound feature on a training manikin.

After a series of tests, Alpha concluded to pursue with the built-in feature option. Ambiguity was hence reduced, and the development project was concluded based on this single product interpretation.

4.1.2. *Beta storyline*

Patient compliance is defined in the medical industry as the degree to which patients adhere to a prescribed treatment scheme. A major problem in medical treatment is that chronically ill patients who need to take medications in specific amounts and at specific time intervals often fail to do so. This led to a clinical problem as non-complying patients would fail to achieve optimal treatment, but it also led to a commercial problem for the drug companies as they did not achieve their intended revenues. There was an interest in the pharmaceutical industry to provide a form of intelligent drug delivery device together with their drugs which would ensure a patient's compliance to the treatment scheme. One specific drug company — PillCo — was interested in being the first major customer and asked Beta, a medical device manufacturer, to develop a product solution. Ambiguity developed throughout the project as follows:

- **Cue: The compliance problem**

Ambiguity arose as the cue could be interpreted as a clinical problem or a commercial problem, as described above. Beta chose to sustain this ambiguity, as the two interpretations represented two important stakeholder needs.

- **Cue: A product concept to improve patient compliance**

Ambiguity arose as there were two main competing product interpretations: one (called low-end) emphasized simplicity and low cost and promoting the drug through branding. The other (called high-end) was a high-end, high-tech concept with multiple features of data logging, communication, and reporting.

- **Cue: The market associated with the compliance problem**

When the alternative product concepts were discussed, more ambiguity arose, as the target market for each product concept was re-interpreted. Supporters of the low-end concept focused on solving the clinical problem of patients in the consumer market. Supporters of the high-end concept wanted to focus initially on the professional clinical trial market, since they believed it would be easier to penetrate a professional market segment first and then later move into the consumer market segment.

Ambiguity was sustained as Beta decided to develop both ideas in a concept development phase and then later decide which to pursue before entering an engineering phase.

- **Cue: Users of the low-end concept**

In pursuit of the low-end concept, multiple interpretations emerged of who the main users would be. They were eventually identified as three main stakeholder groups: the patients, general practitioners (i.e., family doctors), and the drug companies. Ambiguity was sustained as each was considered important stakeholder groups, and one would have to consider the needs of all of these.

- **Cue: The needs of the stakeholder group**

Ambiguity increased further as the Beta team interpreted the needs of the various stakeholder groups. A workshop was held in which these were discussed and the team could conclude on a short list, thus reducing some ambiguity.

- **Cue: The product concept of the low-end option**

Ambiguity arose as the team developed a series of product ideas, each representing a different interpretation of the concept and emphasizing different perceived stakeholder needs. In discussions with a focus group of patients and doctors, some ideas were rejected and some were encouraged for further development. Ambiguity was thus first reduced, and increased again when the selected ideas were considered further in various forms. This process went through cycles of ambiguity generation as new ideas arose (called "divergence" by one informant) and ambiguity reduction as preferred ideas were selected for further development (called "convergence" by the same informant). Finally, ambiguity was reduced when the process resulted in a physical prototype representing one interpretation.

- **Cue: A product to meet PillCo's business interest**

Ambiguity was still present as there were two product and market interpretations: Low-end for the consumer market and High-end for a professional market. A final test was performed as Beta at the end of the concept phase could present prototypes of both product concepts to PillCo. Although PillCo had an interest in both markets, they selected the Low-end interpretation, even for the professional market segments. Ambiguity was then reduced to one interpretation (i.e., the final Low-end concept) and the development project transitioned into an engineering phase.

4.1.3. *Gamma storyline*

Gamma Medical is a small company, specializing in ultrasound-based monitoring equipment used in cardiac and vascular surgery, cardiac bypass operations in particular. In such operations, it is a recommended procedure to assess the blood flow at the joint (anastomosis) where the inserted vein is connected to the coronary artery to verify its quality before closing the patient. Gamma offered an existing product — the Verifier — that allowed the cardiac surgeon to perform such assessment by interpreting various displayed curve shapes and indicator values. Gamma however wanted to offer a new product — the Imager — based on a different kind of ultrasound technology that would provide a dynamic color image with more information for easier and faster blood flow assessment.

Ambiguity in this case was mainly related to market issues and user perceptions. It developed throughout the project as follows:

- **Cue: The application area of the new product**

Ambiguity arose when Gamma considered two different product concept interpretations based on the new technology. One concept would be targeted for cardiac bypass surgery; the other product concept would be for vessel surgery. Gamma chose to reduce ambiguity by selecting the cardiac bypass surgery option and focus their further efforts on developing this concept into a product.

- **Cue: Blood flow assessment during the cardiac bypass operation procedure**

For clinicians using the Verifier or similar products on the market, blood flow assessment in cardiac bypass surgery meant interpreting a combination of waveforms and numbers on the unit's display. To make use of the Imager, clinicians would have to assess blood flow by interpreting a picture with color codes. There was therefore ambiguity among the users as "blood flow assessment" meant one thing to them when using the Verifier, another thing when using the Imager. This ambiguity was considered undesirable by Gamma, and Gamma's marketing manager therefore put much effort into explaining the product concept and educating the users, thus reducing ambiguity.

- **Cue: Main customer group**

Within Gamma, ambiguity arose when they discussed who the main target customer group for the Imager would be. One interpretation was that the main target group would be users who had not yet embraced instrument-based quality control during bypass operations, since this was fairly complicated using the Verifier but would be easier with the Imager. Another interpretation was that the main target group would be those already familiar with quality control using the Verifier. Ambiguity was reduced when the marketing manager investigated among potential users and concluded that the first interpretation was unfounded. The second interpretation therefore became Gamma's basis for further efforts of marketing the Imager.

- **Cue: Roles and responsibilities during cardiac bypass operations**

Since the Imager represented a new piece of equipment and a new component in the surgical procedure that did not fit into the established roles of the members of the clinical operating team, there were several interpretations of who the operator of the device would be. This was an important issue, since optimal design of the user interface would depend on who the operator was and what other roles in the procedure the operator would have. At the time of this research project's end, the Imager had not yet been introduced for clinical testing in user environments; hence, this ambiguity was not resolved.

4.1.4. *Delta storyline*

Delta Medical is a small company that originated in the technological research environment of a Norwegian university. Its business idea was based on a product for ultrasound Doppler guidance during laparoscopic surgery. Since blood vessels under the organ tissue surfaces can't be seen by the optical technique used in laparoscopy, they may accidentally be cut during the operating procedure. Delta's idea for solving this problem was to develop a product — the LapDop — using a sheath fitted with an ultrasound probe attached to the operating instrument and wired to a control unit on the outside of the patient, thus enabling the surgeon to detect blood vessels through audible feedback. In the first phase, the project was driven by the inventor in cooperation with a laparoscopic surgeon, representing a "lead user", and together they developed a prototype of the product. Later, a formal project manager was appointed. Ambiguity in this case was mainly related to product functionality and developed as follows:

- **Cue: Product functionality**

When demonstrating the prototype of the product to potential users, the functionality of the product was interpreted in widely different ways. Some users interpreted the product as easy to use, time-saving, and essential for quality assurance. Others interpreted it as cumbersome to use, time-consuming, and unnecessary for quality assurance.

In response to this ambiguity, Delta conducted user surveys and performed clinical tests in six European countries. However, user perceptions still varied to such an extent that the results from this clinical testing were inconclusive. Delta therefore chose to continue the project based on the inventor's and the lead user's interpretation of what the product concept ought to be.

During the clinical trials, the project manager at Delta had noticed that many of the sophisticated features of the product were never used by the surgeons testing the device. They had a different interpretation of how to use the product which only necessitated a much simpler version of the product. The inventor and lead user argued, however, that the sophisticated features were the very essence of the product concept. They were not willing to interpret the product concept in a new and different way. Their original product idea was brought to launch, but did not meet sales objectives and was discontinued. During the last interview, the project manager of Delta expressed that he believed that a re-interpreted, simplified product concept would have had a good chance of becoming successful. And interestingly, a few years later, a competitor successfully launched a product with features similar to what a simplified version of Delta's device could have been.

4.2. *Results of content analysis of storylines and selective coding*

The results of the content analysis and selective coding can be summarized in Figure 2.

The content analysis revealed that opening behaviors were associated with the development teams generating ambiguity related to the product and market options. Occurrences of ambiguity generation that originated from the external environment were however not associated with opening behaviors, since this ambiguity was not generated by the teams as a part of their search for ideas and new solutions. However, the teams had to respond both to the internally and externally generated ambiguity, and their efforts to reduce this ambiguity were associated with closing behaviors.

Alpha and Beta showed the highest occurrence of opening behaviors, all of which were associated with allowing generation

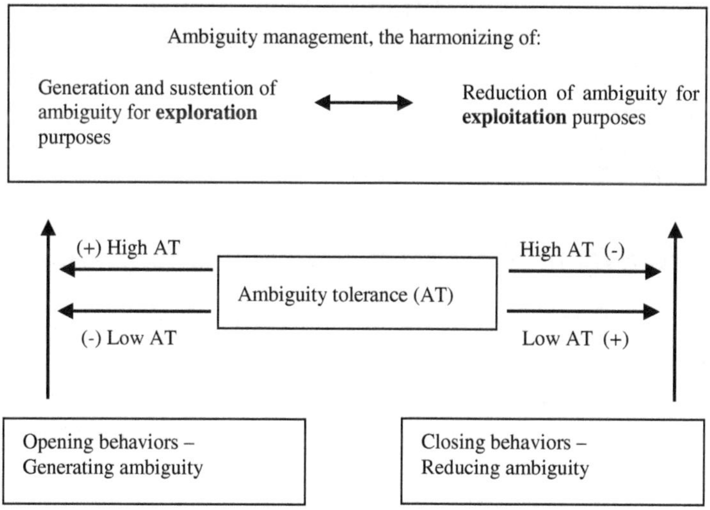

Figure 2. Management of ambiguity through opening and closing behaviors.

of ambiguity to explore and experiment with product and market ideas. Both companies managed ambiguity as a shifting between generation and reduction to harmonize exploration and exploitation and eventually launched a successful product. The teams in both companies exhibited high AT in the early phase of the project, thus emphasizing the left-hand side of Figure 2, allowing generation of ambiguity about product and market options to be explored — and gradually shifted toward a lower AT throughout the project, thus emphasizing the right-hand side of Figure 2, reducing ambiguity and concluding on which options to exploit.

Gamma showed a moderate degree of opening behavior in the early phase of the project, in considering different product concept interpretations, but overall both Gamma and Delta mainly responded to externally generated ambiguity with low AT. They emphasized closing behaviors and reduction of ambiguity in order to adhere to their project plan, as represented by the right-hand side of Figure 2. Delta, in particular, were unwilling to tolerate ambiguity (as represented by the left-hand side of Figure 2) to explore the alternative product interpretation that emerged. The result was the launch of an unsuccessful product and a missed opportunity to redirect their project in a way that might have improved their chance of succeeding.

4.3. *Diversity in NPD team and ambiguity generation*

The display in Table 2 shows the diversity within the NPD team and their generation of ambiguity.

As Table 2 shows, the most diverse team (Alpha) generated more ambiguity than the teams with medium (Gamma) or low (Delta) diversity. Interestingly, the Beta team — although low in diversity — still had the second highest count of ambiguity generation occurrences.

Table 2. Case team characteristics and generation of ambiguity.

Case company	NPD project team generating ambiguity	Characteristics of team	Number of occurrences of ambiguity generated about product or market
Alpha	• VP business development • VP training market • VP for R&D • Project director • Project manager R&D • VP1 marketing • VP2 marketing	**High diversity:** Multitude of representatives from marketing and business development with insights from a variety of market user segments, the rest representing technical and project management functions.	11
Beta	• CEO • VP R&D • Concept development manager • Design engineer1 • Designer 1 • Designer 2 • Marketing manager	**Low diversity:** The majority representing R&D and design functions were main drivers of the project. CEO and Marketing manager represented business and market concerns, but were less involved.	7
Gamma	• CEO • R&D Director • Marketing manager • R&D engineer 1 • R&D engineer 2	**Medium diversity:** The majority representing R&D and engineering expertise were the main drivers of the project. Marketing manager was however also highly involved. CEO was less involved.	5
Delta	• R&D engineer (inventor) • Project manager • Marketing manager • Lead user (laparoscopic surgeon)	**Low diversity:** Market insight was limited to lead user's field. Engineering focus was on the inventor's chosen approach.	4

5. Discussion

5.1. *Generating ambiguity*

As described in the previous sections, Alpha and Beta both generated more ambiguity than Gamma and Delta and also exhibited more behavior than Gamma and Delta of shifting between generating and reducing ambiguity for exploration and exploitation purposes, respectively. As seen in Table 2, Alpha's team was also the one with the highest degree of diversity. This aligns with the discussion in Section 3.2, suggesting that a team exhibiting a variety of reference frames may be more innovative than a homogeneous team. Beta's team, on the contrary, was fairly homogeneous but was still able to generate ambiguity by considering the patient compliance issue from the vantage points of the various stakeholders. Each team, thus, had a different basis for generating ambiguity. These bases can be understood through the terms *requisite variety* in Alpha's case and *perspective-taking* in Beta's case. Each of these will be discussed in the following sections.

5.1.1. *Requisite variety*

Ambiguity arises when project participants ascribe different meanings to a cue based on their differing reference frames. The literature review section referred to research claiming that heterogeneity of the development team plays an important role in innovation. Forming intellectually diverse groups (Leonard and Sensiper, 1998) is one way to enable generation of ambiguity through the diversity of knowledge possessed by the individuals partaking in the NPD project.

Diversity in itself is however not sufficient to generate useful ambiguity; the *kind* of diversity is critically important. Some groups of people or partners with differing sets of reference frames will be more able to produce useful ambiguity than other groups. In the context of NPD, the multitude of interpretations created by the participants in the process needs to be *relevant* to the market. To meet this requirement, the diversity of reference frames represented in the NPD team must in some way match the diversity of reference frames out in the company's market. Relevant diversity as a basis for generating useful ambiguity in NPD is, thus, a form of *requisite variety* (Ashby, 1956; Nonaka, 1994; Weick, 1979). Weick (1979) and later Nonaka (1994) argued that *requisite variety* arises only when the diversity within an organization matches the diversity in the organization's environment. In Weick's (1979) words: "It's because of requisite variety that organizations have to be preoccupied with keeping sufficient diversity inside the organization to sense accurately the variety present in ecological changes outside it" (p. 188) and "... the inability of people in organizations to tolerate equivocal processing may well be one of the most important reasons why they have trouble. It is their unwillingness to meet equivocality in an equivocal manner that produces failure ..." (p. 189). Sadly, this is what was seen in the Delta case when they were unwilling to re-interpret their product concept as a response to the market's interpretations.

Requisite variety in the NPD team, thus, constitutes a basis to generate ambiguity, as shown in Figure 2. Requisite variety can, for example, be achieved by including team members with knowledge similar to users and other important stakeholders in the company's environment. This was indeed so in the Alpha case, which showed the highest count of incidents where ambiguity was generated about the product or market, as shown in Table 2. Their development team consisted of members representing engineering, management, and marketing representatives with insights in a variety of market segments.

5.1.2. *Perspective-taking*

Requisite variety within the NPD team is however not the only basis for generation of useful ambiguity. The NPD team on the one hand and the user community on the other hand are still likely to represent two different *communities-of-knowing*

(Boland and Tenkasi, 1995), i.e., communities of actors with specialized knowledge domains. Another route to generation of useful ambiguity is available if the participants in the NPD team are able to understand the perspective of other stakeholders through *perspective-taking*, defined by Boland and Tenkasi (1995) as "communication that improves (a firm's) ability to take the knowledge of other communities into account" (p. 351).

In contrast to Alpha's team, Beta's development team was fairly homogeneous, consisting mainly of designers and design engineers. However, the team members made considerable efforts to identify and understand the needs of their key stakeholder groups (i.e., pharmaceutical companies, general practitioners, and the patient) and then to use that understanding to interpret the product ideas from the stakeholders' perspectives. The Beta case exemplifies that even a fairly homogenous NPD team can create useful ambiguity if the participants master the skill of perspective-taking.

5.2. *Ambiguity management and contextual ambidexterity*

Based on the foregoing discussion, the model presented in Figure 2 can be expanded to a model, shown in Figure 3, illustrating the link between ambiguity management and contextual ambidexterity.

The following sections will explain the model and discuss its elements in relation to relevant theory.

5.2.1. *Managing ambiguity*

As illustrated in Figure 1, ambiguity is generated and reduced in ongoing cycles throughout the NPD process. Generation of ambiguity occurs through an *interpretive* process, i.e., when a cue is interpreted by the involved participants.

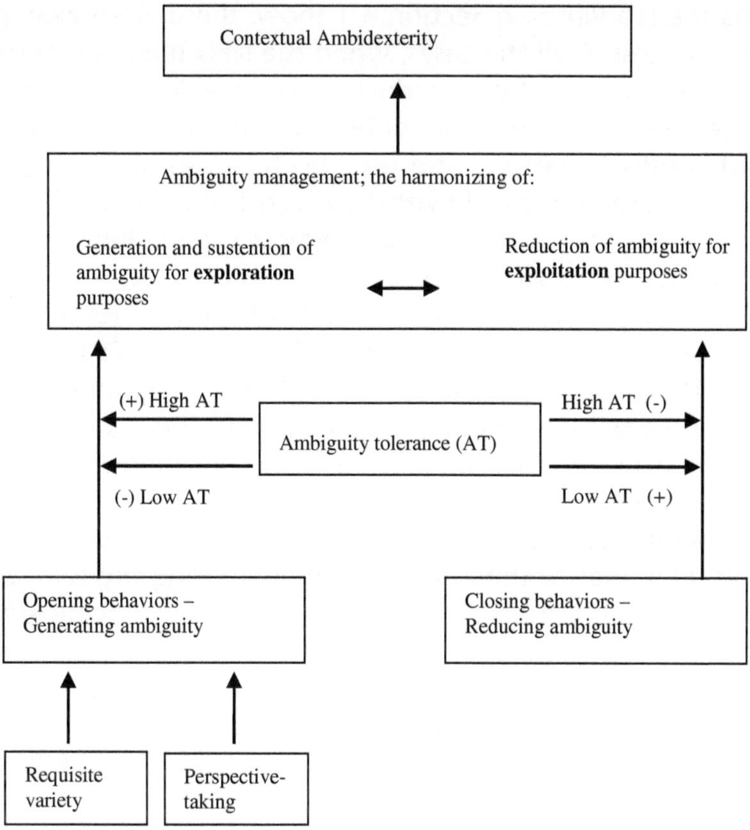

Figure 3. Management of ambiguity and contextual ambidexterity.

Brun and Sætre (2008) have shown that ambiguity reduction in NPD projects can be effectively achieved through a hypothetical-deductive approach, by identifying the competing interpretations of a cue, treating each interpretation as a hypothesis and subsequently testing each hypothesis as well as the assumptions underlying those hypotheses. To succeed with such an approach, the NPD team must be capable of explicating the differing interpretations and their underlying assumptions, formulate each of these as hypotheses, and then perform tests to decide whether to maintain or reject these hypotheses and assumptions.

As the storylines in Section 4.1 show, there were examples of this process in all the cases, when the NPD teams performed tests of prototypes of the products they were developing. These tests served to confirm or disconfirm the companies' hypotheses about product features and user preferences. In Alpha, one informant used the word *hypothesis* consistently when describing the ideas they wished to test against the market. This process can best be described as rational, and *analytic*.

Each cycle, thus, requires two sets of quite different intellectual skills. The opening behaviors (Rosing *et al.*, 2011) associated with generating and making use of ambiguity require interpretive skills, whereas the closing behaviors (Rosing *et al.*, 2011) associated with reducing ambiguity require analytical skills. To manage ambiguity throughout the NPD project, the team members need to alternate between the interpretive and analytical modes of thinking and between using the two skills. This alternating process accords with Rosing and her colleagues' claim that "...in terms of ambidextrous leadership, behavioral complexity refers to the capability to of having a repertoire of both opening and closing leader behaviors as well as the temporal flexibility to switch between them" (2011, p. 968). The dual need for interpretive and analytical skills also accords with Lester and Piore's (2004) claim that NPD processes must be understood according to two approaches, the interpretive and the analytical.

5.2.2. *AT and ambidexterity*

The concept of AT captures this duality. It is reflected in Figure 4, which is a further development of the model in Figure 1, of how ambiguity develops in the NPD project.

The horizontal dimension represents the progression through time of the product development process. At each step, when the team considers multiple interpretations of the product idea or concept (i.e., ambiguity is generated), they are seeking new knowledge — i.e., exploring — how to progress.

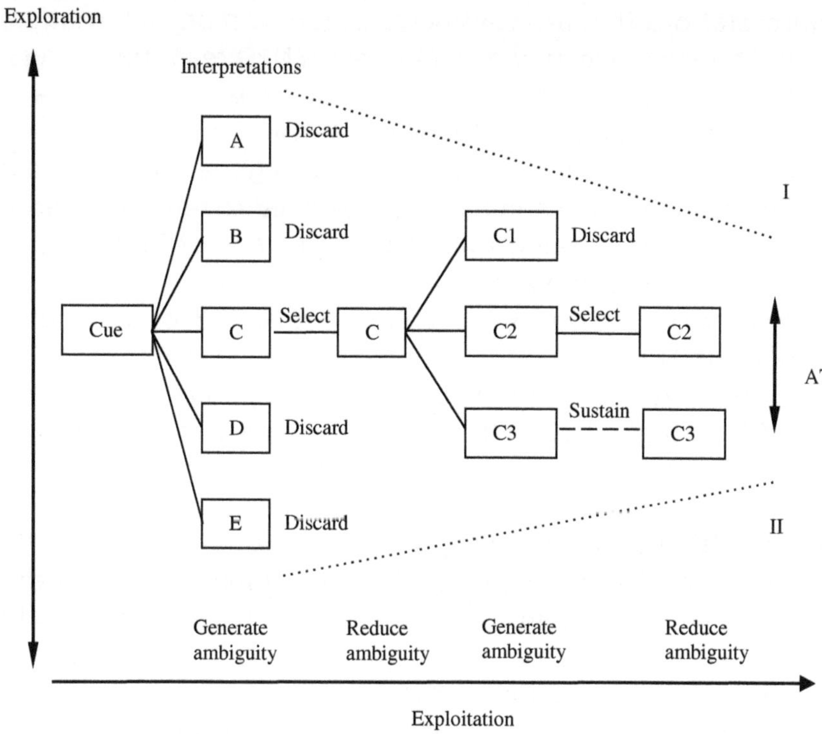

Figure 4. Development of ambiguity relative to exploration and exploitation.

The vertical dimension hence represents *exploration*. When a specific interpretation is selected by the NPD team (i.e., ambiguity is reduced), and they move rightward, the team exploits this knowledge to refine the product concept. Rightward movement, thus, represents *exploitation*. The process will proceed in cycles where ambiguity fluctuates by increasing and decreasing. The NPD team will however decide how much ambiguity — i.e., how many differing interpretations — to tolerate in each step of the process. AT, then, manifests itself along the vertical dimension, reflecting the amount of exploration done at each step, i.e., the *search scope* (Katila and Ahuja, 2002). The level of AT represents the amount of alternative interpretations that are considered and how many alternatives are kept open while moving forward. An NPD team following a strategy of high AT will thus "spread out" more along the vertical dimension than a team following a strategy of low AT.

However, when balancing the need to generate or sustain ambiguity on the one hand against the need to reduce ambiguity on the other, a team following a strategy of high AT will emphasize generation and sustention, whereas a team following a strategy of low AT will emphasize reduction of ambiguity, as shown in Figure 2.

Alpha and Beta were examples of companies following a high-AT strategy. They both allowed ambiguity to be sustained by pursuing competing product concepts in parallel and did not select a preferred product concept (i.e., fully reduce this ambiguity) until later in the NPD project. During an interview at a later stage of the project, an informant at Alpha stated "everything is being kept open" (referring to both target markets and product solutions). In the Delta case — by contrast — a new and competing interpretation of the product idea arose from the user environment during clinical prototype testing, but Delta was not willing to increase ambiguity by considering this interpretation and assessing it as an alternative to the one they had already chosen to pursue.

A main purpose of an NPD project is to develop a new and innovative product concept. To serve this purpose, assessing a variety of ideas by generating and making use of ambiguity is important. However, an NPD project must also conclude on a defined product to launch in a defined market, therefore ambiguity must eventually be reduced toward the end of the project. Ambiguity is thus more useful in the early phase than in the later phase of NPD. Whatever initial strategy the NPD team follows to manage ambiguity — be it high, moderate, or low AT — it therefore needs to shift toward lower AT when approaching the end of the NPD project. The fluctuations along the vertical dimension of the model in Figure 3 will thereby gradually decrease, as illustrated by the two dotted lines marked I and II. As AT decreases, so does contextual ambidexterity as the emphasis shifts from balancing exploration and exploitation toward pure exploitation near the end of the project. As the storylines in Section 5.1 indicate, the identified occurrences of ambiguity mainly appeared in the early phases of the NPD projects, with fewer occurrences near the end of the projects.

Ambiguity and AT are, thus, necessary to achieve ambidexterity. Absence of ambiguity in a project will greatly facilitate operational efficiency and exploitation, but will greatly jeopardize exploration and flexibility. Presence of ambiguity and tolerance for ambiguity allow for exploration and flexibility, but ambidexterity is only achieved when generation and sustention of ambiguity is combined with reduction of ambiguity in an alternating manner. The higher the level of AT, the wider the span of ambidexterity becomes as more exploration activities and more options for flexibility can be combined with exploitation. The model in Figure 3 complies with Sætre and Brun's (2012) concept of "targeted creativity" and broadens their discussion to include the concepts of AT and ambidexterity.

5.3. *Relations to other conceptions of ambidexterity*

Gibson and Birkinshaw (2004) have argued that contextual ambidexterity is achieved by creating a context that enables and encourages staff members to use their own judgments on how to divide their time between the conflicting demands of adaptation and alignment. I contend that such a context is indeed created when a working process is established within an NPD team where ambiguity is tolerated, but where the team understands when to shift between generation/suspension and reduction of ambiguity in the interest of advancing the innovation process. Such a context promotes a behavioral ability to simultaneously pursue both exploration and exploitation within the same organizational unit (e.g., the NPD team) and hence falls within what Simsek and colleagues (2009) have described as *harmonic ambidexterity* in their typology of OA. They refer to Bierly and Daly (2007) who argue that human resources practices that promote creativity will help sustain simultaneous pursuit of exploration and exploitation. I would add that the model shown in Figure 3 where ambiguity fluctuates as the product concept is developed aligns well with the view found in creativity literature of how ideas develop through steps of divergence and convergence (e.g., Basadur *et al.*, 2000; Lerdahl, 2001).

The model presented in Figure 3 views exploration and exploitation as orthogonal dimensions in accordance with the argument of Katila and Ahuja (2002), rather than being two ends of a one-dimensional scale. The model is also consistent with their operationalization of exploration as *search scope* and exploitation as *search depth*. When an NPD team allows generation of ambiguity by considering multiple interpretations of product concepts, then the span of interpretations that the NPD team allows represents their search scope. The greater the level of AT, the greater the search scope will be; but both will need to decrease toward the end of the innovation process. Similarly, when the NPD team reduces ambiguity by selecting an interpretation and moves rightward in the model in order to develop the product concept in more detail, then this movement represents an increase in *search depth*. The model also supports He and Wong's (2004) argument that an interaction between exploration and exploitation is needed to achieve innovation. The relation between ambiguity management and contextual ambidexterity shown in the presented model helps understand the nature of this interaction and how the balance between exploration and exploitation shifts throughout the innovation process.

Raisch *et al.* (2009) have discussed the issue of OA along a variety of dimensions. Among them are the individual vs organizational dimension and the static vs dynamic dimension.

5.3.1. *Static versus dynamic ambidexterity*

Brun and Sætre (2009) argued that managing ambiguity requires a harmonization between the need to sustain ambiguity for the sake of innovativeness and the need to reduce ambiguity for the sake of operational efficiency in the NPD project. From the discussion above, I argue that this harmonization is not a trade-off between two incompatible alternatives, nor is it a simple spatial or temporal separation of exploration and exploitation, as in what Gibson and Birkinshaw (2004) refer to as *structural ambidexterity*.

Admittedly, when managing ambiguity in innovation processes, the generation and the reduction of ambiguity are temporally separate rather than simultaneous. However, as seen in the storylines in Section 4.1, the NPD team had to be flexible in switching between ambiguity generation and reduction as the *situation* in the project evolved; hence, an organizational or process-related separation would be impractical. I therefore contend that managing ambiguity in innovation is a component of *contextual ambidexterity*.

Gibson and Birkinshaw (2004) define contextual ambidexterity as a capacity to *simultaneously* combine alignment and adaptability. Still, as Raisch and colleagues (2009) point out, Gibson and Birkinshaw (2004) do acknowledge that contextual ambidexterity has a dynamic component of alternating sequences, in that "individuals make their own judgments on how to best divide their time between the conflicting demands for alignment and adaptability" (p. 210). Raisch and colleagues (2009) suggest the term "sequential ambidexterity" (p. 688) to denote such a cyclical approach to ambidexterity, involving a dynamic, temporal sequencing of actions of exploration and exploitation. They do, however, suggest that such cycles of explorative and exploitative activities at an individual level are shorter and more tightly coupled than the exploration–exploitation cycles that have been described at the corporate level (e.g., Nickerson and Zenger, 2002; Siggelkow and Levinthal, 2003). This conception of *sequential ambidexterity* aligns well with the medium-range rate of ambiguity generation and reduction at NPD team level that was observed in the four cases in this study.

5.3.2. *Individual versus organizational ambidexterity*

According to Raisch and Birkinshaw (2009), in most studies addressing organizational mechanisms of ambidexterity, the tensions created by ambidexterity are considered resolved at a lower organizational level. Therefore, although the unit of analysis in this study was the project team, it is in order to suggest implications at the individual level.

The sequential nature of exploration–exploitation cycles with generation and reduction of ambiguity accords with Schön's (1983, pp. 241–254) account of how managers practice *reflection-in-action*. Reflection-in-action, he claims, involves *interpreting* market phenomena, *interpreting* organizational troubles and *learning* (i.e., developing new knowledge) about product development. But it also involves experimentation (Schön, 1983, pp. 141–156). One category of experimentation is *exploratory* experiments which, he exemplifies, is what a newcomer does when wandering around in a new neighborhood. This, I will add, involves sensing cues and interpreting them, i.e., an interpretive process, which in turn can lead to ambiguity if multiple participants sense the same cues. Another category of experiments Schön (1983) presents is *hypothesis-testing* experiments, which he claims the practitioner uses to discriminate among competing hypotheses. This accords with Brun and Sætre's argument (2008) of how NPD project participants reduce ambiguity, since ambiguity has the form of competing hypotheses. Schön (1983), thus, contends that managers solve problems as reflective practitioners by framing the problem, conducting experiments, and then reframe the problem and continue in cycles of reframing and experimenting, which I contend is similar to the process illustrated in the model in Figure 4. Since the reflective process involves both interpretation and hypothesis testing, it requires alternating between interpretive and analytic skills.

In all of the cases in this study, the project manager was an important informant. A project manager typically needs to act across organizational units and hierarchical levels to ensure that project goals are met. In this position, the project manager has an important role in managing ambiguity. He or she will be faced with cues both from higher and lower organizational levels, from different business units, and from the company's external environment. He or she needs to interpret these cues and forward the meaning intended by the sender to a receiver. The sender and the receiver will be from different organizational levels or units and, hence, represent different thought worlds. The project manager, hence, has an important role as an *interpreter* in the NPD process, a role that requires a sensitivity to identify differences in meaning, i.e., ambiguity. The project manager also has the main responsibility to determine when to sustain ambiguity in the project for the sake of achieving innovation and flexibility and when to reduce ambiguity for the sake of efficiency. The project manager must possess a high tolerance for ambiguity in order to achieve innovation, but must lower his or her tolerance for ambiguity when operational demands for project efficiency need to take priority. This view of the project manager's important role in maintaining ambidexterity through generation, sustention, and reduction of ambiguity aligns with the findings by Mom *et al.* (2009); that a manager's participation in cross-functional interfaces and his/her connectedness to other organization members are positively related to ambidexterity.

Raisch and colleagues (2009) refer to studies (e.g., O'Reilly and Tushman, 2004; Probst and Raisch, 2005) that observe that some managers are more able than others to take on contradictory tasks, but they also claim that these studies do not offer explanation of *why* these managers — as opposed to others — are able to do so. Such explanations, they suggest, may be found in the personal characteristics of managers. They refer to the work of Smith and Tushman (2005) who argue that effectively managing strategic contradictions is associated with paradoxical cognition and suggest that a manager's ability to engage in paradoxical thinking may play a vital role in managing exploitation and exploration. Smith and Tushman's (2005) study draws on organizational literature on paradox, contradiction, and conflict including the research of Lewis (2000) who, interestingly, repeatedly refers to *ambiguity* in her account of the paradox concept, although she does not specifically tie her discussion to the concept of AT.

5.4. *Limitations*

There are some notable limitations to this study. Two of the cases (Alpha and Gamma) were studied in real time, whereas the two others (Beta and Delta) were studied retrospectively. Common sources of error in retrospective studies are memory loss and retrospective rationality, which may have contributed to finding fewer occurrences of ambiguity in the retrospectively studied cases. On the other hand, it can be argued that the informants in these cases were able — in hindsight — to speak with greater clarity of what actually happened than they could have while the project was ongoing. This effect may then have contributed to finding more occurrences of ambiguity in the retrospective cases. It is therefore difficult to say whether the results of the analysis would have been different had all cases been studied in real time.

In this study, the unit of analysis has been the NPD project, which has limited the ability to study AT characteristics and ambidexterity at the individual manager level. However, since idea development in an NPD project is a team effort and not just the result of managerial decisions, I would argue that the level of AT at the team level results not only from the AT level of the team's manager but possibly also from the AT levels of team members in a variety of roles. I therefore suggest future research to study how AT among individuals in both managerial and non-managerial roles contribute to contextual ambidexterity.

Gibson and Birkinshaw (2004) suggest that there may be different paths to ambidexterity; hence, in a study of contextual ambidexterity, the context of the study is of particular importance. The context of this study was limited to NPD projects in established Scandinavian medical device companies. Although the findings did not show any clear links to characteristics of the medical device industry, one may expect that choosing case companies in other industry contexts could have yielded somewhat different results. Other industry contexts that could be explored include other industry types (e.g., consumer goods, software, and energy) and companies of different ages and sizes (e.g., start-ups versus small and large established businesses). Also, since AT may differ across organizational and national cultures (Furnham and Ribchester, 1995; Hofstede, 2001), the influence of company culture and management style should be explored, both within the chosen geographical region (Scandinavia) and across national boundaries.

Being based on qualitative analysis of a contextually limited sample of four cases, the findings cannot be generalized to be valid across all industry contexts. However, having followed prescribed procedures for the GT method and classical content analysis, the presented model is well grounded in the case data. Also, as far as possible, the research process from data to conclusion has been made as transparent as possible, in accordance with recommended trustworthiness-building measures in qualitative studies (Miles and Huberman, 1994), to enable the reader to judge whether the findings are transferrable to other contexts. The presented findings should therefore provide a well-founded basis for further research in other contexts and for further scrutiny through quantitative methods.

6. Conclusion

This chapter has presented a model by which the relation between ambiguity management and contextual ambidexterity can be understood. The model contends that ambiguity management is an underlying process supporting ambidexterity and that the level of AT determines the potential to exercise ambidexterity: The higher the AT, the greater the span of ambidexterity that can be exercised. Contextual ambidexterity in NPD is achieved by generating and sustaining ambiguity and reducing it in cycles throughout the innovation project, and this nature of the process aligns with Raisch and colleagues' (2009) conception of sequential ambidexterity. Requisite variety, interpretive capability, and capability of perspective-taking are factors leading to the generation of ambiguity, while analytic capability is needed to reduce ambiguity.

The research in this chapter contributes to meet the need for theory to better understand the phenomenon of contextual ambidexterity. First, this research adds to the sparse research literature on ambidexterity at the project team level, thus complementing the predominant corporate or top management level focus of previous ambidexterity research. Furthermore, introducing AT and ambiguity management as new parameters in the behavioral approach to contextual ambidexterity provides a more detailed understanding of the phenomenon of contextual ambidexterity compared to earlier research. Grounded in the empirical data, it suggests and explains relationships between — on the one hand — AT, ambiguity management and — on the other hand — different conceptions of ambidexterity as well as concepts in extant ambidexterity research, such as exploration versus exploitation, search scope, and search depth.

This research can be useful to managers to understand in more specific detail than earlier how to achieve ambidexterity in their project team. By first composing project teams with requisite variety and selecting team members who possess perspective-taking ability, AT, and a combination of interpretive and analytic skills, and second alternating between ambiguity generation and reduction as the project situation requires, they will be better able to exercise contextual ambidexterity in their innovation projects.

References

Ahmed, P. K. (1998). Culture and Climate for Innovation, *European Journal of Innovation and Management*, 1, 30–43.

Aldrich, H. (1999). *Organizations Evolving*, Sage Publications, Thousand Oaks, CA.

Ashby, W. R. (1956). *An Introduction to Cybernetics*, John Wiley & Sons Inc.,

Basadur, M., Pringle, P., Speranzini, G. and Bacot, M. (2000). Collaborative problem solving through creativity in problem definition: Expanding the pie, *Creative and Innovation Management*, 9, 54–76.

Begley, T. M. and Boyd, D. P. (1987). Psychological characteristics associated with performance in entrepreneurial firms and smaller businesses, *Journal of Business Venturing*, 2, 79–93.

Benner, M. J. and Tushman, M. L. (2003). Exploitation, exploration, and process management: The productivity dilemma revisited, *Academic Management Review*, 28, 238–256.

Bierly, P. E. and Daly, P. S. (2007). Alternative knowledge strategies, competitive environment, and organizational performance in small manufacturing firms, *Entrepreneurship: Theory & Practice*, 31, 493–516.

Boland, R. J. and Tenkasi, R. V. (1995). Perspective making and perspective taking in communities of knowing, *Organization Science*, 6, 350–372.

Brown, S. and Eisenhardt, K. (1995). Product development: Past research, present findings, and future directions, *Academic Management Review*, 20, 343–378.

Brun, E. and Sætre, A. S. (2008). Ambiguity reduction in new product development projects, *International Journal of Innovation Management*, 12, 573–596.

Brun, E. and Sætre, A. S. (2009). Managing ambiguity in new product development, *Creative and Innovative Management*, 18, 24–34.

Brun, E., Sætre, A. S. and Gjelsvik, M. (2008). Benefits of ambiguity in new product development, *International Journal of Innovation and Technology Management*, 5, 303–319.

Brun, E., Sætre, A. S. and Gjelsvik, M. (2009). Classification of ambiguity in new product development projects, *European Journal of Innovative Management*, 12, 62–85.

Budner, S. (1962). Intolerance of ambiguity as a personality variable, *Journal of Personality*, 30, 29.

Burgelman, R. A. (1983). A process model of internal corporate venturing in the diversified major firm, *Administrative Science Quarterly*, 28, 223–244.

Burns, T. and Stalker, G. M. (1961). *The Management of Innovation*, Tavistock, London.

Burrell, G. and Morgan, G. (1979). *Sociological Paradigms and Organisational Analysis*, Heinemann, London.

Carmeli, A. and Halevi, M. Y. (2009). How top management team behavioral integration and behavioral complexity enable organizational ambidexterity: The moderating role of contextual ambidexterity, *The Leadership Quarterly*, 20, 207–218.

Cegarra-Navarro, J. G. and Dewhurst, F. (2007). Linking organizational learning and customer capital through an ambidexterity context: An empirical investigation in SMEs, *International Journal of Human Resource Management*, 18, 1720–1735.

Daft, R. L. and Lengel, R. H. (1986). Organizational information requirements, media richness and structural design, *Management Science*, 32, 554–571.

Dougherty, D. (1992). Interpretive barriers to successful product innovation in large firms, *Organization Science*, 3, 179–202.

Eisenberg, E. (1984). Ambiguity as strategy in organizational communication, *Communication Monograph*, 51, 227–242.

Eisenhardt, K. M. and Tabrizi, B. (1995). Accelerating adaptive processes: Product innovation in the global computer industry, *Administrative Science Quarterly*, 40, 84–110.

Furnham, A. and Ribchester, T. (1995). Tolerance of ambiguity: A review of the concept, its measurement and applications, *Current Psychology*, 14, 179.

Galbraith, J. (1974). Organization design: An information processing view, *Interfaces*, 4, 28–36.

Gibson, C. B. and Birkinshaw, J. (2004). The antecedents, consequences, and mediating role of organizational ambidexterity, *Academic Management Journal*, 47, 209–226.

Griffin, A., Hoffmann, N., Price, R. L. and Vojak, B. A. (2007). How serial innovators navigate the fuzzy front end of new product development, *ISBM Report*, Institute for the Study of Business Markets, The Pennsylvania State University, 3.

Gupta, A. K., Smith, K. G. and Shalley, C. E. (2006). The interplay between exploration and exploitation, *Academic Management Journal*, 49, 693–706.

Harvey, O. J., Hunt, D. E. and Schroder, H. M. (1961). *Conceptual Systems and Personality Organization*, Wiley New York, NY.

He, Z.-L. and Wong, P.-K. (2004). Exploration vs. Exploitation: An empirical test of the ambidexterity hypothesis, *Organization Science*, 15, 481–494.

Hofstede, G. (2001). *Culture's Consequences: Comparing Values, Behaviors, Institutions and Organizations across Nations*, 2nd edn., Sage Publications, Thousand Oaks, CA.

Janis, I. L. (1982). *Groupthink: Psychological Studies of Policy Decisions and Fiascoes*, Houghton Mifflin, Boston.

Katila, R. and Ahuja, G. (2002). Something old, something new: A longitudinal study of search behavior and new product introduction, *Academic Management Journal*, 45, 1183–1194.

Khurana, A. and Rosenthal, S. R. (1997). Integrating the fuzzy front end of new product development, *Sloan Management Review*, 38, 103–120.

Khurana, A. and Rosenthal, S. R. (1998). Towards holistic front ends in new product development, *Journal of Product Innovative Management*, 15, 57–74.

Lane, D. and Maxfield, R. (1996). Strategy under complexity: Fostering generative relationships, *Long Range Planning*, 29, 215–231.

Leonard, D. and Sensiper, S. (1998). The role of tacit knowledge in group innovation, *California Management Review*, 40, 112–132.

Lerdahl, E. (2001). Staging for creative collaboration in design teams; models, tools and methods, PhD thesis, Dept. of Product Design, Norwegian University of Science and Technology, Trondheim.

Lester, R. and Piore, M. (2004). *Innovation — The Missing Dimension*, Harvard University Press, Cambridge, MA.

Lewis, M. W. (2000). Exploring paradox: Toward a more comprehensive guide, *Academic Management Review*, 25, 760–776.
Lubatkin, M. H., Simsek, Z., Ling, Y. and Veiga, J. F. (2006). Ambidexterity and performance in small- to medium-sized firms: The pivotal role of top management team behavioral integration, *Journal of Management*, 32, 646–672.
MacCormack, A. and Verganti, R. (2003). Managing the sources of uncertainty: Matching process and context in software development, *Journal of Product Innovative Management*, 20, 217–232.
Magnusson, M. G. and Martini, A. (2008). Dual organizational capabilities: From theory to practice — The next challenge for continuous innovation, *International Journal of Technology Management*, 42, 1–19.
Magnusson, M. G., Boccardelli, P. and Börjesson, S. (2009). Managing the efficiency-flexibility tension in innovation: Strategic and organizational aspects, *Creative and Innovative Management*, 18, 2–7.
March, J. G. (1991). Exploration and exploitation in organizational learning, *Organization Science*, 2, 71–87.
Miles, M. B. and Huberman, A. M. (1984). *Qualitative Data Analysis*, Sage Publications, Beverly Hills, CA.
Miles, M. B. and Huberman, A. M. (1994). *Qualitative Data Analysis*, 2nd edn., Sage Publications, Thousand Oaks, CA.
Moenaert, R. K., De Meyer, A., Souder, W. E. and Deschoolmeester, D. (1995). R&D/marketing communication during the fuzzy front-end, *IEEE Transactions on Engineering Management*, 42, 243–258.
Mom, T. J. M., van den Bosch, F. A. J. and Volberda, H. W. (2009). Understanding variation in managers' ambidexterity: Investigating direct and interaction effects of formal structural and personal coordination mechanisms, *Organization Science*, 20, 812–828.
Neuliep, J. W. and Hazleton, V. (1986). Enhanced conversational recall and reduced conversational interference as a function of cognitive complexity, *Human Communication Research*, 13, 211–224.
Nickerson, J. A. and Zenger, T. R. (2002). Being efficiently fickle: A dynamic theory of organizational choice, *Organization Science*, 13, 547–566.
Nonaka, I. (1994). A dynamic theory of organizational knowledge creation, *Organization Science*, 5, 14–37.
Nonaka, I. and Takeuchi, H. (1995). *The Knowledge -Creating Company. How Japanese Companies Create the Dynamics of Innovation.* Oxford University Press, New York, NY.

O'Reilly, C. A. and Tushman, M. (2004). The Ambidextrous Organization. *Harvard Business Review*, 82; 74–81.

Probst, G. and Raisch, S. (2005). Organizational Crisis: The Logic of Failure. *Academy of Managament Executive*, 19; 90–105.

Putnam, L. L. (1983). The interpretive perspective: An alternative to functionalism, in Putnam, L. L. and Pacanowski, M. E. (eds.), *Communications and Organizations: An Interpretive Approach*, Sage Publications, Thousand Oaks, CA.

Raisch, S. and Birkinshaw, J. (2008). Organizational ambidexterity: Antecedents, outcomes, and moderators, *Journal of Management*, 34, 375–409.

Raisch, S., Birkinshaw, J., Probst, G. and Tushman, M. L. (2009). Organizational ambidexterity: Balancing exploitation and exploration for sustained performance, *Organization Science*, 20, 685–695.

Reid, S. and de Brentani, U. (2004). The fuzzy front end of new product development for discontinuous innovations: A theoretical model, *Journal of Product Innovative Management*, 21, 170–184.

Rosing, K., Frese, M. and Bausch, A. (2011). Explaining the heterogeneity of the leadership-innovation relationship: Ambidextrous leadership, *The Leadership Quarterly*, 22, 956–974.

Sarasvathy, S. D. and Dew, N. (2005). New market creation through transformation, *Journal of Evolutionary Economics*, 15, 533–565.

Satish, U. (1997). Behavioral complexity: A review, *Journal of Applied Social Psychology*, 27, 2047–2067.

Schere, J. L. (1982). Tolerance of ambiguity as a discriminating variable between entrepreneurs and managers, *Annual Meeting of the Academy of Management*.

Schön, D. A. (1983). *The Reflective Practitioner*, Basic Books.

Siggelkow, N. and Levinthal, D. A. (2003). Temporarily divide to conquer: Centralized, decentralized, and reintegrated organizational approaches to exploration and adaptation, *Organization Science*, 14, 650–669.

Simsek, Z. (2009). Organizational ambidexterity: Towards a multilevel understanding, *Journal of Management Studies*, 46, 597–624.

Simsek, Z., Heavey, C., Veiga, J. F. and Souder, D. (2009). A typology for aligning organizational ambidexterity's conceptualizations, antecedents, and outcomes, *Journal of Management Studies*, 46, 864–894.

Smith, W. K. and Tushman, M. L. (2005). Managing strategic contradictions: A top management model for managing innovation streams, *Organization Science*, 16, 522–536.

Strauss, A. and Corbin, J. (1998). *Basics of Qualitative Research. Techniques and Procedures for Developing Grounded Theory*, 2nd edn., Sage Publications, Thousand Oaks, CA.

Sutcliffe, K. M., Sitkin, S. B. and Browning, L. D. (2000). Tailoring process management to situational requirements; beyond the control and exploration dichotomy, in Cole, R. E. and Scott, W. R. (eds.), *The Quality Movement and Organization Theory*, Sage Publications, Thousand Oaks, CA.

Sætre, A. S. and Brun, E. (2012). Strategic management of innovation: Managing exploration-exploitation by balancing creativity and constraint, *International Journal of Innovation and Technology Management*, 9.

Thompson, J. D. (1967). *Organizations in Action*, MacGraw-Hill, New York, NY.

Tushman, M. L. and O'Reilly, C. A. (1996). Ambidextrous organizations: Managing evolutionary and revolutionary change, *California Management Review*, 38, 8–30.

Tushman, M. L. and O'Reilly, C. A. (1997). *Winning Through Innovation: A Practical Guide to Leading Organizational Change and Renewal*, Harvard Business School Press, Boston, MA.

Verganti, R. (1999). Planned Flexibility: Linking Anticipation and Reaction in Product Development Projects. *Journal of Prod. Innovation Management*, 16, 363–376.

Weick, K. E. (1979). *The Social Psychology of Organizing*, 2nd edn., McGraw-Hill, New York, NY.

Weick, K. E. (1995). *Sensemaking in Organizations*, Sage Publications, Thousand Oaks, CA.

Zhang, Q. and Doll, W. (2001). The fuzzy front end and success of new product development: A causal model, *European Journal of Innovation Management*, 4, 95–112.

Chapter 11

Benefits of Ambiguity

Eric Christian Brun[*,§], Alf Steinar Sætre[†,¶] and Martin Gjelsvik[‡,||]

[*]*Department of Safety, Economics and Planning,*
University of Stavanger, Norway

[†]*Department of Industrial Economics and Technology Management,*
Norwegian University of Science and Technology, Norway

[‡]*NORCE Norwegian Research Centre, Norway*

[§]*eric.brun@uis.no*

[¶]*alfs@iot.ntnu.no*

[||]*martin.gjelsvik@iris.no*

Abstract

In this chapter, we challenge the traditional notion of ambiguity as an undesirable element in New Product Development (NPD) and explore how companies sometimes sustain or even increase ambiguity during their NPD projects. Based on qualitative analysis of case data from four NPD projects in the medical devices industry, we present a model by which this process can be better understood. We identify four ways that NPD projects can benefit from temporarily sustaining ambiguity: retaining fallback options, saving costs, saving time, and retaining ideas.

Keywords: New product development, ambiguity, qualitative research.

1. Introduction and Background Theory

Numerous researchers over the past few decades have sought to help us understand and manage New Product Development (NPD) processes (e.g., Cooper, 1993, 1994; Griffin, 1997; Rothwell, 1994). Many of the models in use are variants of the so-called "stage-gate" models (Cooper and Kleinschmidt, 1993). But traditional stage-gate models, with their formal, sequential, and linear nature, have been argued to be less than suitable for managing projects in contexts of high levels of uncertainty and rapidly changing environments, characteristics that typify many innovation projects (Eisenhardt and Tabrizi, 1995; MacCormack *et al.*, 2001; Poolton, 2000; Veryzer, 1998). The problem is especially prevalent in the earliest stage of development, which is characterized by considerable uncertainty and ambiguity, characteristics that don't fit well with the requirement for accurate up-front information that's needed for a sequential process of planning and subsequent execution. This phenomenon is commonly recognized in literature as the "Fuzzy Front End" of NPD (Kim and Wilemon, 2002; Koen *et al.*, 2001; Reid and Brentani, 2004).

A common approach to managing the Fuzzy Front End of NPD has been to try to significantly reduce, or ideally eliminate, the uncertainty and ambiguity inherent in NPD processes, in order to enable the use of sequential and linear models (Montoya-Weiss and O'Driscoll, 2000; Zhang and Doll, 2001). An alternative approach taken by several authors emphasizes the accommodation of flexibility in the NPD processes. Eisenhardt and Tabrizi (1995) and MacCormack (1998) have argued that in environments with high levels of uncertainty, projects tend to adopt processes with greater flexibility. MacCormack and colleagues (MacCormack *et al.*, 2001; MacCormack and Verganti, 2003) have further shown that in one such environment — the Internet software industry — constructs that support a more flexible process are associated with better performance. Such a flexible process is characterized by iteration, learning, and adaptation, together with the ability to generate and respond to new information for a longer proportion of the development cycle, in contrast to the commonly used stage-gate models, characterized by a sequential process of planning and execution. Specifically, the term "investment in architectural design" (MacCormack and Verganti, 2003) entails enabling the product architecture to accommodate to changing requirements, an issue addressed earlier on a more general level by Rothwell (1994). Another alternative approach has been presented by Lester and Piore (2004), who contend that NPD involves two fundamental processes. The first one is analysis, understood as rational problem-solving, which — they claim — dominates management and engineering practice. The second process is interpretation, understood as coping with and even exploiting ambiguity, a process not widely understood but, according to their argument, crucial to innovation.

Several theoretical contributions comment on the important distinction between uncertainty and ambiguity (Daft and Lengel, 1984, 1986; March, 1994; Weick, 1995). They argue that uncertainty can be understood as lack of information; hence, uncertainty can be reduced by providing more information. In contrast, ambiguity can be understood as different interpretations of the same piece of information, caused by actors interpreting the information from different frames of reference. Hence, ambiguity isn't reduced by providing more information but rather through a communicative process that allows stakeholders to arrive at a common interpretation. We believe that ambiguity according to this description represents much of the "fuzziness" as experienced by practitioners at the "Fuzzy Front End" of NPD. We also suggest that ambiguity isn't limited to the Front End, but may be present throughout the NPD process. We do, however, expect the likelihood of encountering ambiguity to be highest in the early phases of NPD.

Previous research on NPD has emphasized the terms "uncertainty" and "flexibility", but, as indicated by Lester and Piore (2004), there is a lack of theory specifically addressing management of ambiguity, as distinct from uncertainty, in NPD projects.

A common assumption in management literature is that ambiguity is undesirable and should be reduced to provide clarity. An alternative view, offered by Eric Eisenberg (1984), contends that clarity isn't necessarily a sensible standard of organizational effectiveness. He says that maintaining a "strategic ambiguity" serves an important function of maintaining flexibility and maneuverability in unstable, changing situations. We ourselves contend that NPD processes often take place under unstable, unpredictable, and changing situations, especially when developing radically new products and that this warrants our researching whether NPD processes may actually benefit from not fully clarifying all ambiguous issues.

Evolutionary approaches to innovation argue that innovations develop through processes of variation and selection (Aldrich, 1999; Burgelman, 2002), implying that the innovation process may not always be steadily moving toward lesser and lesser ambiguity. Ambiguity may actually increase variation by developing a higher number of new combinations. Similarly, creativity theory describes how innovation processes can go through stages of divergence and convergence (Basadur *et al.*, 2000; Lerdahl, 2001). Aldrich (1999) and Burgelman (2002), however, address organizational and strategic business innovation processes and not NPD processes at the project level.

The objective of this chapter is to explore whether and how sustaining ambiguity may play a role in managing NPD projects.

2. Method

2.1. *Research design*

Our research design is a holistic multiple-case study design (Yin, 1994) with the NPD project being our unit of analysis. Each case was an NPD project in its early phase, being run by an established company in the medical devices industry. We applied this constraint both to limit the number of extraneous variables and to collect data where we expected to find most of what we were studying (Eisenhardt, 1989). For our purposes, cases from the medical devices industry were appropriate because this industry is characterized by (1) a high rate of NPD, (2) a high degree of knowledge and complexity within both the R&D and engineering functions and the clinical customer environment (hence a greater likelihood of encountering ambiguity), and (3) a high degree of structured NPD methodology. Further, we focused our study on the earliest phases of the selected NPD projects, because that was where we expected to find most occurrences of ambiguity.

We studied four cases — three cases in Norway and one in Denmark. Two of the cases were followed in real time as they evolved, and we collected data by interviews, observations, and document review. The two other cases were studied retrospectively; hence, direct observations weren't possible, so we collected there solely through interviews and document review. Our data, collected over three years from March 2004 to August 2007, consists of 46 interviews, 7 hours of meeting observation, 913 pages of archival data, and 17 video files. To preserve confidentiality, we have substituted pseudonyms for all names in the following case narratives and in all references to case data.

2.2. *Analysis method*

For the purpose of this study, we define *ambiguity* as "the existence of two or more interpretations of a single cue". A "cue" in this respect can be a piece of oral or written information, a physical artifact, or a situation. The first step of our analysis was to build a conceptual framework based on our definition of ambiguity, to guide our data analysis.

Figure 1 shows the conceptual framework that we used as the starting point for our analysis. The lines represent the *act of interpreting* the cue, and each box at the right end of the line

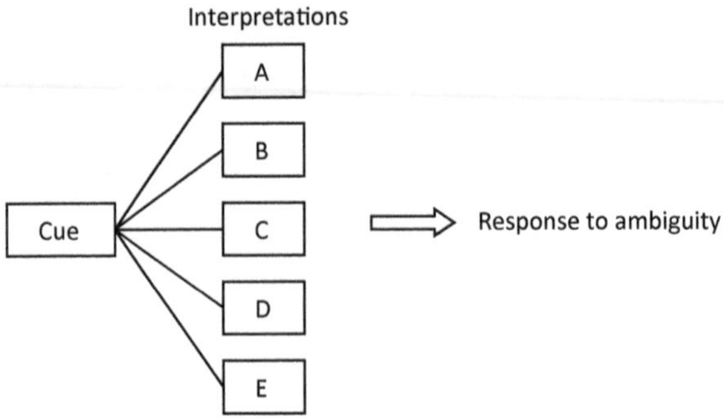

Figure 1. Conceptual framework.

represents *the resulting interpretation* of the cue. Several actors participating in the NPD process may interpret a cue, and so the cue may be assigned various interpretations, illustrated as A–E in our conceptual model.

The ambiguity in the situation is represented by the presence of these multiple interpretations, and the participants in the project will need to respond to this ambiguity.

When utilizing the conceptual model to analyze our data, we first searched the data for cues that were interpreted with two or more meanings, thus, identifying occurrences of ambiguity based on our definition of the term. We then coded these occurrences according to how the participants in the projects had responded to the occurrences of ambiguity. The findings fell into two broad categories: (1) actions that led to reduction of ambiguity, and (2) actions that led to sustention or increase of ambiguity. This chapter focuses on the second of these two categories.

Actions that sustained ambiguity were further coded by constant comparison to data and to informing theory (Charmaz, 2006; Eisenhardt, 1989; Glaser and Strauss, 1967; Orton, 1997; Strauss and Corbin, 1998), using the software tool NVivo7 to structure the analysis process. Analysis was performed in cycles, each cycle consisting of four steps: (1) identifying and comparing occurrences of ambiguity, (2) identifying and comparing actions that sustained ambiguity, (3) coding these actions, and (4) refining the conceptual framework. The comparisons in steps 1 and 2 were performed within each case as well as across the four cases. We repeated the cycles until no new findings occurred and until our conceptual framework had developed into a model that was simple yet still fit our data.

3. Case Descriptions

3.1. *Case 1: Project "The Snapper" at Alpha Medical*

Alpha Medical is a globally operating company that develops, manufactures, and markets products for emergency medical treatment and training. Alpha perceived two needs in the market. The first one was related to first aid treatment. When giving first aid to patients, rescuers often need to perform certain compression maneuvers, but there was a growing concern in the market that the rescuers often didn't perform these compressions with sufficient quality. The second need was related to first aid training; organizations providing first aid training expressed a need to deliver their courses in a more cost-efficient manner. Alpha therefore pursued two product ideas. The first one was a device, called "the Snapper", that could be placed on a patient during the compression maneuver. Each time the rescuer had performed a compression correctly, the Snapper would provide audible feedback. The rescuer could also use the device while being trained in a first aid course and then include it in a first aid kit and use it on a real patient when needed. The other product idea was a new complete training system that would radically reduce training time in first aid courses. This system could potentially include the Snapper.

Alpha experienced several challenges within its project: One was to create a device that performed both accurately and consistently, yet was also reasonably priced. Creating a single product solution that served the needs optimally for both the training and the therapy application also proved problematic.

Multiple interpretations of product alternatives arose as Alpha considered what different market segments to target. Whether aiming at the training or the therapy market, Alpha had to provide evidence of the product's effectiveness. The operating principle of the device became an issue of controversy, too. The US Food and Drug Administration (FDA) interpreted the Snapper's operating principle as conflicting with a current requirement that had to be met to allow access to the US therapy market. Alpha's project was organized with many parallel activities, so internal communication proved a challenge, too. On top of all this, there was a considerable sense of urgency within the project.

3.2. *Case 2: Project "Patient compliance" at Beta Medical*

Beta Medical is a globally operating company offering product solutions for drug delivery to ensure "patient compliance", which can be defined as the degree to which patients adhere to a prescribed treatment scheme. Prior to 2001, Beta's experience included product solutions for patient compliance to treatments with inhaled and injected drugs. Beta now wanted to develop a product for treatments requiring pill medication. Pursuing their ambition, Beta developed a multitude of product ideas. Two of these (here designated Hi-tech and Lo-tech) were chosen for development independent of each other. Lo-tech was to be a very user-friendly and inexpensive device that could be carried by the patient as a pill container including a very simple but effective reminder and feedback function. Hi-tech represented a pricier product solution with more advanced data management and reporting features. Thus Hi-tech and Lo-tech were alternative interpretations of a product solution.

The main stakeholder groups in the market were the patients, the general practitioners, clinical research organizations, and the pharmaceutical companies. To develop the

Lo-tech idea into a product, it was necessary to arrive at a product concept that had the necessary emotional appeal to a sensitive patient group, while being both efficient in ensuring patient compliance and relatively cheap. Adding to the challenge, the Lo-tech idea was developed into a product concept through a novel development process that previously hadn't been tried at Beta Medical.

Although Hi-tech was the product concept favored by top management, it turned out that Lo-tech was the product concept preferred by the pharmaceutical customers. Once this preference was clear, Beta urgently had to develop the Lo-tech concept further into a final product and start delivery to its customers.

3.3. *Case 3: Project "cardiac surgery imaging" at Gamma Medical*

Gamma Medical is a small company specializing in ultrasound equipment for quality control in cardiac and vascular surgery. Gamma Medical wanted to address a problem related to cardiac bypass operations. During such operations, it's a recommended procedure to verify the quality of the new blood-flow pattern before closing up the patient. This is done by measuring the blood flow at specific points in the coronary arteries and assessing a combination of curve shapes and numeric data on a monitor. In practice, this quality control is not always performed. Gamma Medical's idea was to provide the cardiac surgeon with an improved diagnostic tool in the form of an ultrasound two-dimensional color image for easier and quicker clinical assessment of the blood-flow quality. To achieve this, Gamma needed to develop a new graphic user interface and introduce it to a group of users (cardiac surgeons) who weren't accustomed to interpreting images as part of their medical procedures. Interpretation of images related to bypass surgery is usually done by cardiologists (before and after — not during — the operation) and anesthetists (who have a different role from the cardiac surgeon during the operation). Implementing the innovation would therefore necessitate a certain shift in roles and expertise among the physicians — a potential area of conflict. Also, even though the innovation would enable better quality control over the operation, the idea was perceived as somewhat threatening to some cardiac surgeons who by habit didn't emphasize such quality control.

Gamma developed its technology in partnership with other small companies. This gave rise to a heavy technology focus from the start of the project, with simultaneous technology and concept development; there was no clear division between a concept development and a product development phase.

3.4. *Case 4: Project "Laparoscopic surgery" at Delta Medical*

Delta Medical is a small company that originated in a technological research environment. Their business plan was based on two product ideas. The first one, called the "LapDop", was a product for ultrasound Doppler guidance during laparoscopic surgery. The other one, called the "BrainSound", was a product for ultrasound guidance during brain surgery. The first invention became the subject of this case study.

Laparoscopic surgery, commonly called "keyhole surgery", is a technique that allows the surgeon to operate through very small incisions in the patient's skin. A rod equipped with a light source and a video lens is introduced through one incision, and operating instruments are introduced through the other incisions. The surgeon can then perform the operation while watching an image on a television monitor. However, blood vessels residing under tissue surface can't be seen by this optical technique, so there is a risk of accidentally cutting them during the operating procedure. The LapDop represented Delta's idea to solve this problem. The LapDop concept included using a sheath fitted with an ultrasound probe that could be attached at the end of the operating instrument. This would enable the surgeon to detect hidden blood vessels through sound feedback.

Delta developed the product concept and prototype in close cooperation with a leading laparoscopic surgeon and conducted several trials of the LapDop to document its clinical usefulness. Still, the response from the market was less than enthusiastic — clinicians quoted a variety of objections to the device. It also became clearer to Delta that the actual customers of the product would be the hospitals' purchasing officers, rather than the clinicians — who were the users.

Complicating matters further, Delta did not have the resources to take both their new products to market simultaneously. Both products were based on ultrasound technology, but their target market segments and business models were very different. Delta's investors favored pursuing the "BrainSound", so early in 2003, Delta's board decided to give priority to that product. Delta made a last attempt to find a way to commercialize LapDop in cooperation with other medical devices suppliers, but did not succeed. Consequently, the project was shelved in early 2006.

4. Analysis

Our analysis revealed that the occurrences of ambiguity sustention fell into four categories, the common characteristic of which was a benefit achieved by sustaining ambiguity. The categories were as follows: (1) retaining fallback options, (2) saving costs, (3) saving time, and (4) retaining product ideas.

4.1. *Retaining fallback options by sustaining ambiguity*

Faced with ambiguity and the need to reduce it, the actors in a situation will discuss, test out alternative interpretations, or negotiate in order to arrive at a commonly agreed interpretation. Ambiguity may also be reduced without this process of dialogue if a leader or expert exercises his or her authority and unilaterally decides on one interpretation. Either way, the selection process is based on assumptions held by the involved actors, and these assumptions may or may not be valid. If they later prove invalid, and if all other interpretations have been eliminated, the company will have no options for further progress in its NPD process. By not fully reducing ambiguity, however, and instead by leaving certain interpretations open, the project will retain these as fallback options, should the assumptions underlying the selected interpretation fail.

In the Alpha case, the Snapper was considered in several options for product solutions for a considerable length of time. Some of these options proposed different measurement principles; another proposed using the Snapper as a separate device; still another proposed using the Snapper as a device built into a training manikin. All of these proposals were held open throughout the early phase of development, resulting in a product concept flexible enough to cater to multiple options. In addition, there were multiple interpretations of the target market, based on assumptions of customer perceptions, sales volumes, and diffusion dynamics. This, too, was an ambiguity that was kept open to maintain flexibility, should they need to adjust their launch strategy. During an interview at a later stage of the project, the Product Director for therapy products stated, "Everything is being kept open" (referring to both target markets and product solutions), indicating that this was a deliberate strategy by Alpha.

In the Beta case, its two alternative interpretations of the patient compliance product solution, Hi-tech and Lo-tech, were pursued as parallel development efforts. This was a sustention of ambiguity in order to keep strategic options open. If one concept failed, then the other would still be an available option.

4.2. *Saving costs by sustaining ambiguity*

Our analysis revealed a category of ambiguity sustention occurrences that was associated with cost savings. Developing two or more alternative concepts in parallel is normally more costly than developing only one, so logic would suggest that a company would seek to reduce ambiguity in a project to cut costs. But measures taken to reduce ambiguity may also incur costs. Such costs could involve, for example, performing external tests or convening people from different locations for meetings. Full reduction of ambiguity might therefore prove cost-prohibitive, or at least not cost-effective. Participants in the Alpha case continually assessed the cost of clarifying an ambiguous issue against the benefit of clarifying. Alternative interpretations of a cue were occasionally left open because eliminating them, while deemed desirable, was considered too costly compared to the benefit that would be achieved by clarification. But even this assessment was performed at regular intervals throughout the project, so any decision to sustain ambiguity might be reversed later, in light of new information or a new situation.

Cross-case analysis revealed differences between the companies as to how they had allocated resources to certain activities aimed at reducing ambiguity. Alpha, for instance, ran several resource-consuming research projects and focus-group sessions in the external stakeholder community to resolve ambiguity about the product's user-friendliness, effectiveness, and attractiveness. Delta, for the same purpose, conducted clinical tests in 6 European countries in which development staff from Delta attended close to 100 operations where product prototypes were tested. By contrast, Gamma conducted clinical tests at only one user site, and Beta performed such external activities to a very limited degree during the concept development phase. By choosing these routes, Beta and Gamma sustained more ambiguity than Alpha and Delta related to external stakeholders' perception of the product concept, but on the contrary, Beta and Gamma also avoided the costs that the other two companies incurred with these activities.

Saving costs is, thus, a second category of benefit that may be obtained by sustaining ambiguity.

4.3. *Saving time by sustaining ambiguity*

Measures such as experiments, market research tasks, and internal discussions that are taken to reduce ambiguity not only incur costs but also take time to perform. Alternative interpretations may be left open not because they are considered useful fallback options or too costly, but because eliminating them will be too time-consuming and will jeopardize the progress of the project. Our analysis revealed that saving time and maintaining project progression is a third category of benefit that can be obtained by sustaining ambiguity.

This category was identified in the Alpha and Beta cases as well as by analysis across the four cases. At Alpha, time-to-market was heavily emphasized, with significant pressure on meeting milestones and a specific launch date. Fully reducing the ambiguity related to the product's acceptance in the US therapy market would have involved a series of time-consuming tests to strengthen Alpha's arguments for its interpretation when communicating with the FDA. One option Alpha considered, therefore, was to launch the product initially in other geographical markets before reducing this ambiguity, rather than delaying the worldwide launch until all ambiguity related to the US market issues had been reduced.

At Beta, there was a sudden increase in urgency as soon as the first pharmaceutical customer had selected concept Lo-tech, and Beta committed to ship the first production units within a year. The concept team handed over concept Lo-tech to the NPD team. The NPD project manager pointed out that a number of remaining ambiguities should have been eliminated during the concept phase, but these were carried into the NPD phase since the engineering phase had to start without further delay in order to meet the commitment to the pharmaceutical customer.

Cross-case analysis revealed differences between the cases as to how time had been allocated to certain activities aimed at reducing ambiguity. Despite time pressure in the Alpha case, the company did perform a number of external time-consuming, ambiguity-reducing activities that it considered necessary. By contrast, Gamma and Beta performed fewer such external activities and, thus, sustained more market-related ambiguity than Alpha, but on the contrary, they at least temporarily saved time in their projects by their courses of action.

4.4. *Retaining ideas by sustaining ambiguity*

Viewing our conceptual model in Figure 1 from left to right, one can see that a cue can have many interpretations. In a process of complete ambiguity reduction, a commonly agreed-on interpretation will be selected, upon which further progress of the process will be based. In the further development process, this interpretation may be subject to additional scrutiny and, thus, become a new cue that will be interpreted in different ways by different actors. One of these interpretations may then be selected for further progress, and the process can iterate toward the right. Our analysis revealed a category of ambiguity sustention that exhibited a unique trait. In this category, an interpretation emerging in the NPD process may be found to include *components* from previous interpretations that were thought to be discarded. This gives rise to the question of whether these older interpretations actually *have* been discarded. Hence, components of interpretations that are in rivalry with the selected interpretation are carried forward, and ambiguity isn't fully clarified.

This category of ambiguity sustention was found when analyzing Beta's concept-development process. During this process, the initial Lo-tech concept idea was explicated in a number of competing alternatives, with the concept names of "picture frame", "note pad", "calendar", and "handheld unit". These alternatives represented four different interpretations of the product idea, of which "handheld unit" was selected for further development. This concept was then considered in a number of more detailed interpretations for further discussion and selection. But these interpretations often incorporated ideas that had originated in the three discarded concept interpretations. Some of these discarded concepts had included details representing useful ideas that were not inherent in the original "handheld unit" concept alternative. Although the concepts in which these idea details had emerged had been discarded, Beta didn't want to discard the idea details, but instead wanted to seek new use for them when further developing the "handheld unit" concept.

In this analytical category, retention of valuable creative ideas in the innovation process, thus, represents a fourth possible benefit of ambiguity sustention.

5. A Model for Benefits of Sustaining Ambiguity

Based on our analysis, we developed our conceptual framework into a model explaining how ambiguity can be sustained in product innovation projects and the benefits of doing so. Figure 2, which represents the main model, illustrates sustention of ambiguity to retain fallback option, save costs, and save time.

Following the logic of our conceptual model and viewing it from left to right, one sees that a cue can have a multitude of interpretations, designated A, B, C, D, and E in Figure 2. The cue can, for example, be a product idea, and interpretations A–E are different interpretations of that idea. A process of complete reduction of ambiguity would select a commonly agreed-on interpretation, denoted by C in Figure 2, upon which further progress of the process is to be based, and

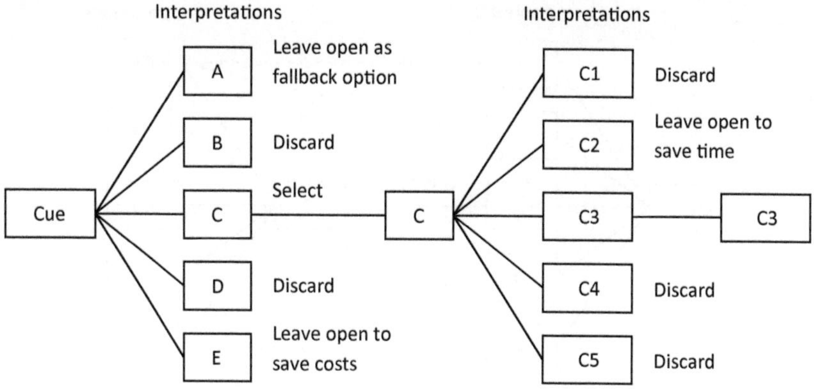

Figure 2. Sustaining ambiguity to retain fallback options, save costs, or save time.

discard A, B, D, and E. In the further development process, interpretation C will be subject to additional scrutiny and, thus, become a new cue that will be interpreted in different ways by different actors, for example, as product ideas brought to a more defined level of detail. These differing interpretations are designated C1, C2, C3, C4, and C5. Again, a process of complete reduction of ambiguity would select a commonly agreed-on interpretation, denoted by C3 in Figure 2, and discard C1, C2, C4, and C5. C3 can again become a cue subject to further interpretation, and the process can continue for further steps onward to the right.

When ambiguity is not completely reduced, interpretation C may be selected as a commonly agreed-on interpretation to be used as the basis for further work, but interpretations A and E have not been eliminated and still represent alternatives to the selected interpretation C. Similarly, although interpretation C3 has been selected as a basis for further progress, C2 has not been eliminated and still represents an alternative interpretation. As described in our previous section and as shown in Figure 2, the alternatives may be left open to retain fallback options, save costs, or save time.

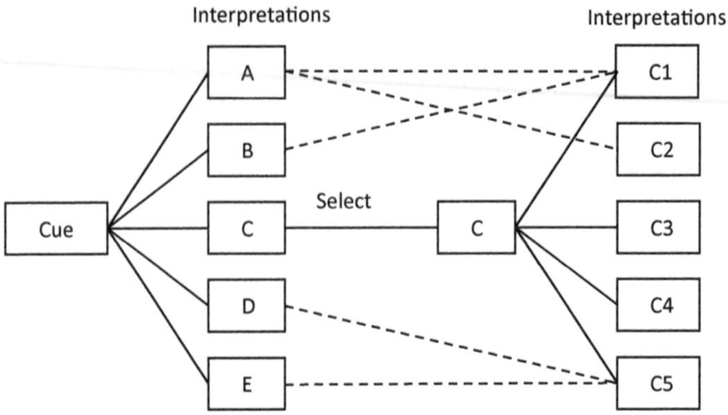

Figure 3. Sustaining ambiguity to retain ideas.

Figure 3 shows how the model illustrates sustention of ambiguity to retain valuable creative ideas.

As in our conceptual model in Figure 1, the solid lines represent the act of interpreting a cue at the left, resulting in its interpretation at the right. The dotted lines indicate that an interpretation at the right includes certain *components* from a cue at the left, rather than from the entire cue. The alternatives C1–C5 include interpretations of these components that were not inherent in C, but were inherent in the discarded alternatives A, B, D, and E. Hence, components of interpretations other than the selected interpretation C are carried forward, and ambiguity is not fully clarified.

6. Discussion

We have shown that companies may not consistently seek to reduce ambiguity in NPD projects, a finding contrary to common assumptions in management literature.

According to Eisenberg's argument (1984), clarity is a measure of effectiveness only if the organization views it as an objective. In NPD projects, this may be the case if surprises from the outside aren't expected — surprises related to technology, customers, competitors, and regulators. Measures of effectiveness are, however, related to all the objectives that the organization seeks to achieve, and clarity is only one such objective. In NPD projects, organizations also seek to minimize costs and time-to-market, maintain maneuverability through fallback options, and make optimal use of creative ideas that emerge within their projects. In a balance between these objectives, we see that some of them might be given priority at the expense of others. Just as a company may yield the cost objective and thereby accept higher costs to give priority to another objective it believes more important, such as time-to-market, the company may yield the clarity objective and thereby sustain ambiguity to give priority to another important objective, be it cost-saving, time-saving, retention of fallback options, or retention of ideas. Cost and time are always important performance factors of a company's operational undertaking, and so it's not surprising that savings of cost and time may be a benefit sought by sustaining ambiguity. Fallback options and creative ideas are, however, factors of more specific importance to the NPD process. Sustaining ambiguity to retain fallback options and creative ideas according to our model is consistent with Eisenberg's argument that strategic ambiguity enables flexibility, creativity, and adaptability to context and environmental change (Eisenberg, 1984). Sustaining ambiguity to retain fallback options for the product's functionality can take the form of building ambiguity into the product design to keep options open, which is akin to the notion of "investments in architectural design" (MacCormack and Verganti, 2003). The principle of sustaining ambiguity to retain fallback options is also in alignment with the theory of real options as presented by MacMillan and colleagues (MacMillan and McGrath, 2002; MacMillan *et al.*, 2006). As they present it, a real option represents an opportunity, but not a commitment, to make an investment. For example, a company may choose to invest in limited development and testing of a new technology, but not commit to further development until the technology has been proven. Companies may retain and invest in real options as learning platforms. This may be the case when the technological uncertainty is high, as in periods where a "dominant design" has yet to emerge (Utterback, 1996). Investments in real options allow the company to build knowledge in more than one future. Since ambiguity by its nature doesn't lend itself well to quantification and expression as risk, the traditional present-value calculations as selection mechanism have limited value. The use of real options acknowledges the true ambiguity in such cases and facilitates further testing and learning by doing until the ambiguity is reduced and more substantial investments can be made.

The iterative nature of our model can be understood as an ongoing process of variation and selection, the variation being the generation of multiple interpretations of a cue, from which one interpretation is selected. According to organizational evolutionary theory, variation emerges in the form of new combinations (Burgelman, 2002), and this is also what our model demonstrates, most clearly in Figure 3, where components of interpretations and cues are combined to retain ideas. In Schumpeter's (1934) account of innovation, he defined innovation in terms of entrepreneurial actions, where entrepreneurs carry out new combinations of productive resources. This notion of innovation also aligns well with our model, showing how ambiguity resulting from the innovation process manifests itself as new combinations which need to be sustained to retain a scope of ideas and options, particularly in the early phase of an NPD project. Our model relates to the variation–selection–retention theme from evolutionary theory that Burgelman (2002) applied to innovation processes at that firm level and that Weick (1979) applied to sensemaking at an individual level. In both contributions, variation is seen as a basis to achieve a broad field of alternatives for selection. Weick (1979) stressed the actual need for such a variety through the term "requisite variety".

Reducing ambiguity will eventually become necessary at a certain time during the innovation process. One consequence of the above arguments, however, is that ambiguity is a natural companion to innovation and that at least in the early phase of the process a certain degree of ambiguity is absolutely necessary to achieve innovation.

The focus of this chapter has been to explore how sustaining ambiguity can play a role in managing NPD processes. An important question worthy of further investigation, however, concerns the nature of the selection processes — i.e., how ambiguity is reduced. Brun and Sætre (2008) address this topic in a separate paper and we suggest further research to explore the nature of ambiguity reduction in NPD processes.

Our model doesn't explain all occurrences of ambiguity sustention but only those where an identifiable benefit of doing so contributed to the four categories. Thus, the model merely explains four potential benefits of sustaining ambiguity in NPD projects. Our model furthermore makes no distinction as to whether ambiguity is sustained as an effect of a deliberate choice. Through the categories that were found, the model explains what benefits may be achieved by sustaining ambiguity, intentionally or unintentionally. In our empirical material, we found some clear occurrences of intentional ambiguity sustention. In the occurrences of ambiguity sustention, we found by cross-case analysis that, however, there was no empirical evidence that these occurrences were intended, but still our data identified how the companies in these occurrences had benefited from sustaining ambiguity. As an explanation of the potential benefits of ambiguity sustention, however, the model provides practitioners with increased awareness upon which they can make deliberate choices of ambiguity sustention in their NPD projects.

Since the model is based on an empirical sample of only four case studies, we cannot conclude that it applies generally to NPD projects. But the four analytical categories that were identified are not specific to the limiting characteristics of our sample, i.e., established companies in the medical devices industry in Norway and Denmark. The objectives to save costs, save time, retain fallback options, and retain product ideas are expected to be essential in NPD projects, regardless of the company size, age, industry segment, and geographical location, so we believe that our model has applicability even outside the limitations of our study. Further research is needed, however, to determine that further applicability.

7. Conclusion

We have explored how sustaining ambiguity can play a role in the management of NPD projects and presented a model to understand this process. We have identified four categories of benefit that can be obtained from sustaining ambiguity in NPD processes: retaining fallback options, retaining ideas, saving costs, and saving time. Our model contrasts with the implicit assumption common to mainstream management literature that ambiguity is undesirable and should consistently be eliminated, wherever possible. The model aligns with previous research arguing for the importance of flexibility and options in innovation processes. We have also pointed out its alignment with theories seeing innovation as processes of variation resulting from new combinations and selection.

There are many useful questions for further research to be pursued. Some examples are as follows:

(a) Are there other benefits from sustaining ambiguity besides the four categories we have identified?
(b) Does intentional and unintentional sustention of ambiguity result in different processes? If so, what are they?
(c) Does the model presented here apply to other industries and other geographical locations?
(d) What is the nature of ambiguity reduction in NPD projects?

Our research has managerial implications by showing that companies in certain situations can benefit from sustaining ambiguity in NPD projects. The results presented in this study provide practitioners with an increased awareness of the potentially positive effects of ambiguity; thus, the findings we have presented can enable practitioners to more efficiently manage their NPD projects.

References

Aldrich, H. (1999). *Organizations Evolving,* Sage Publications, Thousand Oaks, CA.

Basadur, M. *et al.* (2000). Collaborative problem solving through creativity in problem definition: Expanding the pie, *Creative and Innovative Management*, 9, 54–76.

Brun, E. and Sætre, A. S. (2008). Ambiguity reduction in new product development projects, *International Journal of Innovation Management*, 12, 573–596.

Burgelman, R. (2002). *Strategy is Destiny: How Strategy-Making Shapes a Company's Future*, The Free Press, New York, NY.

Charmaz, K. (2006). *Constructing Grounded Theory: A Practical Guide through Qualitative analysis: Methods for the 21st Century*, Sage Publications, London.

Cooper, R. G. (1993). *Winning at New Products. Accelerating the Process from Idea to Launch*, 2nd edn., Addison-Wesley, Reading, MA.

Cooper, R. G. (1994). Third generation new product processes, *Journal of Product Innovative Management*, 11, 3–14.

Cooper, R. G. and Kleinschmidt, E. J. (1993). Stage-gate systems for new product success, *Marketing Management*, 1, 20–29.

Daft, R. L. and Lengel, R. H. (1984). Information richness: A new approach to managerial behavior and organizational design, in Staw, B. M. and Cummings, L. L. (eds.), *Research in Organizational Behavior*, Jai Press, Greenwich, CT.

Daft, R. L. and Lengel, R. H. (1986). Organizational information requirements, media richness and structural design, *Management Science*, 32, 554–571.

Eisenberg, E. (1984). Ambiguity as strategy in organizational communication, *Communication Monograph*, 51, 227–242.

Eisenhardt, K. (1989). Building theories from case study research, *Academic Management Review*, 14, 532–550.

Eisenhardt, K. and Tabrizi, B. (1995). Accelerating adaptive processes: Product innovation in the global computer industry, *Administrative Science Quarterly*, 40, 84–110.

Glaser, B. and Strauss, A. (1967). *The Discovery of Grounded Theory: Strategies for Qualitative Research*, Aldine de Gruyter, New York.

Griffin, A. (1997). PDMA research on new product development practices: Updating trends and benchmarking best practices, *Journal of Product Innovative Management*, 14, 429–458.

Kim, J. and Wilemon, D. (2002). Focusing the fuzzy front-end in new product development, *R&D Management*, 32, 269–279.

Koen, P. *et al.* (2001). Providing clarity and a common language to the 'Fuzzy Front End', *Research-Technical Management*, 44, 46–55.

Lerdahl, E. (2001). Staging for creative collaboration in design teams; models, tools and methods, PhD thesis, Department of Product Design, Norwegian University of Science and Technology, Trondheim.

Lester, R. and Piore, M. (2004). *Innovation — The Missing Dimension,* Harvard University Press, Cambridge, MA.

MacCormack, A. (1998). Towards a contingent model of product development: A comparative study of development practices, in *5th International Product Development Management Conference*, Lake Como, Italy.

MacCormack, A. and Verganti, R. (2003). Managing the sources of uncertainty: Matching Process and context in software development, *Journal of Product Innovative Management*, 20, 217–232.

MacCormack, A. *et al.* (2001). Developing products on 'internet time': The anatomy of a flexible development process, *Management Science*, 47, 133–150.

MacMillan, I. C. and McGrath, R. G. (2002). Crafting R&D project portfolios, *Research-Technical Management*, 45, 48.

MacMillan, I. C. *et al.* (2006). Using real options discipline for highly uncertain technology investments, *Research-Technical Management*, 49, 29–37.

March, J. G. (1994). *A Primer on Decision Making: How Decisions Happen,* The Free Press, New York, NY.

Montoya-Weiss, M. M. and O'Driscoll, T. M. (2000). From experience: Applying performance support technology in the fuzzy front end, *Journal of Product Innovative Management*, 17, 143–161.

Orton, J. D. (1997). From inductive to iterative grounded theory: Zipping the gap between process theory and process data, *Scandinavian Journal of Management*, 3, 49–438.

Poolton, J. (2000). New developments in innovation, *Journal of Management Psychology*, 15, 795–811.

Reid, S. and Brentani, U. d. (2004). The fuzzy front end of new product development for discontinuous innovations: A theoretical model, *Journal of Product Innovative Management*, 21, 170–184.

Rothwell, R. (1994). Towards the fifth-generation innovation process, *International Marketing Review*, 11, 7–31.

Schumpeter, J. A. (1934). The theory of the economic development: An inquiry into profits, capital, credit, interest and the business cycle, Harvard University Press, Cambridge, MA.

Strauss, A. and Corbin, J. (1998). *Basics of Qualitative Research. Techniques and Procedures for Developing Grounded Theory,* Sage Publications, Thousand Oaks, CA.

Utterback, J. (1996). *Mastering the Dynamics of Innovation,* Harvard Business School Press, Brighton, MA.

Veryzer, R. W. (1998). Discontinuous Innovation and the New Product Development Process, *Journal of Product Innovative Management*, 15, 304–321.

Weick, K. (1979). *The Social Psychology of Organizing,* 2nd edn. McGraw-Hill, New York, NY.

Weick, K. (1995). *Sensemaking in Organizations,* Sage Publications, Thousand Oaks, CA.

Yin, R. (1994). *Case Study Research — Design and Methods,* 2nd edn. Sage Publications, Thousand Oaks, CA.

Zhang, Q. and Doll, W. (2001). The fuzzy front end and success of new product development: A causal model, *European Journal of Innovative Management*, 4, 95–112.

Chapter 12

Managing Exploration–Exploitation*

Alf Steinar Sætre[†,§] and Eric Christian Brun[‡,¶]

[†]*Department of Industrial Economics and Technology Management, Norwegian University of Science and Technology, Trondheim, Norway*

[‡]*Department of Safety, Economics and Planning, University of Stavanger, Norway*

[§]*alf.steinar@iot.ntnu.no*

[¶]*eric.brun@uis.no*

Abstract

This chapter offers a model for effectively managing ambiguity at the fuzzy front end of innovation projects. The innovation process is characterized by cycles of expensive (explorative) activities where ambiguity increases,

*This chapter is based on two previously published articles. (1) Sætre, A. S. and Brun, E. (2012). Strategic management of innovation: Managing exploration–exploitation by balancing creativity and constraint. *International Journal of Innovation and Technology Management*, 9(4), 1–24. (2) Sætre, A. S. and Brun, E. (2013). Ambiguity and learning in the innovation process: managing exploration–exploitation by balancing creativity and constraint revisited. *International Journal of Innovation and Technology Management*, 10(4), 1–9.

and constrictive (exploitative) activities where ambiguity decreases. We argue that ambiguity oscillates in the short run and decreases in the long run while learning increases. These fluctuations in the opportunity space are driven by the balancing of creativity and constraint. We conducted in-depth studies of four new product development projects from the medical device industry. Through the abductive process of iterative grounded theory, we built a model for the management of ambiguity. The model we propose shows that innovation teams that have a higher tolerance for ambiguity are better able to exploit it. The successful management of ambiguity in innovation projects rests upon the balancing of opposing needs.

Keywords: Managing ambiguity, exploration and exploitation, balancing, learning, targeted creativity.

1. Introduction

Exploration of new opportunities and exploitation of their potential is at the heart of organizational competitiveness (Jansen *et al.*, 2006; Lavie *et al.*, 2010). This chapter presents a model for understanding and managing ambiguity in the fuzzy front end of product development. The successful management of ambiguity takes place through balancing the need for ambiguity reduction with bursts of ambiguity sustension. Our model is based on research conducted in four medical device companies. Ambiguity is understood as multiple interpretations of a cue, which fits nicely with Weick's (1979) term, equivocality. We claim that ambiguity is not only present in innovation projects but is in fact a requisite ingredient for successful innovation and new product development. It is important to understand and manage ambiguity effectively and productively. Management of ambiguity is of importance to scholars and practitioners alike.

2. Ambiguity and the Need for Balance in NPD Processes

Any firm hoping to maintain its competitiveness must learn to manage its product innovation wisely. Several research contributions over the last few decades have sought to clarify how new product development (NPD) can best be done (Cooper, 1993, 1994; Griffin, 1997; Rothwell 1994). Many of the models they have created, which are now in common use, are variants of the so-called "stage-gate" models (Cooper, 1990; Myrup Andreasen and Hein, 1987). Such models typically posit a decidedly rational, sequential process that emphasizes up-front data-gathering, planning, and subsequent execution. But the earliest stage of the NPD process typically exudes considerable uncertainty and ambiguity, neither of which fit well with the tidy, sequential nature of the stage-gate approach or with its requirement for accurate, up-front information. For this reason, the earliest stage of NPD is now often referred to in the literature as the "Fuzzy Front End" of NPD (Brun and Sætre, 2009; Khurana and Rosenthal, 1997; Moenaert *et al.*, 1995; Reid and Brentani, 2004; Reinertsen, 1999). The term "fuzzy" is itself fuzzy. It signals the need for a better understanding of what that fuzziness is and how best to cope with it in order to manage innovation processes.

As several scholars have helped us to distinguish between two of its presumed components, *uncertainty* and *ambiguity* (Daft and Lengel, 1984, 1986; March, 1994; Weick, 1995), a now common view is that *uncertainty* stems from, and betokens, lack of information; and management can reduce it simply by acquiring more data. *Ambiguity*, meanwhile, is typically viewed as different interpretations of the same information, which implies that acquiring more data won't necessarily reduce it; in fact, it might increase it.

"True uncertainty" has been understood to signify a lack of probabilities attached to outcomes (Knight, 1921; Shackle, 1961). One might, therefore, argue that true uncertainty and ambiguity are identical, but true uncertainty is focused on *ex post* effects, whereas ambiguity is focused on interpreting *ex ante* cues as well as potential outcomes of these interpretations. Corley and Gioia (2004) argue that ambiguity exists when multiple interpretations of a situation or cue are possible. We believe that the notion of ambiguity captures much of the fuzziness experienced at the front end of new product development, ascribing to Brun and Sætre's (2009) definition of *ambiguity* as *the existence of two or more interpretations of a single cue*, which here is synonymous with Weick's (1979) understanding of equivocality. The cue being subject to interpretation could be an idea, a piece of oral or written information, a physical artifact, even a situation — in short, any sort of stimulus or signal to perception. We further believe that ambiguity is not limited to the front end, but will in fact often be present throughout the NPD process — and that it is not necessarily a just bad thing, quite the contrary.

Important theoretical contributions have addressed the issue of ambiguity and how an organization can reduce it (Daft and Lengel, 1986; March, 1994; Weick, 1979, 1995). Their common assumption is that ambiguity is undesirable; that it must be reduced to provide clarity, which, once achieved, will then help propel the NPD project forward. Aldrich (1999) and Burgelman (2002) have argued that innovations develop through a process of variation and selection, implying that the innovation process may not always be steadily moving toward lessened ambiguity. While we concede that ambiguity in an NPD project must eventually be reduced before launching a specific product at a specific market, we contend that the reduction may not always occur in a sequential, continuous manner — nor should it. Eisenberg (1984), as well as Brun *et al.* (2008), maintain that transiently sustaining or even increasing ambiguity can be a useful strategy for various communication-based processes in organizations.

Organizations need to balance two fundamental needs — the need to maintain order (i.e., the need for clarity through reducing or even eliminating ambiguity) and the need for creativity (i.e., the use of constructive chaos maintained through continued ambiguity). Here, creativity refers to "the production of novel and useful ideas by an individual or a small group of individuals working together" (Amabile, 1988, p. 126). Many will recognize the need and the sentiment, expressed by one of our interviewees that "we must tighten up the development process, we must gain control over development cost, and we must finish in a timelier manner", nicely illustrating what we will call "constraint". Holbek (1988) and March (1991) contend that without constraint, clarity, and order, it's difficult for a firm to move forward with a solution. While we agree, our research also showed us that clarity, or constraint, is in itself not enough for successful innovation.

Balancing opposing needs is central to organized innovation with tensions like the outside (market-based) and inside (technology and operations), new and old, determination and emergence, and freedom and responsibility (Dougherty, 1996). She continues, noting that established organizations tend to emphasize inside over outside, old over new, determination over emergence, and responsibility over freedom, concluding that: "These tensions must be balanced throughout the organization because the activities of innovation extend beyond a project, and are inextricably bound up with the organization as a whole" (Dougherty, 1996, p. 430). Traditionally, scholars have recommended focusing on either exploration or exploitation (Barney, 1991; Ghemawat and Ricart I Costa, 1993; Porter, 1985) to avoid the risk of being mediocre at both (March, 1991). More recently however, scholars (Atuahene-Gima and Ko, 2001; Hamel and Prahalad, 1994; Levitt and March, 1988; Slater and Narver, 1994; Smith and Tushman, 2004; Tushman and O'Reilly III, 1996, 1997) have argued that balancing opposing needs can increase organizational performance.

The notion of balancing opposing forces is not new. Balancing opposing needs or forces is a fundamental management skill. Chester Barnard stated it aptly, "It is precisely the function of the executive to facilitate the synthesis in concrete action of the contradictory forces, to reconcile the conflicting forces, instincts, interests, conditions, positions and ideals" (1938/1968, p. 21). Early management thinker Mary Parker Follett agrees, noting that, "as conflict — difference — is here in the world, as we cannot avoid it, we should I think, use it" (1925/1996, p. 67). We could not agree more.

Returning to ambiguity, it is clear that without ambiguity it is difficult for a firm even to think new thoughts or generate solutions to new problems. We contend that firms that manage ambiguity through the balancing of creativity and constraint are apt to be the most successful at new product development and that the tension between creativity and constraint is akin to the balance between exploration and exploitation (March, 1991).

> Exploration and exploitation are fundamentally different logics that create tensions. They complete for firms scarce resources, resulting in the need for firms to manage the trade-offs between the two, however, there may be a synergistic effect between the two as well, and hence there is a need for firms to manage the balance between the two (He and Wong, 2004).

Balancing creativity and constraint, and exploration and exploitation is, in essence, the crucial and fundamental balance between current viability and long-term survival (Levintal and March, 1993). Our focus in this chapter is not on an oft-used temporal shift between these two activities (Holbek, 1988; Puranam *et al.*, 2006) but on how one can manage both simultaneously.

In keeping with Corley and Gioia's (2004) understanding of ambiguity, Spender (1996) has promoted the term *interpretive flexibility* as a useful heuristic in knowledge-based organizations. Interpretive flexibility entails flexibility with respect to how a cue can be interpreted and has become a central term also in the theory of social construction of technology (Bijker *et al.*, 1987) where it's viewed as the key to achieving agreement among stakeholders in technological innovation processes. Recent NPD research has also argued that NPD processes emphasizing iterations and flexibility are more suitable than the sequential process of stage-gate models in uncertain and dynamic environments (Eisenhardt and Tabrizi, 1995; MacCormack and Verganti, 2003; MacCormack *et al.*, 2001; Verganti, 1999). However, these contributions address uncertainty in NPD without distinguishing between uncertainty and ambiguity.

There has been a lack of theory, then, explicitly addressing the nature and management of *ambiguity* in the early phase of NPD projects. Over the last few years, Brun and his associates have sought to rectify that lacuna (Brun and Sætre, 2008, 2009; Brun *et al.*, 2008, 2009). Our claim here is that managing ambiguity entails balancing two opposing needs. On the one hand, there is a need for clarity to achieve operational efficiency in the NPD project — in which case ambiguity should be reduced. On the other hand, there is a need for novelty and flexibility to achieve innovation — in which case it may be useful to sustain ambiguity temporarily. In this chapter, we will present a model illuminating this balancing act.

Focusing on the constraining and creative aspects of structure, Anthony Giddens (1979) speaks of the duality of structure, arguing that structure is both the outcome and the medium of the reproduction of social practices. In much the same way, we can speak of the duality of ambiguity, that is, its constraining and creative aspects. If a firm isn't able to accommodate enough ambiguity to perceive new problems and generate new solutions, it will be left behind in the ever-evolving marketplace of ideas. If a firm isn't able to constrain ambiguity enough to decide on solutions to these problems, it won't be able to translate its new ideas into practice and move them into the marketplace of products and services that generate financial rewards. Firms need to manage ambiguity by balancing creativity and constraint, and communication is the key to this balancing. It is through the communication of diverging social realities that ambiguity is generated, and it is through communication that these ambiguities are resolved.

March (1991, p. 71) reminds us that exploration "includes things captured by terms such as search, variation, risk-taking, experimentation, play, flexibility, discovery, innovation", all of which hinge upon a certain amount of ambiguity. The presence of ambiguity is thus indispensable in all innovative processes in organizations. But March also states that exploitation includes "refinement, choice, production, efficiency, selection, implementation, execution" (1991, p. 71). These processes require the absence of ambiguity to be engaged and have effect. It follows that effective organizations need to strike a balance between sustaining ambiguity and reducing it. Our initial purpose was to explore how firms handle ambiguity at the fuzzy front end and to develop mid-range theory to this end. What we found was a balancing act. Organizations do, to varying degrees, both reduce ambiguity and sustain it in a continual, cyclical manner. It is this balancing act we explicate here.

3. Methodology

As ambiguity arises from an interpretive process, we employ a qualitative approach to best explore aspects of interpretation. Using the methodology of iterative grounded theory development (Gephart, 2004; Orton, 1997; Sætre *et al.*, 2007), we establish a middle-range theory (Daft and Lewin, 1993; Weick, 1974, 1992) of managing ambiguity in innovation projects. Mid-range theory allows for the study of only a few aspects of the organization, such as decision-making, communication structures, and technology, managing specific processes, leadership. Daft and Lewin wrote: "We believe that researchers can profitably apply midrange methods by studying a limited number of case examples or innovative outliers to understand and develop the labels, variables, and models to explain and define the phenomenon"

(1993, p. ii). Theories generated in this manner have a limited range (as opposed to grand theories) (Weick, 1974). Analyzing case data from a limited number of NPD projects, we built a full model of how teams manage ambiguity to guide a more general discussion (Weick, 1992).

Our data are drawn from case studies of NPD projects in four medical devices companies, three in Norway and one in Denmark. Heeding Eisenhardt's (1989) principle of collecting data wherever one might expect to find the most of what one is studying, we focused on the front end of these NPD projects. We felt this was where it would be most likely to encounter ambiguity. We followed two of the cases for the duration of their projects; the other two we were able to study only retrospectively. Data were collected over 3 years and consisted of 46 semi-structured interviews, 7 hours of meeting observations, 913 pages of document data, and 17 video files. We then developed a conceptual model, followed by qualitative analysis of the case data using constant comparisons and theoretical comparisons, thereby building a model grounded in empirical data (Charmaz, 2006; Glaser and Strauss, 1967; Strauss and Corbin, 1998).

Strauss and Corbin (1998) discuss three archetypes of qualitative data coding: *open coding* (where categories are discovered), *axial coding* (where categories are conceptually arranged), and *selective coding*, which includes integration of concepts, refinement, and validation of theory. We analyzed the data through the process of selective coding. The techniques used included the use of draft diagrams, draft manuscripts, and conceptual discussions (Strauss and Corbin, 1998). During the selective coding process, we moved inductively in iterations between integration and refinement of our analysis and extant literature. The inductive nature of this study can best be described as iterative grounded theory (Orton, 1997, 2000; Sætre *et al.*, 2007), an approach whereby the researcher, using an iterative process, gradually moves from primarily dealing with data and theoretical categorization to focusing primarily on analysis (Orton, 2000). Our approach to data and data analysis is also similar to that used by Hargadon and Sutton (1997). In our analysis process, we worked with data and theory simultaneously, because theory and data inevitably feed off each other. Van Maanen *et al.* (2007) stated:

> What seems apparent to those who have carried out organizational research is that method can generate and shape theory, just as theory can generate and shape method. There is a back-and-forth character in which concepts, conjectures, and data are in continuous interplay. If one thinks of concepts and conjectures as existing on a conceptual plane and of data residing on an empirical one, the more links and the more varied the links between the two planes, the more promising the research" (p. 1146).

The new ideas in our model stem from the interplay of deduction with induction, a process which Peirce (1995/1903) termed abduction; abduction being the "process of forming an explanatory hypothesis". Peirce went on to say that abduction "is the only logical operation which introduces any new idea" (Peirce, 1995/1903, p. 216). Abduction is present in the grounded theory approach through moving between deduction and induction while making constant comparisons (Suddaby, 2006). Strauss and Corbin (1998) argue that grounded theory is moving between induction and deduction. "In fact, there is an interplay between induction and deduction (as in all science)" (p. 137). This abductive interplay between theory and data, between deduction and induction, aptly describes our research process and is the process through which our models are generated.

Iterations occurred between both the conceptual and theoretical analysis. It also occurred with the data itself, as we revisited the categories during the development of our models. Our analysis gained power through these iterations since we considered the multiple implications of each of these theories for our focal issue. The methodologist Donald T. Campbell rightly observed that if a social scientist tries out multiple theories to explain the focal issue before finding one that fits, "he has tested the theory with degrees of freedom coming from the multiple implications of any one theory" (1975, p. 182). Herein lies the strength of iterative grounded theory. Iterative grounded theory operates as a reflexive practice whereby naturalistic data drawn from the field inform theoretical concepts already in place. It is also designed to inform the understanding of practice by applying those same theories to the understanding of practice.

3.1. *The cases*

To ensure anonymity, we have replaced all names with pseudonyms in references to case data. The heavy regulation of the medical device industry can at least partially explain the similarities we found in the companies studied. All used multifunctional teams and organized product development on a project bases. All four companies also used some version of a stage-gate model.

Case #1 was an NPD project at Alpha Medical. Alpha Medical was established in 1940 and has substantial international presence employing over 2,200 people worldwide (including subsidiaries) and an annual turnover of about US$350 million. Alpha Medical was seeking to develop a new product that would improve the efficiency of a specific first aid treatment procedure. Ideally, the product would be used both in first aid treatment and in first aid training courses, two segments with widely differing requirements. In developing their innovative product idea, they ran up against established regulatory standards. Complicating matters further, Alpha knew that there would also be widely differing potential user groups involved: lay people, instructors, and professional rescuers. A problematic fact was that to achieve a profitable product, Alpha had to keep its production costs extremely low. This requirement inevitably conflicted with a medical need for an accurate measurement principle, something that usually implies expensive technology.

Case #2 was an NPD project at Beta Medical. Beta Medical was established in 1930 and employed 2,500 people with a turnover of about US$720 million. Beta Medical sought to develop a new product that could help patients with chronic illness adhere to their drug treatment scheme, a principle called "patient compliance". Since a variety of potential stakeholders were involved — patients, general practitioners, clinical research organizations, pharmaceutical companies — Beta's main challenges were to define which segment to target and to define an appropriate product concept for it. In the end, Beta elected to develop two product concepts in parallel. One they called "Hi-Tech" for the clinical research market segment, the other was called "Lo-Tech" for the consumer segment. Beta Medical also elected to develop the Lo-Tech concept through a process that it hadn't previously tried.

Case #3 was an NPD project at Gamma Medical. Gamma Medical is a relatively young company established in 1984 and has a turnover of about US$25 million and employs 70 people. Gamma Medical wanted to develop a new product to improve quality control of blood vessel surgery during cardiac bypass operations. Gamma's new product was to be based on an existing ultrasound product in its product line, but with the added functionality of 3D imaging. The company faced some serious challenges. It lacked experience in developing ultrasound imaging applications, and the potential users — cardiac surgeons — themselves lacked experience in using imaging as part of their surgical procedure. As a small company, Gamma depended heavily on other RandD partners and external suppliers, and its early phase of the NPD project had a strong technology focus.

Case #4 was an NPD project at Delta Medical. Delta Medical was established as recently as 1998 and employs 20 people with a turnover of about US$3 million. It sought to develop a product to improve safety during laparoscopic surgery by combining the standard laparoscopic operating instrument with a probe that could detect hidden blood vessels so that they wouldn't be accidentally snipped during the operation. Using the product implied a slight change in the technique traditionally employed in that surgical procedure. Though the product was developed in close cooperation with a laparoscopic surgeon and tested in numerous clinical trials, gaining the users' acceptance of that change in surgical technique as well as their acceptance of the actual need for the product proved problematic. Meanwhile, Delta was also developing another new product targeting a different market, pitting both projects against each other to compete for the company's limited financial and human resources.

4. Balancing Creativity and Constraint: A Model of Ambiguity Management in New Product Development

Much has been written on how best to manage the processes of exploration and exploitation in organizations. One recent proposal recommends the temporal and spatial separation of these processes (Puranam *et al.*, 2006). Though there are similarities to the management of ambiguity and therefore lessons to be learned, there are also important conceptual differences that make the management of ambiguity unique. For example, once you find what you think is a solution and move forward with it, you often discover that things aren't what they seemed, or something changes that render your solution inadequate, requiring one to move "backward" in the process — that is, toward greater ambiguity. This process was apparent in all of our cases as teams generated ideas and pursued them to various extents that were later rejected. Therefore, while firms need to reduce ambiguity in the innovation process, they often find they need to sustain it, or re-admit it, even as they make moves toward exploitation to discover a genuinely viable product solution. Only when a new product or solution is finally successful in the marketplace are the last remnants of ambiguity removed. Figure 1 illustrates this process.

Inside the gray box, a firm typically experiences competing needs. On the one hand, getting to Launch requires it to reduce ambiguity to be clear about what its product will do, and for whom, and at a reasonable production cost. Because there are invariably unforeseen hitches, it needs to retain or allow for, and sometimes even sustain ambiguity, which will facilitate moves from right to left whenever these become required. Our case studies show that *right-to-left moves* are not only reasonable in new product development processes but also are required in product development projects. A firm that is effective at new product development retains ambiguity to facilitate these *right-to-left moves*. The ability to move effectively through the new product development process to a successful product launch requires a firm not only to be effective at reducing ambiguity but also to be good at sustaining ambiguity. Beta Medical is an excellent example of this. They had an idea for a "patient compliance" product and decided to develop a high-tech solution for the medical testing market. But one engineer at Beta Medical insisted they also develop a low-tech mass market solution, on the back-burner, that the pharmaceutical company preferred in the end. Instead of cutting all other options at once, they had decided to go for the high-tech solution. They sustained ambiguity by allowing a very different

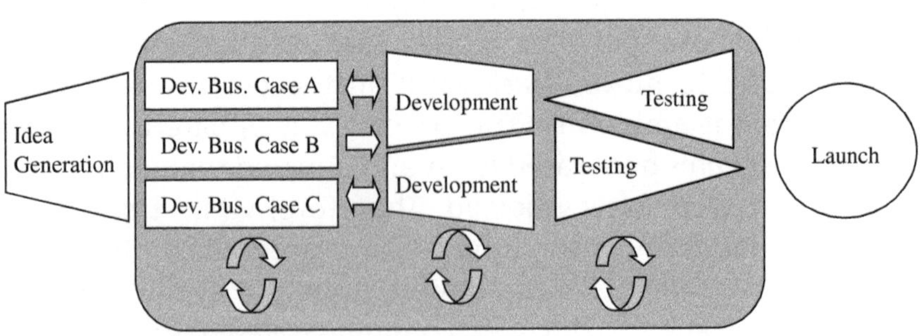

Figure 1. The iterative nature of NPD.

solution to be pursued by another team. Alpha Medical did not pursue multiple options in parallel but was quick to integrate what they had learned from their failed effort into a different product. The dual capacity of reducing and sustaining ambiguity enables and facilitates all necessary moves throughout the new product development process.

Even when engaged in activities that increase ambiguity (*right-to-left* moves), a project can still be moving forward toward a successful product launch, though admittedly project participants may temporarily feel otherwise. This paradox can create tensions (Lewis, 2000). The process — from the development of alternative business cases through development, validation, and testing — is highly dynamic (as illustrated in Figure 1). There is a certain extent to which visual models such as Figure 1 and language fail us in this regard. We contend that moving from right-to-left — that is, when an option is explored and rejected — is not ultimately a backward move, though it certainly involves going back to revisit other options initially left unexplored. And why? Because learning has increased irreversibly. In the words of Thomas Edison, "If I find 10,000 ways something won't work, I haven't failed. I am not discouraged, because every wrong attempt discarded is another step forward".[1] An example from our data further illustrates this. At Beta Medical, while two prototypes were developed in parallel and one was later abandoned in favor of the other, significant learning from the rejected project had occurred. Some of this learning was applied to developing the prototype that was chosen. As Hargadon and Sutton (1997) have pointed out, "Project teams will often develop alternative solutions throughout the project that, while not used in the final product, represent viable alternatives for subsequent projects" (p. 734). It is not insignificant this point that meaningful learning can take place even from right-to-left moves or from failures.

[1]http://en.wikiquote.org/wiki/Thomas_Edison.

Part of the key to balancing creativity and constraint in new product development is to move *left-to-right* with the most promising option quickly instead of exhaustively rejecting all other options before moving on. Due to the diminishing returns of information (Blair, 2002; Howson, 1977; Lohmann, 1998), this significantly increases the speed with which companies can move forward. We would argue that due to the diminishing returns of information, new information will eventually have a negative marginal utility, $\Delta U = U(S_2) - U(S_1)$ — that is, the utility of a subsequent state (S_2), given you have more information than you have in a preceding state (S_1), has less utility (is less useful to you) simply because the costs (financial and time) outweigh the benefits of that extra piece of information. This is especially true if we also consider the importance of time-to-market. The total utility will usually increase as a firm spends more time and resources on gathering new information. The marginal utility will soon be decreasing, though remaining positive for quite some time, and will eventually become negative. Figure 2 illustrates this. Utility is shown along the *Y*-axis, and the quantity of time, or alternatively, of money and effort, is shown along the *X*-axis.

If we compare a company that spends 13q (quantities) of time or effort, to a company that spends 20q, we see that the 13q company achieves a utility of 76, whereas the 20q company achieves a utility of 82. In this example, a 53.8% increase in input yields only a 7.9% increase in utility. Further along in the process, extra effort yields negative utility.

Uncertainty and ambiguity are different, since the relationship between information and ambiguity isn't uniformly proportional, as it is assumed to be between information and uncertainty. That is, a piece of new information doesn't necessarily lead to less ambiguity (as it does uncertainty, Daft and Lengel, 1984); on the contrary, it often leads to greater ambiguity because interpretations of the new information diverge and some of it may contradict previous information and assumptions. But it seems reasonable to assume that on average; that

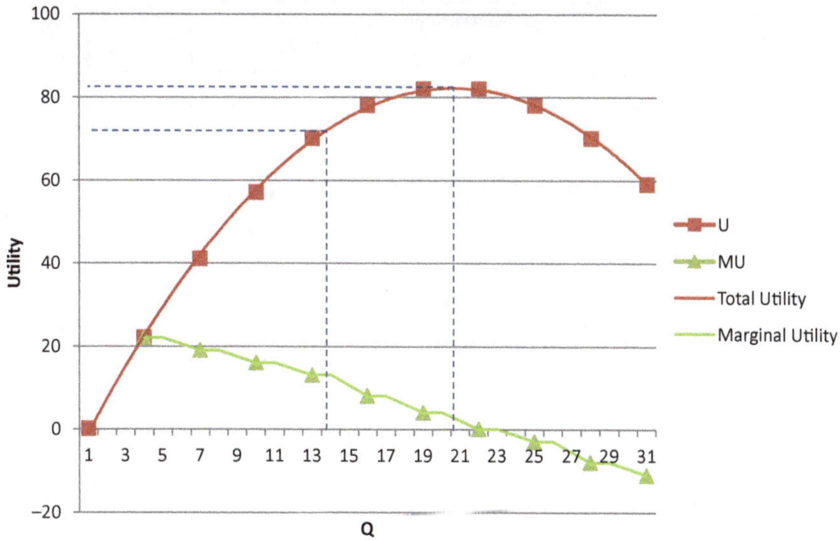

Figure 2. Marginal utility of information.

is over time, and across multiple projects, the relationship will assume a form similar to that shown in Figure 2. This illustrates well the advantages in time or cost (*Q*) that can be obtained by retaining some ambiguity and moving forward early, even though missteps might be slightly more frequent. The retained ambiguity enables and facilitates subsequent *right-to-left* moves and further helps accelerate overall product development.

Figure 3 shows the tensions of managing ambiguity in NPD projects. In Figure 3, we have revised and extended Brun and Sætre's (2008) notion of reducing ambiguity (the left-hand side of the figure) and joined it with their argument that ambiguity has benefits (Brun *et al.*, 2008) (the right-hand side of the figure). The matrix in the middle of Figure 3 illustrates how ambiguity can be classified in terms of what is the ambiguity about — represented in the columns — and what has caused the ambiguity to arise — represented in the rows (Brun *et al.*, 2009).

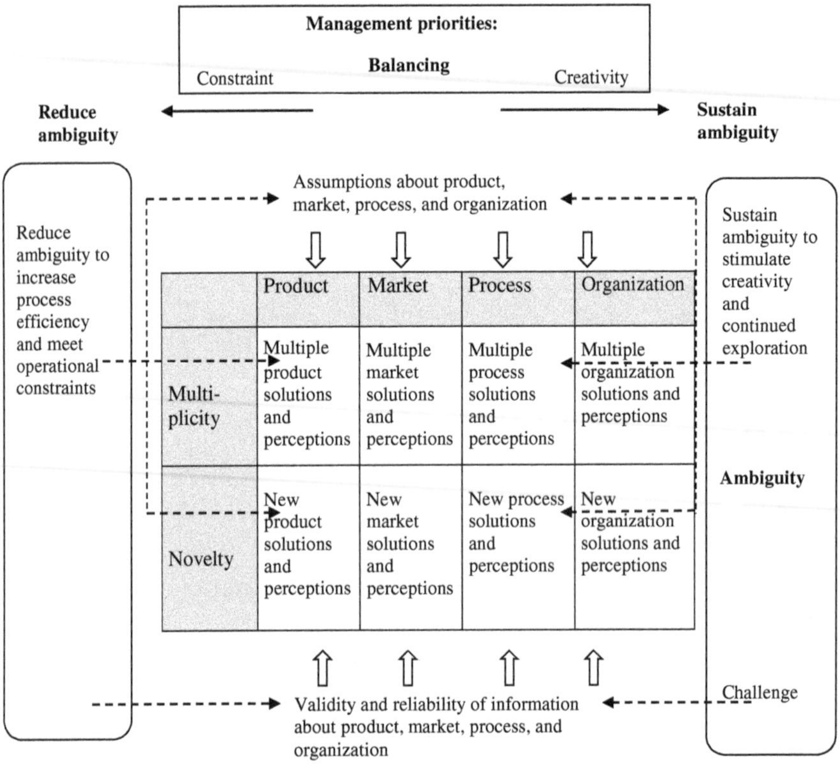

Figure 3. Managing ambiguity through balancing creativity and constraint.

The connection between ambiguity and innovation is strong. Ambiguity resulting from *multiplicity* will contribute to the variance that is important for innovation. To achieve innovation with more than a minimum of newness, some ambiguity resulting from *novelty* must be accepted. Thus, innovation is closely tied to ambiguity. Ambiguity may be either useful or desirable for providing novelty and variance to the innovation process, and as such, it should be exploited; or it may be undesirable, caused by excessive novelty and multiplicity in the project, or by unreliable or unrepresentative information sources. In the latter cases, ambiguity should be reduced.

4.1. *Sustaining ambiguity*

Our study of new product development projects in the medical device industry showed that ambiguity is regularly sustained or even increased in these projects. Furthermore, innovation projects profit by temporarily sustaining and increasing ambiguity. The benefits fall into two main categories: (1) retaining flexibility of action and (2) savings of scarce resources (cost and time primarily). Both flexibility and savings help ensure the project's progression.

4.1.1. *Sustaining ambiguity to retain flexibility*

Faced with ambiguity and desiring clarity, the participants in a situation will discuss and test alternative interpretations to arrive at some commonly accepted interpretation. The selection process is based on assumptions held by the participants — assumptions that later may be tested and strengthened or rejected. If all alternative interpretations have been eliminated and then, later in the process, one or more key assumptions underlying the selected interpretation also get rejected, the company will hit at least a temporary wall, having no options for further progress in its NPD process. By not fully eliminating ambiguity and instead leaving certain interpretations open, the project will retain these as fallback options, should the assumptions underlying the selected interpretation fail (Brun *et al.*, 2008). At Alpha Medical, alternative interpretations of both product concepts and market segments were upheld to retain fallback options throughout the process. Alternative concepts of Beta Medical's patient compliance product idea were pursued in parallel to maintain fallback options, as well as to retain what it considered promising innovative ideas that they hoped to find ways of using later in the NPD process. A counterexample is provided by Delta Medical who failed to sustain ambiguity when they saw, but failed to notice, how surgeons actually used their product.

Progressing by retaining fallback options will also accelerate the development process, by not spending too much time completely eliminating options that initially look weak. An interpretation that is different from the selected one may contain some promising ideas that management wishes to retain and utilize when further developing new alternatives of the selected interpretation. This implies that the alternative interpretation is at least partially open and ambiguity is sustained.

4.1.2. *Sustaining ambiguity to preserve resources*

Our analysis revealed a category of ambiguity sustention that was associated with cost savings. Developing two or more alternative concepts in parallel is more costly than developing only one, so consistent ambiguity reduction would seem a cost-effective strategy in any NPD project.

At Gamma Medical, the management had no choice. While it encountered considerable ambiguity about what the relevant market segments were and about the potential users' attitudes toward the product concept, Gamma, being a small company, just didn't have the resources to perform sufficient actions to reduce this ambiguity early in the project, so ambiguity was sustained, and the company moved forward with its choices. Beta Medical also only performed a minimal amount of external testing, retaining ambiguity but saving cost.

At Alpha, the NPD project carried a considerable sense of urgency to reach a given launch date. There just wasn't time to clarify all the ambiguous issues in sequence if this launch date was to be achieved. At Beta, there was a sudden increase in urgency as soon as the Lo-Tech concept was selected, and Beta committed to shipping the first production units within a year. The NPD project manager pointed out that a number of remaining ambiguities should have been eliminated during the concept phase, but these were carried into the NPD phase since the engineering phase had to start without further delay to meet their commitment to the pharmaceutical customer.

Time constraints made it too costly to eliminate the remaining ambiguities.

Full reduction, or elimination, of ambiguity, may therefore *not* be cost-effective. Measures were taken to reduce ambiguity, such as experiments, building and testing a prototype, market research tasks, and internal discussions, which not only incur costs but also take time to perform. Therefore, alternative interpretations may be left open not to retain flexibility or to save costs but simply because eliminating them will be too time consuming and retard, if not jeopardize, the progress of the project.

4.2. *The balancing act*

Balancing creativity and constraint, then, involves being able to successfully launch new products by reducing ambiguity during product development to move projects forward and rein in cost; *while simultaneously* sustaining ambiguity during these stages to increase the innovativeness of the product through creativity stimulation and continued option exploration. Success stems from this simultaneity of opposing processes (Jansen *et al.*, 2006; March, 1991). This balancing act is the real management of innovation. Discussing why success is so often followed by failure, Tushman and O'Reilly III (1996, p. 10) concluded that "Senior managers in these firms fell victim to their previous success and their inability to play two games simultaneously". Playing two games simultaneously is an apt description of what balancing creativity and constraint involves. The challenge for organizations today may not be a lack of ideas or a lack of technology, but rather a lack of innovation process capability and management talent to translate new ideas and technologies into market impact (Govindarajan and Trimble, 2010).

Another way of stating this is to say that innovative organizations, or at least those parts of the organizations that deal most directly with innovation and new product development, need to be simultaneously tight and loose (Andriopoulos and

Lewis, 2009, 2010). Tightness, or constraint, which seeks stability and predictability by resolving ambiguity, is often the default mode of most for-profit businesses. Looseness, or creativity, is playful and explorative, thriving on ambiguity, and is frequently found in creative organizations such as theaters, advertising agencies, and jazz ensembles (Ligus, 1994; Weick, 1998). The challenge is that the skills required for, and the personality traits conducive to, reducing ambiguity (constraint) are opposed to those needed for sustaining ambiguity (creativity). Organizational actors' typical responses to tensions or paradoxes are defensive, tending toward wanting to eliminate the tension or to move toward their default behavior (Andriopoulos and Lewis, 2009; Lewis, 2000). In innovation, as in most cases, the traps are one-sided, escalating efforts either toward exploration at the expense of exploration or vice versa (Andriopoulos and Lewis, 2009; Gupta *et al.*, 2006; Tushman and O'Reilly III, 1996).

Most managers are accomplished in behaviors associated with constraint — that is, in behaviors associated with reducing ambiguity, such as finding, evaluating and categorizing information, and making decisions. They, like most people, prefer certainty and can handle only moderate amounts of ambiguity before becoming uncomfortable. The resulting reticence toward ambiguity in general, and toward increasing ambiguity in particular, results in organizational members actively resisting such *right-to-left* moves. It is here that those organizations that are skilled at managing ambiguity through balancing creativity and constraint differ from more traditional organizations. Instead of resisting increased ambiguity, successful ambiguity managers embrace it. This enables them to make *right-to-left* moves much more decisively and effectively than their more hesitant counterparts, which in turn enables them to start making new *left-to-right* moves all the more quickly. We argue that the balancing act that follows from embracing ambiguity is a pivotal foundation for contextual ambidexterity (Birkinshaw and Gibson, 2004; Gibson and Birkinshaw, 2004).

Furthermore, organizations that have a higher tolerance for ambiguity are better able to pursue multiple alternatives in parallel. At Alpha, for example, two different concepts of a first aid training product emerged that represented alternative interpretations of the product idea. At Beta, two alternative interpretations of the product idea emerged — the Hi-Tech and the Lo-Tech product concept — each of which targeted alternative interpretations of the market. In both these cases, the simultaneous pursuit of multiple solutions significantly reduced the time it took to launch a final product, as the organizations applied what they had learned from one potential solution to the other.

If organizations only focus on one or even overemphasize one at the expense of the other, they may experience short-term success, but they will fail in the long run. With too much focus on constraint, the innovativeness or newness of NPD projects will suffer, and the firm will lose out to more innovative competitors (March, 1991; Tushman and O'Reilly III, 1996). With too much focus on creativity, time-to-market will suffer as firms find it difficult to move the NPD process forward and lose market share to more efficient and agile competitors. Organizations who manage NPD processes successfully repeatedly make the transitions from constraint to creativity and back again. It is *not* a two-step process. Rather, the balancing of constrictive (constraint) and expansive (creativity) processes occurs in a recursive cycle. Throughout this cycle, learning increases steadily, even when ambiguity temporarily increases.

The causes for reducing ambiguity — that is, constraint — are closely linked not only to the cost of time and resources but also to the requirements of user needs and time-to-market pressures. On the other hand, the sustention of ambiguity is the basis for creativity. Without ambiguity, there is little room or even need, for creativity. It is when the reduction of ambiguity (constraint) and the sustention of ambiguity (creativity) are properly balanced that one gets what we call *targeted creativity*. The clarity often associated with ambiguity reduction is needed to propel a project forward, whereas the innovative elements of the project stem from ambiguities. Targeted creativity is not only effective but it is as efficient as innovation can get. By this, we mean that effective innovation processes contain the requisite, but not excessive amounts of both ambiguity and constraint; to create value in competitive marketplaces, both are needed. This is illustrated in Figure 4.

The narrower the process depicted in Figure 4, the more constricted the creativity, but the greater the risk of missing creative opportunities. Companies skilled at managing ambiguity then need to be able to make the transition from creativity to constraint and back again — not once, not twice, but continuously. This is the balancing of creativity and constraint. One of the critical challenges is to manage the transition between these two opposing processes. Figure 4 illustrates the constricting-and-expanding iterations — reducing ambiguity–sustaining and increasing ambiguity — inherent in the innovation process. The innovation process is often illustrated by a funnel with smooth edges. In reality, it is a funnel with the jagged edges of a crocodile's jaw, which can serve as an effective reminder of the many hazards and ups-and-downs of the innovation process (Cooper, 1993; Van de Ven *et al.*, 2008).

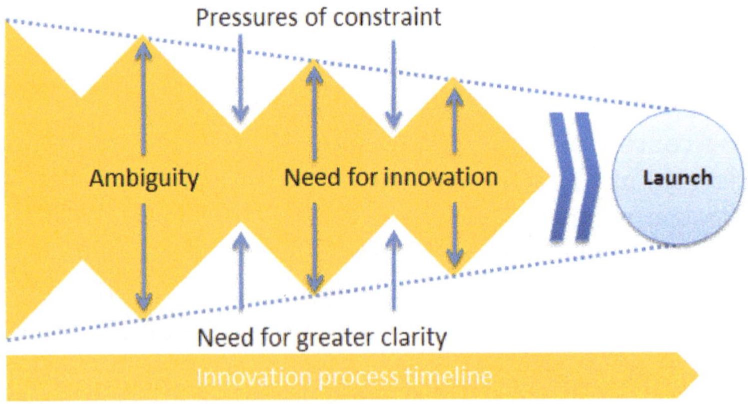

Figure 4. Targeted creativity: Balancing opposing pressures.

The balancing of creativity and constraint — the *jeu d'aller et retour* of reducing and retaining ambiguity — is how an organization adapts, integrates, and reconfigures organizational skills and resources (Teece *et al.*, 1997) and senses, seizes, and shapes opportunities (Teece, 2007). For our purposes, however, it is perhaps more natural to relate our work to absorptive capacity than to dynamic capabilities. Dynamic capabilities' main focus is on organizational assets and a firm's ability to "integrate, build, and reconfigure internal and external competences" (Teece *et al.*, 1997, p. 516). Dynamic capabilities thus have more of a "macro-level" emphasis that we do in our research. Absorptive capacity (Cohen and Levinthal, 1989, 1990), on the contrary, focuses more on the "ability to recognize the value of new information", from outside sources of knowledge — external both to the organization and to the unit innovating — "assimilate it, and apply it to commercial ends" (Cohen and Levinthal, 1990, p. 128); and is, thus, more directly relevant to our research.

We argue that the successful balancing of creativity and constraint undergirds an organization's absorptive capacity. To sense opportunities based on recognizing the potential value of outside information depends on being attuned to technology, product, and market ambiguities; as well as heterogeneous information distribution where an organization's prior knowledge and skills give it "sensory" advantages in some areas and disadvantages in other areas. To acquire or seize such opportunities requires tolerance of, and an ability to handle, ambiguity. Combining and reconfiguring not only stem from ambiguity but are also ways to deal with it. Sensing and acquiring information and opportunities are usually expansive activities, especially in the initial stage; that is, these activities expand not only the opportunity space but also increase the inherent levels of ambiguity.[2] Successfully coping with exploring and

[2]In subsequent stages, sensing and acquiring additional information and opportunities can also potentially have a constrictive effect in that the additional information contradicts or disconfirms previously perceived opportunities.

fruitfully exploiting this increased opportunity space — that is, innovating — requires at a minimum a high tolerance of ambiguity. Acquisition and assimilation of new external (to the innovating unit or the organization) information are primarily driven by the need for newness and the desire to innovate. Transformation is accomplished through iterative stages of expansion and constriction of ambiguity in such a way that ambiguity is reduced over time. Successful innovation rests on the requisite reduction, though not complete removal, of ambiguity. The critical issue here is the manner, or process, through which this reduction in ambiguity is achieved.

Shaping opportunities begin with embracing ambiguity and continues through iterative cycles of expanding and constricting the opportunity space. It is only over time, after repeated cycles, that the average opportunity space gradually narrows. Throughout these iterative cycles, innovators figure out what direction to take the opportunity: how to integrate it to existing technologies, products, processes, and markets, or now to fashion new products, processes, technologies, or markets. The driving forces of the expansive phases in this iterative process are perceptions of new opportunities and possibilities that create a "desire for newness". The pressures driving the constricting phases are pressures of constraint; stay on budget, meet deadlines, and "keep moving forward".

The expansive phases of Figure 4 are really about retaining options, acquiring and generating new knowledge by expanding the space where the innovation team searches for solutions. In short, it is about expanding the opportunity space. The constrictive phases are about assessing and taking advantage of the increased opportunity space created in the expansive phase, whittling away possibilities and options that seem too time consuming, not technologically feasible, too costly, and so on. Together, these two phases of expansion and constriction are strung together to form a sequence of micro-level exploration and exploitation.

The balancing of the opposing forces of creativity and constraint can also be depicted in a decision tree format. Figure 5 illustrates the choices that have to be made in the course of an innovation or NPD process. Overlaying this decision tree are arrows depicting the choices that are made in a given innovation project. Unidirectional arrows represent *left-to-right* moves. Bidirectional arrows represent *left-to-right* moves that were followed *by right-to-left* moves. *Right-to-left* moves can be one step and multiple step (as represented by the dashed arrow).

There are two separate dynamics at work here. One is the number of moves or steps that are made, and the other is the speed with which these moves are made. First, savvy managers of ambiguity make forward moves at, say, 60% reduced ambiguity (certainty), whereas more ambiguity-averse managers wait until 80% reduced ambiguity — which doesn't take 20% more time but may take as much as twice the time due to the diminishing returns of information. Managers or teams with

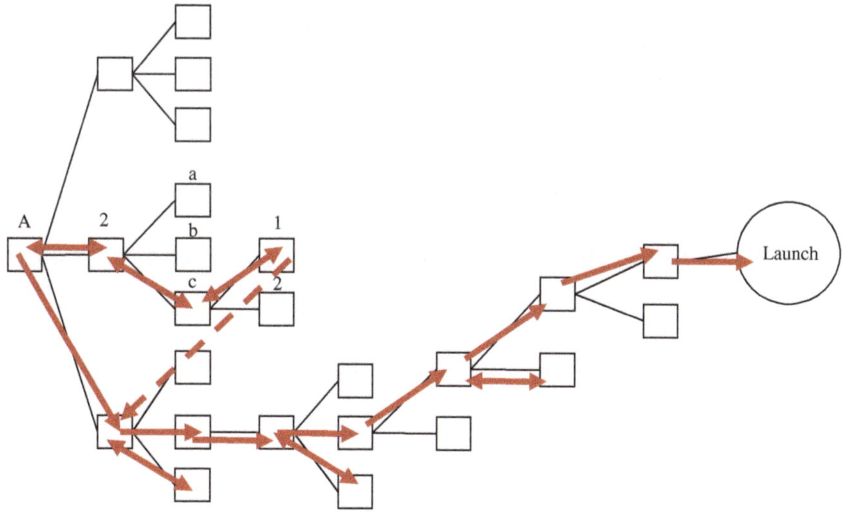

Figure 5. Lateral moves in the NPD process.

a high tolerance for ambiguity make faster forward moves, but the real difference comes when they are making *right-to-left* moves over several steps in the process. Teams with higher tolerance for ambiguity know where the misstep was made and can go back several steps in a single move — say, from A2c1 all the way, back to A in one move (middle of figure) — whereas less skilled handlers of ambiguity first go back to A2c and might even consider A2c2 before retreating to A2 and so on. For high ambiguity tolerance teams, these backward moves happen so fast that to a casual observer it would look as if the team moved directly from say A2c1 to say A3, while innovation teams with less ambiguity tolerance tend to re-explore options at each step. This advantage can become even more pronounced when high-tolerance teams explore multiple interpretations of a product solution in parallel.

Getting to launch requires reduction of ambiguity to increase clarity about critical features of the end product (or service). Unforeseen things invariably happen during an innovation process (Van de Ven *et al.*, 2008) and having retained a certain level of ambiguity will facilitate the exploration of alternative options (Brun and Sætre, 2009; Brun *et al.*, 2008). Our case studies show that *right-to-left moves* are not only reasonable in innovation processes but also essential.

4.3. *Examples of balancing*

Consider Beta Medical; they came to focus on what they called patient compliance. When a doctor prescribes a drug, the effectiveness of the treatment hinges upon the patient taking the prescribed drugs, on patient compliance. The developers at Beta Medical had discussions with several pharmaceutical companies that produced drugs in blister packs (metal foil packs with little bubbles or blisters containing a pill each). Beta decided there was unexplored potential here, and came up with three different interpretations of this perceived opportunity:

(1) *Clinical trial*, an advanced computer-enhanced system for tracking during clinical trials.
(2) *Advanced treatment*, an advanced and computer-enhanced solution focusing primarily on physicians and patients.
(3) *Branding*, a simple, easy-to-use product costing no more than three or four US dollars. A trial concept was started with a pharmaceutical company called PillCo, and it was decided that the clinical trial concept was the one Beta would go for. It was a mature market, and since PillCo was set to launch a new drug, this was thought a useful tool to help them through clinical trials.

The concept manager argued and received permission to develop the branding concept in addition to the chosen clinical trial concept. After several months of development, Beta was ready to present its concept to PillCo. By this time, it turned out, PillCo's new drug was already through clinical trials, and PillCo's interest in their advanced solution was not what Beta Medical had hoped for. PillCo, however, loved the branding solution Beta had termed the Assistant. This Assistant solution was later developed and launched, subsequently winning several design awards.

The substantial ambiguity regarding this opportunity and its potential solutions led Beta Medical not only to generate multiple possible solutions but also to develop two of them in parallel. When they received input from their key client that they preferred the simpler solution, Beta quickly abandoned their primary solution in favor of their alternate. Beta saw the ambiguity surrounding the notion of patience compliance as something to be exploited, not something to be avoided. In the terminology of Figure 5, Beta had a sufficiently high tolerance of ambiguity that they developed two branches in parallel, designating one as a primary and the other as a secondary. When ambiguity regarding a viable solution was effectively reduced, they quickly terminated their primary solution and jumped to the other development branch.

Delta Medical, the small medical device company, had a different approach. Delta's innovative new product concept to improve safety during laparoscopic surgery was developed by an engineer at Delta Medical in close cooperation with a leading laparoscopic surgeon. At the core of their concept were a sophisticated set of controls and the ability to switch between cutting with a pair of remote-controlled scissors and probing the patient with an ultrasound device. The technological sophistication of the product led to a relatively high cost, an issue of potential concern to hospitals and clinics since part of the product was meant to be disposable. Some prototypes were tested in approximately 100 surgeries. During trials, the project manager at Delta Medical saw that the surgeons testing the device never used many of the sophisticated features of the product and that these surgeons had a different understanding of how to use the product.

At Delta Medical, however, the prevailing view was that the sophisticated features were the very essence of their product concept. There was little or no willingness to re-interpret the product concept in a different way. Their inflexibility or lack of ability to notice and exploit this ambiguity (low tolerance) led the Delta team to remain on their branch of the decision tree in Figure 5 never making the backward move required to get on to the branch with the possible solution of a simplified device. Delta instead brought their full-fledged version of the product to market, a product that did not meet sales expectations and was later discontinued. Today a simplified version of Delta's product concept is on the market, manufactured and sold by a competitor. This unfortunate outcome is a result of Delta's propensity to reduce ambiguity too soon (a one-sided trap) (Gupta *et al.*, 2006; Lewis, 2000; Tushman and O'Reilly III, 1996).

Figure 5 has only eight levels of options or decision-making. In reality, there are several dozen if not hundreds of decisions that need to be made and options to be weighed. Firms that focus entirely on reducing ambiguity will be able to move from *left-to-right* but will struggle with *right-to-left* moves. We argue that firms that retain the requisite amount of ambiguity will move effectively throughout the new product development process and will arrive at the launch with a better product than their counterparts. They may also arrive more quickly at product launch, as they are less likely to get stuck in the process. One way of retaining ambiguity is to explore multiple interpretations of the product simultaneously, as exemplified by both Beta Medical with its parallel efforts toward a Lo-Tech and a Hi-Tech solution and by Alpha Medical with its first aid device.

5. Learning in the Innovation Process

It is all too easy to think of the innovation process or the product and service development process, in particular, a process where ambiguity is reduced linearly. Perhaps the best way to illustrate the non-linear dynamics of the NPD process is to imagine a 3D space, where the three critical dimensions are time, ambiguity, and learning. Ambiguity oscillates in the short run but decreases in the long run. There is an inverse relationship between ambiguity reduction and learning. Ambiguity fluctuates in the short run, but the moving average of ambiguity decreases over time. If AMB_t is the level of ambiguity at a given time t, its moving average at t calculated over the last n time periods is mathematically expressed as $VAMB_t(n) = \sum_{i=t-n+1}^{t} AMB_i/n$ (the moving average is not defined unless $t \geq n$). Learning is the empirical inverse of the running average and increases over time: $L_t(n) = (1 - VAMB_t(n))$, where $L_t(n)$ is the level of learning achieved at time t. That is, during the innovation project, the organization is continually learning. This is illustrated in Figure 2; here n is set to 2, so the moving average at each time is based on the two most recent data points. Figure 6 illustrates the relationship between ambiguity and learning. During the NPD phase, the organization is continually learning, particularly from its mistakes.

Learning from "small failures" is central to organizational learning (Hargadon and Sutton, 1997; Huber, 1991; Lounamaa and March, 1987; Sitkin, 1992), and it is critical in all innovation

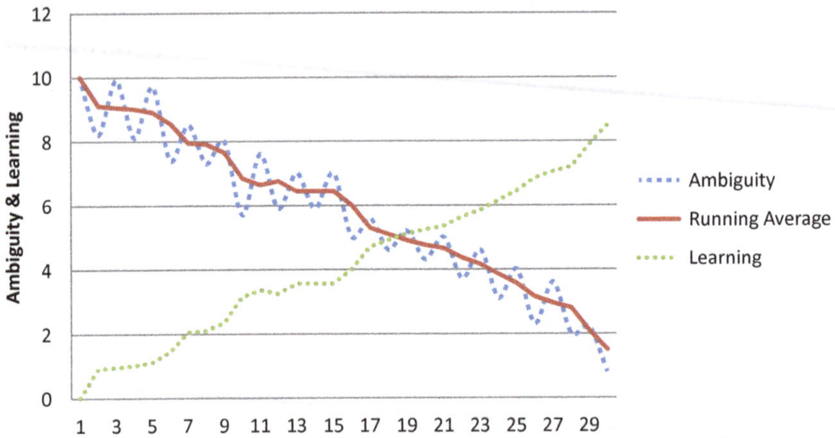

Figure 6. Ambiguity and learning in an NPD project.

efforts. We agree in principle with Huber's (1991) argument that organizational effectiveness does not have to increase for organizational learning to have taken place. He points out that, "Learning does not always lead to veridical knowledge. Sample data are not always representative, and new findings sometimes overturn what was previously 'known to be true.' Entities can incorrectly learn, and they can correctly learn that which is incorrect" (Huber, 1991, p. 89). It is this "overturning what was previously 'known to be true'" that happens when innovation teams have to make "left-to-right moves" (Sætre and Brun, 2012, pp. 10–19). From a learning perspective, this is equivalent to saying that what you thought you knew or learned turned out to be incorrect, or not what you thought it was. You have in effect tested a hypothesis you thought was likely and rejected it.[3] Ruling out plausible solutions, or

[3]Rejecting plausible hypothesis in science (or perhaps more precisely, failing to reject the null hypothesis) is real (scientific) progress; a fact that perhaps is not adequately reflected in today's scientific journals, as editors usually decline to publish such studies. In fact, for studies with a substantial sample size, rejecting the null hypothesis is often fairly trivial; and, little or no real scientific progress is made by retaining the tested hypothesis in the pool of plausible hypothesis explaining the phenomenon under investigation.

explanations is not only learning (though it often feels like a step back), in terms of innovating, it is real progress.

Learning and learning capability are essential for innovative output under a variety of conditions (Hull and Covin, 2010). During innovation processes, it is particularly important to learn from failures and missteps. The well-known IDEO slogan "fail often in order to succeed sooner" is an oft-cited example of learning from small failures (Cannon and Edmondson, 2005; Kelley and Littman, 2001). *Harvard Business Review* dedicated the April 2011 issue to failure and how to learn from it (e.g., Edmondson, 2011; McGrath, 2011).

One might argue that this is a simplistic model and ask: What happens when ambiguity increases over two or more periods in a row? Does learning then decrease? This is equivalent to having multiple *right-to-left* moves in Figure 5. That is, *left-to-right* moves that have been made turn out to be premature and the NPD project needs to revisit these choices. From a learning perspective, this is equivalent to saying that what you thought you knew or learned turned out to be incorrect, or not what you thought it was. You have in effect tested a hypothesis you thought was likely and rejected it. Ruling out plausible solutions or explanations is not only learning but is real progress. When frustrations are mounting due to wrong choices, managers and members of innovation teams will do well to remember that such missteps are also moving the team toward a solution.

We point out that stepping "back" is an integral part of moving forward. Innovation managers and innovation researchers alike will do well to remember that often it is necessary to take one step back to move forward again.

6. Conclusions and Implications

Balancing the two countermanding demands of innovation — creativity and constraint — make it one of the most challenging processes to manage. The ability to balance tensions is found in most, if not all, industries (Lampel *et al.*, 2000; Taylor and Greve, 2006). The capability to not only simultaneously play two games (Tushman and O'Reilly III, 1996) but also to play them both well is of great importance to organizations wishing to remain competitive. We argue that organizations who manage to do this well switch seamlessly and continuously between reducing ambiguity and sustaining it. One of the many challenges facing organizations trying to balance ambiguity reduction and sustention is that management training as well as higher education, in particular in engineering, is geared singularly toward reducing ambiguity. Being able to embrace it periodically and exploit it may seem counterintuitive at first but will yield significant benefits if managed successfully.

Perhaps the biggest challenge for traditionally trained managers is to embrace and exploit ambiguity consistently. A successful balancing act yields what we here have called *targeted creativity*. The promise for those who learn targeted creativity is great. We have argued that this will enable innovation teams to move more quickly through various options in the innovative process. Targeted creativity is the ability to exploit ambiguities to increase the degree of novelty while reducing ambiguities to move the project forward toward a successful market launch.

One may reasonably ask whether it is possible to reduce all ambiguity without reducing innovativeness too. No! Innovation without ambiguity and novelty is self-contradictory. We argue that ambiguity arising from novelty is an inevitable ingredient of innovation and that actions to reduce this ambiguity too early in the NPD project hamper innovation. Our finding that some companies do in fact sustain ambiguity to retain *flexibility* is a key to successfully managing innovation processes in uncertain and dynamic environments (Eisenhardt and Tabrizi, 1995; MacCormack *et al.*, 2001; Verganti, 1999). That is, successful management of ambiguity hinges upon striking a balance between reducing it and sustaining it — balancing creativity and constraint. For managers of innovation processes and product development in established firms, our findings indicate that an awareness of, tolerance of, and willingness to utilize ambiguity can be an essential competitive factor in a firm's innovation strategy.

We have developed a middle-range model through the analysis of case data from our specific sample: four NPD projects in established medical devices companies. We expect ambiguity about any product, market, NPD process, and organization to occur in NPD projects regardless of company size, age, industry segment, and geographical location. We also expect that ambiguity can result from multiplicity, novelty, and low validity or reliability in other NPD projects. How much these ambiguities can successfully be explored and exploited, however, may well vary a great deal from industry to industry.

It seems reasonable to expect that different industries — pharmaceuticals, cellphones, and cement — would be best served with different levels of tolerance for ambiguity in their innovative search strategies. In sectors with very narrow parameters defining a product success (such as pharmaceuticals), a lower tolerance might be the preferred strategy, whereas in industries with broader product solutions, firms might be best served with a high-tolerance innovation strategy. More research is needed to determine under what conditions the different innovation strategies are most successful. Industry differences notwithstanding, we agree with Lubatkin and his colleagues (2006) that executives should reconsider the separation of units focusing on creativity (exploration) and constraint (exploitation) and instead consider fostering units capable of both.

References

Aldrich, H. (1999). *Organizations Evolving,* Sage Publications, Thousand Oaks, CA.

Amabile, T. M. (1988). A model of creativity and innovation in organizations, *Research in Organizational Behavior,* 10, 167.

Andriopoulos, C. and Lewis, M. W. (2009). Exploitation–exploration tensions and organizational ambidexterity: Managing paradoxes of innovation, *Organization Science,* 20, 696–717.

Andriopoulos, C. and Lewis, M. W. (2010). Managing innovation paradoxes: Ambidexterity lessons from leading product design companies, *Long Range Planning,* 43, 104–122.

Atuahene-Gima, K. and Ko, A. (2001). An empirical investigation of the effect of market orientation and entrepreneurship orientation alignment on product innovation, *Organization Science,* 12, 54.

Barnard, C. I. (1938/1968). *The Functions of the Executive* (30th Anniversary edition), Harvard University Press, Cambridge, MA.

Barney, J. (1991). Firm resources and sustained competitive advantage, *Journal of Management,* 17(1), 99.

Bijker, W. E., Hughes, T. P. and Pinch, T. (1987). *The Social Construction of Technological Systems*, The MIT Press, Cambridge, MA.

Birkinshaw, J. and Gibson, C. (2004). Building ambidexterity into an organization, *MIT Sloan Management Review,* 45, 47–55.

Blair, D.C. (2002). Knowledge management: Hype, hope, or help? *Journal of American Society Information Science and Technology,* 53, 1019–1028.

Brun, E. and Sætre, A. S. (2008). Ambiguity reduction in new product development projects, *International Journal of Innovation Management,* 12, 573–596.

Brun, E. and Sætre, A. S. (2009). Managing ambiguity in new product development, *Creativity Innovation Management,* 18, 24–34.

Brun, E., Sætre, A. S. and Gjelsvik, M. (2008). Benefits of ambiguity in new product development, *International Journal of Innovation and Technology Management,* 5, 303–319.

Brun, E., Sætre, A. S. and Gjelsvik, M. (2009). Classification of ambiguity in new product development projects, *European Journal of Innovation Management,* 12, 62–85.

Burgelman, R. (2002). *Strategy is Destiny: How Strategy-Making Shapes a Company's Future*, The Free Press, New York, NY.

Campbell, D. T. (1975). Degrees of freedom and the case study, *Comparative Political Studies,* 8(2), 178–193.

Cannon, M. D. and Edmondson, A. C. (2005). Failing to learn and learning to fail (intelligently): How great organizations put failure to work to innovate and improve, *Long Range Planning,* 38(3), 299–319.

Charmaz, K. (2006). *Constructing Grounded Theory: A Practical Guide through Qualitative analysis: Methods for the 21st Century*. Sage Publications, London.

Cohen, W. M. and Levinthal, D. A. (1989). Innovation and learning: The two faces of R and D, *The Economic Journal,* 99(397), 569–596.

Cohen, W. M. and Levinthal, D. A. (1990). Absorptive capacity: A new perspective on learning and innovation, *Administrative Science Quarterly,* 35(1), 128–152.

Cooper, R. G. (1990). Stage-gate systems: A new tool for managing new products, *Bus. Horizons,* 33, 44–54.

Cooper, R. G. (1993). *Winning at New Products. Accelerating the Process from Idea to Launch*, 2nd edn., Addison-Wesley, Reading, MA.

Cooper, R. G. (1994). Third generation new product processes, *Journal of Product Innovation Management,* 11, 3–14.

Corley, K. G. and Gioia, D. A. (2004). Identity ambiguity and change in the wake of a corporate spin-off, *Administrative Science Quarterly,* 49, 173–208.

Daft, R. L. and Lengel, R. H. (1984). Information richness: A new approach to managerial behavior and organizational design, in Staw, B. M. and Cummings, L. L. (eds.), *Research and Organizational Behavior,* JAI Press, Greenwich, CN, pp. 191–233.

Daft, R. L. and Lengel, R. H. (1986). Organizational information requirements, media richness and structural design, *Management Science,* 32, 554–571.

Daft, R. L. and Lewin, A. Y. (1993). Where are the theories for the 'new' organizational forms? An editorial essay, *Organ. Science,* 4, i–vi.

Dougherty, D. (1996). Organizing for innovation, in Clegg, S. R., Hardy, C. and Nord, W. R. (eds.), *Handbook of Organization Studies*, Sage Publications, Thousand Oaks, CA, pp. 424–439.

Edmondson, A. C. (2011). Strategies for learning from failure, *Harvard Business Review,* 89(4), 48–55.

Eisenberg, E. (1984). Ambiguity as strategy in organizational communication, *Communication Monographs,* 51, 227–242.

Eisenhardt, K. M. (1989). Building theories from case study research, *Academy of Management Review,* 14(4), 532–550.

Eisenhardt, K. and Tabrizi, B. (1995). Accelerating adaptive processes: Product innovation in the global computer industry, *Administrative Science Quarterly,* 40, 84–110.

Follett, M. P. (1925/1996). Constructive conflict, in Graham, P. (ed.), *Mary Parker Follett; Prophet of Management*, Harvard Business School Press, Boston, MA.

Gephart, R. (2004). From the editors: Qualitative research and the Academy of Management Journal, *Academy of Management Journal,* 47, 454–462.

Ghemawat, P. and Ricart i Costa, J. E. (1993). The organizational tension between static and dynamic efficiency, *Strategic Management Journal,* 14(Special Issue).

Gibson, C. B. and Birkinshaw, J. (2004). The antecedents, consequences, and mediating role of organizational ambidexterity, *Academy of Management Journal,* 47, 209–226.

Giddens, A. (1979). *Central problems in social theory: Action, structure, and contradiction in social analysis,* Vol. 241, University of California Press.

Glaser, B. and Strauss, A. (1967). *The Discovery of Grounded Theory: Strategies for Qualitative Research,* Aldine de Gruyter, New York.

Govindarajan, V. and Trimble, C. (2010). *The Other Side of Innovation: Solving the Execution Challenge,* Harvard Business Review Press, Boston, MA.

Griffin, A. (1997). PDMA research on new product development practices: Updating trends and benchmarking best practices, *Journal of Product Innovation Management,* 14, 429–458.

Gupta, A. K., Smith, K. G. and Shalley, C. E. (2006). The interplay between exploration and exploitation, *Academy of Management Journal,* 49, 693–706.

Hamel, G. and Prahalad, C. K. (1994). *Competing For the Future,* Harvard Business School Press, Boston, MA.

Hargadon, A. and Sutton, R. I. (1997). Technology brokering and innovation in a product development firm, *Administrative Science Quart,* 42, 716–749.

He, Z.-L. and Wong, P.-K. (2004). Exploration vs. exploitation: An empirical test of the ambidexterity hypothesis, *Organization Science,* 15, 481–494.

Holbek, J. (1988). The innovation design dilemma: Some notes on its relevance and solutions, in Grønhaug, K. and Kaufmann, G. (eds.), *Innovation: A Cross-Disciplinary Perspective,* Norwegian University Press, Oslo, Norway, pp. 253–277.

Howson, C. (1977). Why once may be enough, *Australasian Journal of Philosophy,* 55, 142–146.

Huber, G. P. (1991). Organizational learning: The contributing processes and the literatures, *Organization Science,* 2(1), 88–115.

Hull, C. E. and Covin, J. G. (2010). Learning capability, technological parity, and innovation mode use, *Journal of Product Innovation Management,* 27(1), 97–114.

Jansen, J. J. P., Van Den Bosch, F. A. J. and Volberda, H. W. (2006). Exploratory innovation, exploitative innovation, and performance: Effects of organizational antecedents and environmental moderators, *Management Science,* 52, 1661–1674.

Kelley, T. and Littman, J. (2001). *The Art of Innovation: Lessons in Creativity from IDEO, America's Leading Design Firm*. Doubleday, New York.

Khurana, A. and Rosenthal, S. R. (1997). Integrating the fuzzy front end of new product development, *Sloan Management Review,* 38, 103–120.

Knight, F. (1921). *Risk, Uncertainty and Profit,* McMuffin, Boston, MA.

Lampel, J., Lant, T. and Shamsie, J. (2000). Balancing act: Learning from organizing practices in cultural industries, *Organization Science,* 11, 263–269.

Lavie, D., Stettner, U. and Tushman, M. L. (2010). Exploration and exploitation within and across organizations, *The Academy of Management Annals,* 4, 109–155.

Levinthal, D. A. and March, J. G. (1993). The myopia of learning, *Strategic Management Journal,* 14, 95–112.

Levitt, B. and March, J. G. (1988). Organizational learning, *Annual Review of Sociology,* 14, 319–340.

Lewis, M. W. (2000). Exploring paradox: Toward a more comprehensive guide, *Academy of Management Review,* 25, 760–776.

Ligus, R. G. (1994). Enterprise agility: Jazz in the factory, *Industrial Management,* 26, 18–19.

Lounamaa, P. H. and March, J. G. (1987). Adaptive coordination of a learning team, *Management Science,* 33(1), 107–123, doi: 10.1287/mnsc.33.1.107.

Lohmann, S. (1998). An information rationale for the power of special interests, *Amer. Political Science Review,* 92, 809–827.

Lubatkin, M. H., Simsek, Z., Ling, Y. and Veiga, J. F. (2006). Ambidexterity and performance in small-to medium-sized firms: The pivotal role of top management team behavioral integration, *Journal of Management,* 32, 646–672.

MacCormack, A. and Verganti, R. (2003). Managing the sources of uncertainty: Matching process and context in software development, *Journal of Product Innovation Management,* 20, 217–232.

MacCormack, A., Verganti, R. and Iansiti, M. (2001). Developing products on 'internet time': The anatomy of a flexible development process, *Management Science,* 47, 133–150.

March, J. G. (1991). Exploration and exploitation in organizational learning, *Organization Science,* 2, 71–87.

March, J. G. (1994). *A Primer on Decision Making: How Decisions Happen*. The Free Press, New York, NY.

McGrath, R. G. (2011). Failing by design, *Harvard Business Review,* 89(4), 76–83.

Moenaert, R. K., De Meyer, A., Souder, W. E. and Deschoolmeester, D. (1995). RandD/marketing communication during the fuzzy front-end, *IEEE Transactions on Engineering Management,* 42, 243–258.

Myrup Andreasen, M. and Hein, L. (1987). *Integrated Product Development,* Springer Verlag, London.

Orton, J. D. (1997). From inductive to iterative grounded theory: Zipping the gap between process theory and process data, *Scandinavian Journal of Management,* 13, 419–438.

Orton, J. D. (2000). Enactment, sensemaking and decision making: Redesign processes in the 1976 reorganization of U.S. intelligence, *Journal of Management Studies,* 37, 213–234.

Peirce, C. S. (1903/1995). In Turrisi, P.A. (ed.), *Pragmatism As a Principle and Method of Right Thinking: The 1903 Harvard Lectures on Pragmatism,* State University of New York Press, Albany.

Porter, M. E. (1985). *Competitive Advantage: Creating and Sustaining Superior Performance*. The Free Press, New York, NY.

Puranam, P., Singh, H. and Zollo, M. (2006). Organizing for innovation: Managing the coordination-autonomy dilemma in technology acquisitions, *Academic Management Journal,* 49, 263–280.

Reid, S. and Brentani, U.d. (2004). The fuzzy front end of new product development for discontinuous innovations: A theoretical model, *Journal of Product Innovation Management,* 21, 170–184.

Reinertsen, D. G. (1999). Taking the fuzziness out of the fuzzy front end, *Research and Technical Management,* 42, 25.

Rothwell, R. (1994). Towards the fifth-generation innovation process, *Interntanional Marketing Review,* 11, 7–31.

Shackle, G. L. S. (1961). *Decision, Order and Time,* Oxford University Press, Oxford.

Sitkin, S. B. (1992). Learning through failure: The strategy of small losses, *Research in Organizational Behavior,* 14, 231–266.

Slater, S. F. and Narver, J. C. (1994). Does competitive environment moderate the market orientation-performance relationship? *Journal of Marketing,* 58, 46–55.

Smith, W. K. and Tushman, M. L. (2005). Managing strategic contradictions: A top management model for managing innovation streams, *Organization Science,* 16, 522–536.

Spender, J.-C. (1996). Making knowledge the basis of a dynamic theory of the firm, *Strategic Management Journal,* 17, 45–62.

Strauss, A. and Corbin, J. (1998). *Basics of Qualitative Research. Techniques and Procedures for Developing Grounded Theory,* Sage Publications, Thousand Oaks, CA.

Suddaby, R. (2006). What grounded theory is not, *Academy of Management Journal,* 49, 633–642.

Sætre, A. S. and Brun, E. (2012). Strategic management of innovation: Managing exploration-exploitation by balancing creativity and constraint, *International Journal of Innovation and Technology Management,* 9(4), 1–24.

Sætre, A. S. and Brun, E. (2013). Ambiguity and learning in the innovation process: Managing exploration-exploitation by balancing creativity and constraint revisited, *International Journal of Innovation and Technology Management,* 10(4), 1–9.

Sætre, A. S., Sørnes, J.-O., Browning, L. D. and Stephens, K. K. (2007). Enacting media use in organizations, *Journal of Information, Information Technologies and Organization,* 2, 133–158.

Taylor, A. and Greve, H. R. (2006). Superman or the Fantastic Four? Knowledge combination and experience in innovative teams, *Academy of Management Journal,* 49, 723–740.

Teece, D. J. (2007). Explicating dynamic capabilities: The nature and microfoundations of (sustainable) enterprise performance, *Strategic Management Journal,* 28(13), 1319–1350.

Teece, D. J., Pisano, G. and Shuen, A. (1997). Dynamic capabilities and strategic management, *Strategic Management Journal,* 18(7), 509–533.

Tushman, M. L. and O'Reilly III, C. A. (1996). Ambidextrous organizations: Managing evolutionary and revolutionary change, *California Management Review,* 38, 8–30.

Tushman, M. L. and O'Reilly III, C. A. (1997). *Winning through innovation: A practical guide to leading organizational change and renewal,* Harvard Business School Press, Boston, MA.

Van de Ven, A. H., Polley, D. E., Garud, R. and Venkataraman, S. (2008). *The Innovation Journey*, Oxford University Press, Oxford.

Van Maanen, J., Sørensen, J. B. and Mitchell, T. R. (2007). The interplay between theory and method: Introduction to special topic forum, *Academy of Management Review,* 32(4), 1145–1154.

Verganti, R. (1999). Planned flexibility: Linking anticipation and reaction in product development projects, *Journal of Product Innovation Management,* 16(4), 363–376.

Weick, K. E. (1974). Middle range theories of social systems, *Behavioral Science,* 19, 357–367.

Weick, K. E. (1979). *The Social Psychology of Organizing,* 2nd edn., McGraw-Hill, New York, NY.

Weick, K. E. (1992). Agenda setting in organizational behavior: A theory focused approach, *Journal of Management Inquiry,* 1, 171–182.

Weick, K. E. (1995). *Sensemaking in Organizations.* Sage, Thousand Oaks, CA.

Weick, K. E. (1998). Introductory essay: Improvisation as a mindset for organizational analysis, *Organizational Science,* 9, 543–555.

Part 5

Technology Adoption Perspectives

Chapter 13

IT Adoption in Healthcare Organizations

Nathasit Gerdsri* and Chonyacha Suebsin

College of Management, Mahidol University, Bangkok, Thailand

nathasit.ger@mahidol.ac.th

Abstract

This chapter addresses the key issues impacting the adoption of information technology (IT) in healthcare organizations. Four case studies were developed from different hospitals through a series of in-depth interviews to determine the factors affecting their IT adoption. The findings reveal that, at the organization level, these hospitals primarily make decisions to adopt new technologies based on project-related costs. At the individual level, the complications in the implementation process play a major role as they are influenced by human-related issues. Apart from the identification of key factors from the case studies, the latter part of this chapter also presents the mental framework of IT adoption for healthcare organizations developed based on the technology acceptance model.

Keywords: Technology Adoption, Healthcare, Information Technology, Cases.

1. Introduction

Recently, healthcare organizations have continuously put tremendous efforts to improve customer satisfaction as well as strengthen their business competence. Technology has become a vital component to address the continuous changes in patient requirements and medical practices. Without a shred of doubt, healthcare institutions rely heavily on several medical technologies and practices as key components to provide services to patients. However, other supporting technologies have played an important role in facilitating organizational workflow and processes. Despite the efforts invested in new technologies, many healthcare providers still face difficulties in successfully adopting the new technologies.

This study aims to identify the key issues impacting the adoption of new technology in healthcare organizations. In particular, we are interested in the case of healthcare organizations in Thailand because of the growing number of technology investments. In this chapter, the literature on healthcare management and the challenges to successful adoption in healthcare organizations are presented in Sections 2 and 3. Sections 4 and 5 discuss the research methodology and represent the case studies conducted with four hospitals in Thailand. The details of interviews with the doctors, medical personals, and hospital management were published in the PICMET 2011 and 2012 conferences. Section 6 represents the mental model of IT adoption for healthcare organizations in which many parts can lead to the future research studies. Finally, Section 7 provides the conclusion.

2. Healthcare Organizations

Healthcare business has been recognized as a knowledge- and information-intensive system which operates under continuous changes of patient requirements and medical disciplines (Effken, 2002; Lenz and Reichert, 2007; Spil *et al.*, 2002). With the great amount of intangible and intellectual assets, the healthcare industry is often viewed as a complex and unique sector compared to other types of businesses. Operating healthcare organizations involves emerging contingencies and requires a great deal of cooperation among different organizational units. Generally, healthcare operations are classified into key functions including finance and accounting, logistics and supply chain management, facilities management, human resources, business planning and performance improvement, and information management (Langabeer, 2008). These operations involve a mix of professional groups in different departments to support clinical, financial, and administrative activities.

The key challenges healthcare organizations face concern how to provide high-quality services in responding to the increasing patient complexity (Helfert, 2009). Even though healthcare institutions are considered as community-served entities that focus on service quality rather than profit maximization, the limitation of resources such as budget, personnel, and facilities forces healthcare organizations to manage their operations efficiently in order to overcome these constraints. Merely focusing on service quality and community benefits might not be sufficient for funding business operations. Moreover, as healthcare organizations are mostly governed by and greatly depend on medical professionals rather than well-trained businesspersons, it might not be easy for healthcare organizations to specify whether the clear goals and strategies focus on the quality of patient care or financial indicators (Langabeer, 2008).

Recent trends in healthcare management have attempted to reduce costs, maximize productivity, and focus more on profit earning to survive the increasing competition (Langabeer, 2008; Ghodeswar and Vaidyanathan, 2007). Unquestionably, the advancement in technology has been considered a key enabler for creating competitiveness for healthcare organizations. On the one hand, healthcare institutions rely heavily on several medical technologies such as devices, drugs, and disciplinary practices as key components to deliver services to patients. On the other hand, other supporting technologies should play an important role in facilitating organizational workflow and processes. For example, due to the business nature, technologies relating to knowledge and information management are vital arms assisting healthcare organizations to retain their standards and streamline business operations.

3. Healthcare Organization in Thailand

In recent years, numerous attempts have been made to improve the healthcare system in Thailand in accordance with the "Healthy Thailand" policy initiated by the Ministry of Public Health (Health Policy in Thailand, 2006). The rapid increase in national healthcare expenditure and the number of service providers are key indicators of the policy execution which focus on the readily accessible and high-quality medical services (Suraratdecha and Okunade, 2006). As a result, Thailand has the reputation of having a well-developed medical system with approximately 700 government and 300 private hospitals (Cohen, 2008).

Apart from the aforementioned facts, the Ministry of Public Health also positions Thailand as the medical hub of Asia by attempting to attract medical tourists by providing high-quality health services at affordable rates. Noticeably, the campaign is predominantly implemented in the private sector and only in some government hospitals. Three key areas of special medical treatments include medical services, such as surgical care, dental care, bone treatment; healthcare services, such as health spa and traditional massage; and Thai herbal products.[1]

4. Technology Adoption in Healthcare Organization

Technology adoption entails a sequence of stages an adopter follows to obtain a new technology and make it available for use. Rogers proposes that individuals adopt a technology by

[1]Sector Overview: The Health Industry in Thailand, Retrieved December 20, 2009, from http://www.ambbangkok.um.dk/nr/rdonlyres/7aff8a36-95b4-4237-b8e4-382297d1b594/0/sectoroverviewhealthindustryjune2006.pdf.

first being aware of the existence of a technology and forming attitudes toward a technology, followed by the decision whether to adopt or reject a technology. After the adoption decision is made, a technology will be used and eventually accepted if it could function as expected (Rogers, 1995). Regarding organization adoption, the process can be generally divided into two main stages: primary adoption and secondary adoption (Darmawan, 2001; Frambach and Schillewaert, 2002; Kamal, 2006). At an organization level, a firm is motivated by its objectives and business conditions. If an organization decides to acquire a new technology, it then takes a further step at an individual level where employees use the acquired technology. Based on this rationale, it can be presumed that the actual adoption is contingent on a prior decision made by an organization (Gallivan, 2001). Without an official decision, employees would not have an opportunity to utilize a new technology. On the other hand, without the acceptance from individuals, a firm would not be able to receive any benefits from investing in that technology.

Due to the continuous changes in patient requirements and medical practices, healthcare business has been considered as a complex and unique sector that relies heavily on knowledge and information. Apart from the quality of care as the key focus, recent efforts have been made to pursue cost-effectiveness and profit maximization (Langabeer Ii, 2008; Ghodeswar and Vaidyanathan, 2007). Technology has become one of the key enablers for healthcare organizations to achieve these goals. Notably, medical technologies and practices are the fundamental components for healthcare organizations to deliver services to patients. Moreover, other technologies supporting organizational processes have been increasingly embraced to facilitate effective operations and management as well. Considering the business characteristics, technologies relating to knowledge and information management should be vital for healthcare organizations to enhance business capabilities. Some examples of the technologies currently integrated in healthcare organizations include electronic medical records, telemedicine technology, radio frequency identification, enterprise systems, and mobile devices (Chau and Hu, 2002; Lee and Shim, 2007; Omary *et al.*, 2009; Trimmer *et al.*, 2002; Wu *et al.*, 2007; Mcgrady *et al.*, 2010).

Despite the tremendous efforts to actively engage in adoption projects, there are numerous reports of resistance, underuse, and premature termination of the invested technologies (Holden and Karsh, 2010). One key challenge healthcare organizations have faced when adopting a new technology is the concern about the costs associated with the projects. Apart from the price of the technology itself, adoption costs also cover personnel time and other resources used to accomplish the adoption. Different clinical standards and practices among healthcare providers sometimes force organizations to choose between customization and process redesigning, which can be costly in both ways. Moreover, the composition of specialized applications utilized in different organization units makes it necessary for the business to have the effective integration attaching the processes together (Woodside, 2007). Therefore, some additional investments might be required to accomplish the adoption (Omary *et al.*, 2009). In this sense, managers need to be cautious with the cost, which might far exceed the cost expected at the initial stage.

Another challenge persisting when healthcare organizations adopt a new technology concerns changes in management issues. Adopting a new practice often leads to change, which requires additional efforts by organization members. Nonetheless, as a healthcare organization comprises several units that have a substantial degree of autonomy, changing or replacing the established practices might not be easy (Chau and Hu, 2002; Adler-Milstein and Bates, 2010; Tsiknakis and Kouroubali, 2009). Besides, the lack of skilled and trained personnel is a significant barrier to successful adoption. However, by fulfilling this requirement, either providing a comprehensive training or recruiting qualified persons can consume a significant amount from the budget. In this sense, management should plan proper intervention strategies to facilitate such changes affected by the adoption (Bhattacherjee and Hikmet, 2007; Chang *et al.*, 2007; Cohn *et al.*, 2009).

5. Research Approach and Findings

The focus of this study is to address the factors associated with the adoption of technology in healthcare organizations. The following research questions arise:

RQ1: What are the strategic issues for initiating the adoption of a new technology in the case organization?
RQ2: What are the issues associated with the decision process for new technology adoption in the case organization?
RQ3: What are the issues affecting users' attitudes toward technology adoption in the case organization?

To fulfill the objective of the research, the case study development technique is applied. Data were collected through a series of in-depth interviews with the individuals participating in adoption projects within four hospitals in Thailand. These persons are representatives of different groups of stakeholders involved in the technology adoption processes. Some of them had been involved in more than one adoption project. The respondents are classified into four groups based on their roles in adoption projects. The first one is the management group which includes the persons who make the decision to adopt a technology. The second group consists of key players in planning and implementation processes. The third one is users who have to use the adopted technology. The last group comprises persons who support the implementation and the use of the technology (see Table 1).

The sets of specific questions were formulated for each group of respondents (see also in appendix). In general, the interviews lasted for 30 minutes and were recorded. A detailed

Table 1. Description of interview respondents.

Case hospital	Respondent
Hospital A	A1: Accounting Director; A2: Hospital Information System Manager; A3: General Accounting Manager; A4: Account Payable Supervisor; A5: Inventory Supervisor; A6: IT staff; A7: IT staff
Hospital B	B1: IT Manager; B2: Project Consultant (Outsource); B3: Head of Radiology Department; B4: Accounting Supervisor; B5: Nurse; B6: Nurse; B7: IT staff; B8: IT staff
Hospital C	C1: Assistant Hospital Director; C2: IT Manager (Outsource); C3: Head of Radiology Department; C4: Nurse; C5: Head of Emergency Department; C6: Pharmacist; C7: Pharmacist; C8: IT staff (Outsource)
Hospital D	D1: Assistant Hospital Director; D2: IT Manager; D3: Radiologist; D4: Pulmonary Physician; D5: IT staff

analysis was carried out through the transcription of the interviews. Specifically, the analysis was carried out based on adoption processes, including initiation, adoption decision, and implementation and usage.

5.1. *Presentation of cases*

5.1.1. *Hospital A*

Hospital A is a private healthcare provider in Thailand. Apart from local patients, many foreigners have visited the hospital because of its quality of service and the affordable prices. To support the recent vision that highlights the finest service and being the leading health service provider, the hospital has strived to improve its operations in many ways, such as the investment in advanced technologies and recruiting specialized personnel. The management of the hospital decided to adopt a new Enterprise Resource Planning (ERP) system to resolve the mismatch issues between the capability of the old system and business requirements.

The implementation of the new system covered only financial and supply chain management modules. As a result, the front-office operation of the hospital would mainly use a medical software application to operate clinical processes. However, the nurses who are responsible for the ordering of medical supplies would have to use the new ERP. Overall, the adoption project was carried out through multiple phases, including initiation and planning, analysis and design, building and transition, and go-live and post-implementation phases. After the project plan was set up, business requirements were gathered from key users. To take account of the gaps that existed between system capabilities and the given requirements, the management preferred process reengineering rather than customization. Therefore, the only major customization was the interface link between the front-office software and the ERP system.

After the ERP system was installed, the vendor team represented the system prototype based on the final solution. Then training sessions were conducted by the ERP consultants. Some sessions had to be repeated depending on users' understanding. After the system was tested for user acceptance, the data from the old system were transferred to the new one. Users started using the new ERP system and the old system was cut off. Initially, the project was planned to be completed within four months but the data preparation could not be completed within the specified time frame. Given that situation, the "go-live" phase was postponed for 2 months from the original plan. After the "go-live" phase, the ERP vendor continued providing subsequent support together with the hospital IT staff. In this case, IT staff together with the ERP vendor set up a "war room" to respond to users' problems. The issues reported by users and the solutions were recorded in a log file for further use in similar cases.

5.1.2. *Hospital B*

Hospital B is a private healthcare provider which has expanded the operations to several branches over the years. The hospital has attempted to reengineer and improve the business through several strategies including investment in new technologies. The first one was the replacement of the patient management system and accounting application due to their outdated functions and platforms that could not serve business requirements. Moreover, the hospital adopted a picture archiving and communication system (PACS), which allowed electronic storage, distribution, display, and interpretation of medical image to improve the medical diagnostic process.

In general, three applications were selected based on costs and their functional capabilities. The hospital also considered vendors' reference sites as another criterion in selecting technology packages. The new systems were implemented only at the largest branch and would be expanded to others in future. For the patient management and accounting application, the implementation of the three applications generally comprised multi-procedures including project planning, analysis and design, developing and implementation, and go-live and post-implementation phases. Nonetheless, the processes taken to accomplish the adoption of PACS were quite different since the technology did not require much analysis. Also, there was no need for customization and data migration. Therefore, the main implementation processes included planning, implementation, deployment, and post-implementation phases. The simultaneous implementation of three applications requires high level of cooperation among different organizational units. Some individuals were involved in more than one adoption project. Moreover, the three technology vendors were required to work together as all three systems needed to be integrated.

After the new applications were installed, training sessions were held for key users of each system separately. Meanwhile, data from the old systems (i.e., patient management system and accounting system) were transferred to the new ones. Then the three applications were tested for user acceptance and in actual use. The vendors of all three systems continue to standby on site for approximately a month to provide the post go-live support. Moreover, users can contact via IT hotline when they face problems while using the new applications.

5.1.3. *Hospital C*

Hospital C is one of the oldest private hospitals in Thailand, which has a long been reputed for its world-class services. Currently, the hospital is an affiliate of a chief medical facilities operator in the country. According to the central policy, the organization has shared the IT outsourcing department, which accounts for the management of most technologies utilized in the organization, with other hospital members. Within the last few years, several technologies have been adopted to reinforce organizational proficiency. In the current study, the interviews focus on the scarcely adopted ones, including telemedicine and PACS.

The hospital adopted telemedicine technology to provide a real-time consultation through interactive audiovisual media. With telemedicine, patients and hospital's partners such as hotels and other medical facilities can assess medical cases from remote locations using videoconferencing. However, the equipments supporting telemedicine were not universally available since they were installed at some areas in the hospital. Therefore, different departments have to share the facilities together. Moreover, the hospital also plans to apply this technology with other operational areas in future. For example, employees can attend training or seminar sessions that are being conducted at other places from the hospital.

Typically, the hospital considers an adoption decision based on relevant costs and its functional capabilities. Some of the technologies that have been adopted have been implemented and have proven their track records in other hospitals within the chain previously. In general, the implementation processes were mainly carried out by the IT outsourcing department. However, these persons were always transferred to some other sites in accordance with their company's policy, which could result in the shortage of user support and the discontinuance of work procedures. For some applications, users had the chance to attend seminar sessions to preview and give feedback to management regarding the prospected technologies before the adoption decision could be made. After the technologies have been installed, training sessions would be conducted by either the IT department or technology vendors.

5.1.4. *Hospital D*

Hospital D is a government healthcare provider located in a province close to Bangkok. Each day, the hospital provides clinical and health services to more than 1,500 patients from both within and outside the area. Despite the government district hospital, the continuous implementation of restructuring and renovating policy is a key enabler for private hospital impression. As well as the expertise of doctors and medical staff, the investment in modern equipments is another important element for providing efficient health services. In the past few years, the hospital has adopted several new applications such as the laboratory information system (LIS), hospital information system (HIS), and PACS. In this study, the interviews focus on the issues relating to the adoption of PACS.

PACS was mainly integrated with the imaging operation of the radiology department and some other image-based units. The project was partially initiated by the users in the radiology department as they had raised issues demonstrating the need to replace the hard film-printing method with the new system. Moreover, these users also became a part of the decision-making process as they had a chance to visit other hospitals that previously adopted PACS implemented by various vendors to judge the package they preferred. Nonetheless, the final decision is made by the management of the hospital. The new system was selected mainly based on costs, functional features, and maintenance services offered by the vendor. After the decision was made, physicians and medical staff in other image-based units were notified approximately four months before the implementation.

As an extension of the main HIS application, the PACS had to be combined with the patient management system to allow retrieval of medical images from patient records. Therefore, the vendors of the two systems had to work together to customize the linkage. Apart from the investment in the system software, the management decided to replace some hardware related to doctors' reading workstations to better support the adopted system. The implementation of the new system was mainly carried out by the PACS vendor with support from the hospital's IT department. The training sessions were held for key users prior to the full utilization of the system. During the transition phase, the existing hard-copy images were transformed into digital format and also collected in the new system by the vendor. After the formal utilization of PACS, the film-printing system was entirely terminated.

5.2. *Issues pertaining to technology adoption in the case hospitals*

Through the interview transcription, the factors identified are summarized and demonstrated with expressed quotations in Table 2.

Table 2. Summary of the issues pertaining to technology adoption in healthcare organizations.

Factors	**Respondents**
Competitive pressure	*With the PACs, we expect to reduce our film-printing cost. Moreover, the application would enable a more efficient analytical process* — IT Manager (B_1).
	When we adopt a new technology, we expect to increase patient satisfaction.... The successful implementation will help us to reduce the operation costs — Assistant Hospital Director (C_1).
Business strategy	*To support our long term goal that we aim to be a listed company in the stock exchange of Thailand, we have to prepare the data to be agreed with the standards required. We also plan to implement some other tools such as business intelligence (BI) system which support the utilization of information ... but before that, we have to change the software in order that it can support BI utilization* — Accounting Director (A_1).
	In the near future, we expect the cases that patients are transferred from one branch to another. Therefore, there is a need for the exchange of information, such as patient records, between branches. The access to data should be able to be done on web-based applications with the same standard. This could help us to improve our proficiency. Unfortunately, the old patient management and accounting programs do not allow us to develop that feature — IT Manager (B_1).
Government policy	*Sooner or later, it is probable that we need to link our systems to centralized public health departments ... so we have to get ready for that* — IT Manager (B_1).

Cost of technology	*With a limited budget, cost is the first thing we consider. Indeed, I do not think the selected ERP system is the best one among all alternatives ... another seems to be better but it is very costly* — Accounting Director (A_1). *Actually, the PACs technology has been available in Thailand for several years. I think the hospital just recently adopts the application because the cost of it is quite high* — Head of Radiology Department (B_3). *We have to weigh between the benefits we would get with the price we have to pay* — Assistant Hospital Director (C_1).
Functionality and capability	*We select this one because its functionality can respond to what we want, with the acceptable price* — Accounting Director (A_1). *As there are several vendors offering different PACs packages, we consider its functionality and capability to arrive at our final solution* — Head of Radiology Department (B_3). *One criteria we use is the functionality of the technology, considering what benefits we could get from it* — Assistant Hospital Director (C_1).
Technology suitability	*In our case, the key determinants are technology suitability and price. In larger organizations, they might use another ERP software ... which is not appropriate for our hospital* — HIS Manager (A_2). *Some technologies are good but do not match with our organization* — Head of Radiology Department (C_3).

(Continued)

Table 2. *(Continued)*

Factors	Respondents
Vendor experience	*Another factor we consider is an implementing team … this group of people we selected has experience in implementing ERP projects in some other hospitals … so they should know hospital business very well* — Accounting Director (A_1). *We also consider site references … get some information and feedback from hospitals utilizing PACs* — Head of Radiology Department (B_3). *Fortunately, the vendor of new ERP was so proficient. They knew how to implement and convince users to participate in such activities* — HIS Manager (A_2). *The accounting application we adopt is a pre-developed package which has been widely used in other industries. However, some functions do not match with our business process … for example, the way we recognize revenues are different. Moreover, the vendor has no experience implementing within hospital. Therefore, it is sometimes difficult for them to understand our workflow* — Accounting Supervisor (B_4).
Change management strategy	*Resistance issue…. Yes, we had this problem. It was like when you change the government. Some people like the new one, some people do not. Employees were worried about change and thought that the new system would make their lives more difficult. Thus, they did not want to use the new ERP. However, at this time, this seems to be less as they are forced by the organization policy, their supervisors, and workflow* — HIS Manager (A_2).

	The training cases could not help much ... real practices are not that easy — Account Payable Supervisor (A_4).
	I think we did not have much time to prepare ourselves to adapt to the new system before the real use. The old process we were familiar with had been radically changed — Inventory Supervisor (A_5).
	Even though we conducted training sessions, not many people attended the classes at first. We had to set up an evaluation process to force them to join the sessions — IT Manager (B_1).
	At first, no one wanted to use the telemedicine because there was no enforcement — IT Manager (C_2).
	It also depends on the communication ... whether there is someone explaining users why they need to use it — Nurse (C_4).
Routine job	*As key users, we had to prepare data for the new system, attend training, and some other tasks to support the project. However, we also had to concentrate on our routine job at the same time.... In this manner, our work could not be perfect* — General Accounting Manager (A_3).
	Sometimes it is not easy for medical staff such as doctors and nurses.... They have to weigh the priority between giving treatments or learning to use the new technologies ... especially in our case when three technologies were implemented at the same time, — Head of Radiology Department (B_3).
	Medical staffs tend to focus more on delivering service. Thus, time is another important issue that impacts adoption process — IT Manager (C_2).

(*Continued*)

Table 2. *(Continued)*

Factors	Respondents
Management involvement and support	*I think that the steering team should have involved more than just listening to the overview report. In our case, the steering team did not pay much attention on the project … no incentive, no penalty … several problems could not be solved because no one could make decision. In this manner, I would say that it makes no difference whether to have the steering committee or not* — Accounting Director (A_1).
	Top management has played an important role in leading a successful adoption. It is easier to implement change when a person with complete power closely looks after the projects — Project Consultant (B_2).
	The management here is well prepared as there were training sessions and support documents that facilitate our learning process — Nurse (B_5).
	Another factor is management team. If they want to introduce change, they need to take the lead and tightly stick with it — Head of Radiology Department (C_3).
Organizational attitude toward change	*I think employees working in this hospital are familiar with changes* — Nurse (B_5).
	In my opinion, the organization that is familiar with changes will adapt to new things easily — Head of Radiology Department (C_3).
Technology change agent	*It is important to identify the change agent … who can persuade and make others realize the benefits of these technologies* — Nurse (B_6).
	We need the doctors acting as change agents … persuade others to accept change — IT staff (C_8).

Availability and capability of IT personnel	*I think our IT staffs were not adequate as there were only two persons who support users. Moreover, they did not understand the hospital process workflow very well so their support was not effective* — Accounting Director (A_1). *Our IT personnel are very helpful. They help fix the problems we encounter and also act like the liaison between user and vendor* — Nurse (B_5). *I think we do not have enough IT personnel to support when the problems occur* — Pharmacist (C_6).
Work employment and autonomy	*Some part-time doctors do not have time to attend the sessions...Frankly, management had to try to persuade them to use the new system* — Nurse (B_5). *I think medical professionals are not much familiar with technology ... the medical education does not focus that much on technology use. Also, medical specialists normally work with high autonomy and focus more on medical practices. Making adoption mandatory is sometimes not that easy ... especially when the persons work on part-time basis* — Assistant Director (C_1).
Individuals' commitment/ congruence with firm's value	*When users gave their requirements at the beginning of the projects, they mostly stick to their old practices ... and not think that the project is important. Many times, we have to ask vendors to modify what they had developed ... and sometimes we have to pay more while prolong our planned schedule* — IT Manager (B_1).

(Continued)

Table 2. *(Continued)*

Factors	Respondents
Supporting technology	*The screen used to display the PACs image is not appropriate. Many doctors always complain that they cannot see things clearly so they refuse to use the system* — Head of Radiology Department (B_3).
	The PACs system was seldom used as doctors cannot see the image clearly on their computers — Nurse (C_4).
	No matter what the real things are, I think users perceive the benefits of technology based on the problems they encounter during usage. If we have high quality hardware and networks, the problems would be less — IT staff (C_8).
Perceived benefits	*It is important to make people perceive what benefits they would get from technology utilization. When they realize the advantage of it, they tend to willingly adopt it* — IT Manager (C_2).
Patient safety	*Most doctors do not want to use the telemedicine because they think it is risky to diagnose patients when they do not have face-to-face meetings* — Assistant Hospital Director (C_1).
Technology complexity	*I was so nervous to use the new ERP system because it was more complicated. If I did some mistakes, others' work might be affected by my action* — Account Payable Supervisor (A_4).
Staff average age	*I think people in different generations have different attitudes towards technology. Some elderly physicians are not familiar with technology so they refuse to use or hardly learn the new systems. We have found that sometimes nurses have to key information for doctors* — IT staff (B_7).
	At the beginning, only young doctor used Pacs — Nurse (C_4).

6. Comparative Study and Discussion

Based on the transcription of the interviews, the descriptions of the four cases are illustrated in Table 3.

Overall, the adoption of new technologies in the case hospitals comprises two main stages. The first one entails the processes a hospital takes to decide whether to adopt a new technology. The second one encompasses multiple steps in which the system is implemented and used by end users. Apparently, adoption projects are mostly initiated by management of organizations as they foresee technology as the tool to enhance organizational capabilities. There were some cases in which the IT department, which is an outsourcing entity, proposed the idea of adopting new technologies in hospital C. It is less likely that adoption projects would be initiated by end users. Nonetheless, it is found that PACS adoption in hospital D was proposed by the end users in the radiology department as they specified the need to replace the film-printing system with the new one. The underlying motivation-provoking adoption project commonly cited is the need to improve business competency and competitiveness. Moreover, some respondents also mentioned the need to comply with such standards and government policies as the factors initiating the adoption plan. Similar criteria were used to finalize adoption decision, including relevant costs, technology potential benefits and functionality, business compatibility, and vendor experiences.

In some adoption projects where the usage was widely applied with many work units, such as ERP and patient management system, the high degree of user involvement was entailed along the implementation processes. In the secondary stage of adoption, time is considered as a crucial issue as most respondents stated that routine tasks prevented them from project activities. In all four cases, some degree of resistance existed among a few groups of users prior to the actual usage, but it seemed to lessen later on after the technologies that had been implemented had been around for a while. Partially,

Table 3. Comparative findings from the four cases.

	Hospital A	Hospital B	Hospital C	Hospital D
Type of technology being adopted	• ERP	• PACS • Patient management system • Accounting system	• PACS • Telemedicine	• PACS
Target users	• Accountant • Inventory staff • Purchasing officer • Nurse	• Accountant • Radiological technologist • Physician • Nurse • Pharmacist	• Radiological technologist • Physician • Nurse • Pharmacist	• Radiological technologist • Physician • Nurse
Adoption motivation	• Business strategy	• Business strategy • Competitive pressure • Government policy	• Competitive pressure	• Competitive pressure
Criteria used to make decision	• Cost of technology • Functionality and capability • Technology suitability • Vendor experience	• Cost of technology • Functionality and capability • Vendor experience	• Cost of technology • Functionality and capability	• Cost of technology • Functionality and capability • Maintenance services

Issues affecting implementation	• Routine job • Management involvement and support • Change management process (policy enforcement, communication, training, evaluation) • Availability and capability of IT personnel • Technology complexity • Vendor experience	• Routine job • Management involvement and support • Change management process (policy enforcement, communication, training, evaluation) • Technology change agent/champion • Organizational attitude toward change • Supporting technology	• Routine job • Management involvement and support • Change management process (policy enforcement, communication, training, evaluation) • Technology change agent/champion • Organizational attitude toward change	• Routine job • Management involvement and support • Effective integration/ Coordination of vendors • Change management process (policy enforcement, communication, training, evaluation)

(*Continued*)

Table 3. (*Continued*)

	Hospital A	Hospital B	Hospital C	Hospital D
		• Adopters' average age • Vendor experience	• Availability and capability of IT personnel • Supporting technology • Patient safety concern • Work employment and autonomy • Perceived benefits	• Vendor experience • Organizational attitude toward change • Supporting technology • Work employment and autonomy • Adopters' average age • Perceived benefits
Evaluation on adoption success	• Usage volume	• Usage volume • Time taken to complete the project	• Usage volume • Errors occurring during usage	• Time taken to complete the project • Errors occurring during usage

employees eventually had to accept the changes because it was their responsibility to comply with management's decisions. Besides, an effective communication management and implementing team can be another stimulus that fosters employee's willingness to learn to use a new system. The importance of management commitment and involvement can be demonstrated by hospitals B and D. Many respondents commented that adoption projects implemented in hospitals B and D could be achieved by far because the management closely looked after and provided sufficient support during the implementation stage.

The nature of healthcare business itself is an important hindrance for the implementation of such changes. Based on the respondents' comments, it was quite hard to make physicians adopt the new technology that varied from the ones directly used in clinical processes due to their limited time contributing to adoption projects. This issue was found to be more critical in hospitals A, B, and C where most physicians worked on a part-time basis, while it was more convenient to implement such changes in hospital D as the physicians there worked on a full-time basis. In this sense, it implies that the lower degree of work autonomy in government hospitals is a better facilitator for adoption than that in private ones. It is also found that physician champions could help facilitate adoption process as these persons would persuade others to recognize the need for technological change. Moreover, the age of adopters could be another factor impacting adoption behavior. This is obvious when comparing the case of hospital B where some elderly users refused to use new technologies, while the young physicians in hospital D actively engaged with adoption projects. There were also issues concerning patient safety indicated in the case of telemedicine adoption. Most physicians did not want to diagnose a patient through audiovisual media because they were not certain they could make it precisely.

It is also inferred from the cases that organizational readiness is another antecedent of adoption outcomes. Organizational readiness, in a broad sense, refers to the availability of essential resources of the firm to support such organizational activities (Iacovou *et al.*, 1995; Kuan and Chau, 2001). The issue is obvious in the case of hospital C that outsources the IT department. With this strategy, IT persons were not stabilized which occasionally resulted in the shortage of user support and the discontinuance of work procedures. Apart from the human resources aspect, supporting technology is another aspect an organization should consider when adopting new technology. Based on the respondents' comments, some physicians in hospital B preferred film-printing system to PACS because the display screen could not provide clear images.

In general, the success of adoption was evaluated based on usage volume, time consumed to accomplish the project, and problems occurring during usage. However, for all four cases, there were no formal evaluation and follow-up procedures taken after the implementation or installation of new technologies. For hospitals C and D, there were some surveys and informal evaluation conducted after the new technologies had been implemented. However, none of formal processes or reward and punishment policies were strictly applied if the findings were not satisfied.

6.1. *Summary of the key factors affecting the adoption*

Through the analysis, the key issues influencing technology adoption in healthcare organizations are addressed. These factors are categorized into two main groups in accordance with adoption processes. The first one comprises the issues that influence adoption decisions. Obviously, the primary objective of the adoption is to foster organizational competitiveness and to comply with business strategy. The more pressures from intense competition a hospital perceives, the more likely it will adopt new technologies to reinforce its operations. Besides, the direction pointed by government could play an important role in raising awareness or guiding how technology can be used to tackle such business challenges healthcare organizations might face. After an organization recognizes the needs to adopt a new technology, the best-fit solution is selected based on project-related costs, potential benefits, suitability, vendor experience, and maintenance services provided by vendor.

In the secondary stage of adoption, the processes are mostly found to be affected by human-related issues. The resistance existing at early stages can be diminished by the effective change management (i.e., policy enforcement, communication, training, and evaluation). The findings also contend that time management is a crucial issue associated with the success of technology implementation. Moreover, the supportive conditions and directions shaped by management are important when a firm adopts a new technology, especially the sophisticated ones that require lots of resources and high level of cooperation among organization members. Besides, the presence of technology change agents is an antecedent of successful adoption as these persons would help introduce the new idea and persuade others to recognize the need for technological change. It is also found that organizational readiness is another factor that affects adoption outcomes. Some participants highlight the concerns about the lack of resources such as supporting staff and technology as the key inhibitor to the implementation of new technology. The age of adopters is founded to affect adoption process. In general, adoption can be hardly achieved in an organization with elderly adopters.

From the study, it is also asserted that work employment basis can affect adoption outcomes. Full-time staff are more likely to put more effort in learning to use a new technology, while part-time employees contribute less to adoption projects.

6.2. *Integrating technology acceptance model into the analysis framework*

After the key factors are identified, the mental model of the research is developed in this section. The model is drawn upon the technology acceptance model (TAM), which is one of the predominant theories explaining adoption behavior. As an extension of the theory of reasoned action (TRA), TAM postulates two perceived attributes — perceived usefulness and perceived ease of use — as the main determinants of system acceptance (Davis *et al.*, 1989). Perceived usefulness is defined as the degree to which an adopter believes the new technology would improve job performance, and perceived ease-of-use refers to an adopter's perception of the minimum effort required for the use of new technology (Davis *et al.*, 1989). To date, much of the adoption research conducted applies TAM rationale to address the variation in diverse contexts (Adam *et al.*, 1992; Malhotra and Galletta, 1999; Venkatesh and Davis, 2000) (see Figure 1).

Despite the extensive use of TAM in technology adoption research, the model has been mostly incorporated in the studies that focus on individual adoption. As the adoption of a technology in an organization compounds both the organization and the individual, to develop our mental model, TAM's constructs are integrated within the mental model at the secondary stage of adoption as shown in Figure 2.

As demonstrated in the mental model, at the organization level, the adoption project is initiated by such motivations. Then the decisions, including whether to adopt a new technology and which system package will be implemented, will be finalized by an authorized group of persons. At the individual level, after the new technology is acquired, users will have to utilize the technology. The attitudes potential users have toward the technology will be formed as a consequence of perception of such conditions existing in the organization. As TAM was originally developed to explain individual adoption, the constructs perceived usefulness and perceived ease of use are thus integrated in the mental model as the main antecedents of users' attitudes which eventually influence the actual use. However, it is noted from the current study that the

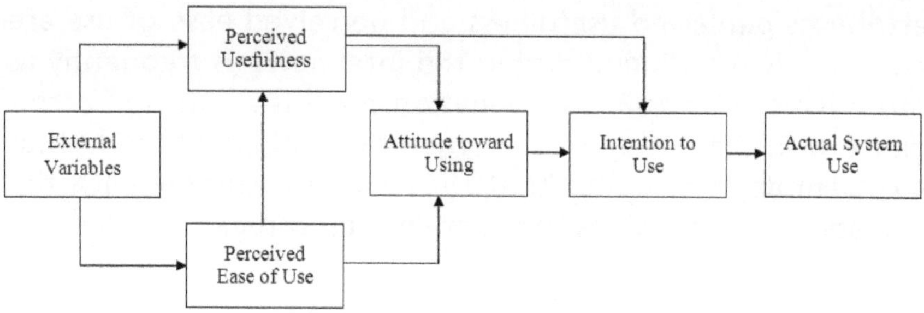

Figure 1. Technology acceptance model.
Source: Adapted from Davis *et al.* (1989).

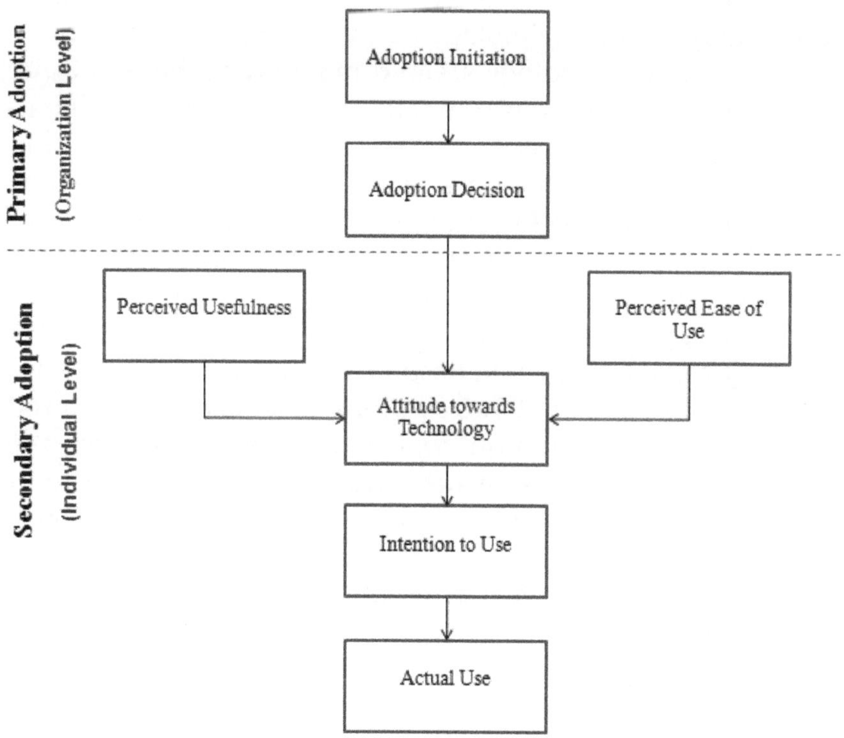

Figure 2. Proposed mental model.

attributes perceived usefulness and perceived ease of use are not directly mentioned during the interviews as frequently as other issues. A possible explanation for this result is in accordance with the nature of the organizational adoption itself as most employees realize that they have to comply with the management's decisions to maintain their career.

7. Conclusion

Through the analysis, the key issues affecting the adoption of new technologies in the case hospitals are addressed in accordance with the main steps that the organizations take to accomplish adoption projects. The first stage of adoption comprises two main processes, including the initiation and the decision to adopt a new technology. The issues motivating hospitals to adopt a new technology are in common with those of other industries, which includes competitive pressure, business strategy, and government policy. In general, the hospitals in this study adopt new technologies with the aim to foster service quality and streamline business processes to enhance customer satisfaction and pursue business competitiveness. Based on the interviews, the cost relevant to the adoption project is the most important factor influencing the adoption decision. However, it is noted from the study that hospitals mainly consider the price of technology and sometimes overlook other expenses incurred during the implementation, which can eventually deter the adoption project. Other issues affecting adoption decisions comprise technology attributes, suitability, vendor experience, and the maintenance services attached with the package.

From the cases, the factors influencing the implementation and usage of new technology are more likely to be human-related issues. Based on the findings, it is suggested that the management should play an important role in shaping organizational attitudes toward change, strictly engaging as part of the project to help overcome such potential barriers for successful adoption. For the adoption of back-office technology such as an ERP system, the factors affecting adoption are quite similar to those of other businesses. Based on the cases, the nature of healthcare business could have more impact on the adoption of technologies relevant to the clinical processes when the changes affect more work units. In particular, the substantial degree of autonomy medical professionals possess is found to be one barrier to change. Noticeably, the issues of work autonomy and medical specialist engagement are more critical in private hospitals than in government hospitals due to the difference in work employment. It even seems that private hospitals should have more opportunities to adopt new technologies, the part-time work employment of physicians and medical specialists sometimes makes it difficult to accomplish the adoption. As most physicians work on a part-time basis, they tend to have limited time for engaging in adoption activities. In this sense, managers who organize the adoption project should foresee this potential issue that could be detrimental to adoption success and draw up the strategy to handle the situation.

Apart from the identification of the issues associated with the adoption, the framework of the TAM is applied to develop the mental organizational adoption framework. Even though TAM's constructs are not directly mentioned by respondents as frequently as some other issues through the interviews, there are some implications that notify the links between TAM's construct and other factors addressed in the study.

Appendix: Questions Asked in the Interview

A. Management Group

- Please briefly explain the general work process before adopting the new technology.
- Why did the hospital decide to adopt the new technology?
- How did the management know that the new technology would solve the problems or limitations of the old system?

- Who was involved in the decision-making process in selecting the new technology?
- How long did the decision-making process take?
- What were the factors determining the final solution/brand/package that was selected among several ones?
- What do you expect from the new technology?
- Please explain the general work process after adopting the new technology.
- What are the facilitating conditions that the management has provided for employees to support the use of the new technology?
- What is the goal of the project? How do you assess project success or follow-up the project progress?
- Do you think the adoption of new technology has succeeded?
- During the project, were there any issues that hindered or obstructed project success?
- What are the important elements that contribute to project success?
- What was the problem-handling strategy?

B. Planning and Implementing Group

- How was the planning and implementing team set up?
- How did you know or gain information about the new technology?
- How did you divide the project into phases?
- What was the role of the technology vendor?
- How did you assign persons to identify the system requirement?
- Were there any changes in requirement? If so, how did you manage the changing requirement?
- How did employees react after they knew they had to use the new system? If the employees resisted using the new technology, what was the plan or strategy to reduce the resistance?

- Do you think the adoption of the new ERP system has succeeded?
- During the project, were there any issues that hindered or obstructed project success?
- What was the problem-handling strategy?
- What are the important parts that contribute to project success?

C. User Group

- Please briefly explain the general work process before adopting the new technology.
- When you knew that the hospital would change to the new system, how did you feel?
- How did the hospital inform you about the use of the new technology?
- How did the hospital prompt or support employees to learn to use the new system? Do you think the support conditions provided were sufficient?
- Please explain the general work process after adopting the new technology.
- Do you think the new technology is useful?
- Are there any problems or issues that cause difficulties using the new technology?
- In case of problems, how did you find the solutions?

D. IT Support Group

- Please briefly explain the general work process before adopting the new technology.
- Please explain the general work process after adopting the new technology.
- What was the role of the support department in adopting the new technology?
- Do you think the adoption of new technology has succeeded?

- During the project, were there any issues that hindered or obstructed project success?
- When users have problems using the new technology, what is the strategy used to find the solution?

References

Adam, D. A., Nelson, R. R. and Todd, P. A. (1992). Perceived usefulness, ease of use and usage of information technology: A replication, *MIS Quarterly*, 16(2), 227–247.

Adler-Milstein, J. and Bates, D. W. (2010). Paperless healthcare: Progress and challenges of an IT-enabled healthcare system, *Business Horizons*, 53, 119–130.

Bhattacherjee, A. and Hikmet, N. (2007). Physicians' resistance toward healthcare information technology: A theoretical model and empirical test, *European Journal of Information Systems*, 16, 725–737, 2007.

Chang, I. C., Hwang, H. G., Hung, M. C., Lin, M. H. and Yen, D. C. (2007). Factors affecting the adoption of electronic signature: Executives' perspective of hospital information department, *Decision Support Systems*, 44, 350–359.

Chau, P. Y. K. and Hu, J. H. (2002). Investigating healthcare professionals' decisions to accept telemedicine technology: An empirical test of competing theories, *Informationa and Management*, 39, 297–311.

Cohen, E. (2008). Medical tourism in Thailand, in *Explorations in Thai Tourism: Collected Case Studies*, Palgrave Emerald, Bingley, UK.

Cohn, K. H., Berman, J., Chaiken, B., Green, D., Green, M., Morrison, D. and Scherger, J. E. (2009). Engaging physicians to adopt healthcare information technology, *Journal of Healthcare Management*, 54(5), 291–300.

Darmawan, I. G. N. (2001). Adoption and implementation of information technology in Bali's local government: A comparison between single level path analyses using PLSATH 3.01 and AMOS 4 and multilevel path analyses using MPLUS 2.01, *International Education Journal*, 2(4), 100–123.

Davis, F. D., Bagozzi, R. P. and Warshaw, P. R. (1989). User acceptance of computer technology: A comparison of two theoretical models, *Management Science*, 35(8), 982–1003.

Effken, J. A. (2002). Different lenses, improved outcomes: A new approach to analysis and design of healthcare information systems, *International Journal of Medical Informatics*, 65, 59–74.

Frambach, R. T. and Schillewaert, N. (2002). Organisational innovation adoption: A multi-level framework of determinants and opportunities for future research, *Journal of Business Research*, 55(2), 163–176.

Gallivan, M. J. (2001). Organisational adoption and assimilation of complex technological innovations: Development and application of a new framework, *The Database for Advances in Information Systems*, 32(3), 51–85.

Ghodeswar, B. M. and Vaidyanathan, J. (2007). Organisational adoption of medical technology in healthcare sector, *Journal of Services Research*, 7(2), 57–81.

Health Policy In Thailand (2006), Retrieved December 20, 2009, from http://www.searo.who.int/en/section1174/section1199/section 1570_13027.htm.

Helfert, M. (2009). Challenges of business processes management in healthcare: Experience in the Irish healthcare sector, *Business Process Management Journal*, 15(6), 937–952.

Holden, R. J. and Karsh, B. T. (2010). Technology acceptance model: Its past and its future in healthcare, *Journal of Biomedical Informatics*, 43, 159–172.

Iacovou, C. L., Benbasat, I. and Dexter, A. (1995). Electronic data interchange and small organizations: Adoption and impact of technology, *MIS Quarterly*, 19(4), 465–485.

Kamal, M. M. (2006). IT innovation adoption in the government sector: Identifying the critical success factors, *Journal of Enterprise Information*, 19(2), 192–222.

Kuan, K. K. Y. and Chau, P. Y. K. (2001). A perception-based model for EDI adoption in small businesses using a technology-organization-environment framework, *Information and Management*, 38(8), 507–521.

Langabeer II, J. R. (2008). *Health Care Operations Management: A Quantitative Approach to Business and Logistics*, Jones and Bartlett, Sudbury, MA.

Lee, C. and Shim, J. P. (2007). An exploratory study of radio frequency identification (RFID) adoption in the healthcare industry, *European Journal of Information Systems*, 16, 712–724.

Lenz, R. and Reichert, M. (2007). IT support for healthcare processes: Premises, challenges, perspectives, *Data & Knowledge Engineering*, 61, 39–58.

Malhotra, Y. and Galletta, D. F. (1999). Extending the technology acceptance model to account for social influence: Theoretical bases and empirical validation, in *Proceeding of the 32nd Hawaii International Conference on System Sciences.*

McGrady, E., Conger, S., Blanke, S., Landry, B. J. L. and Zalucki, P. M. (2010). Emerging technology in healthcare: Navigating risks, evaluating rewards, *Journal of Healthcare Management*, 55(5), 353–365.

Omary, Z., Lupiana, D., Mtenzi, F. and Wu, B. (2009). Challenges to E-Healthcare adoption in developing countries: A case study of Tanzania, in *Proceedings of Networked Digital Technologies Conference.*

Rogers, E. M. (1995). *Diffusion of Innovations*, 4th edn., The Free Press, New York.

Spil, T. A. M., Stegwee, R. A. and Teitink, C. J. A. (2002). Business intelligence in healthcare organizations, in *Proceedings of the 35th Hawaii International Conference on System Sciences.*

Suraratdecha, C. and Okunade, A. A. (2006). Measuring operational efficiency in a health care system: A case study from Thailand, *Health Policy*, 77, 2–23.

Trimmer, K. J., Pumphrey, L. D. K. and Wiggins, C. (2002). ERP implementation in rural health care, *Journal of Management in Medicine*, 16(2/3), 113–132.

Tsiknakis, M. and Kouroubali, A. (2009). Organizational factors affecting successful adoption of innovative eHealth services: A case study employing the FITT framework, *International Journal of Medical* Informatics, 78, 39–52.

Venkatesh, V. and Davis, F. D. (2000). A theoretical extension of the technology acceptance model: Four longitudinal field studies, *Management Science*, 46, 186–204.

Woodside, J. M. (2007). EDI and ERP: A real-time framework for healthcare, *Journal of Medical System*, 31, 178–184.

Wu, J. H., Wang, S. C. and Lin, L. M. (2007). Mobile computing acceptance factors in the healthcare industry: A structural equation model, *International Journal of Medical Informatics*, 76, 66–77.

Chapter 14

Implementation of Electronic Medical Records in Dutch Hospitals

Ferry Koster* and Mattijs Lambooij†

Erasmus University Rotterdam/TIAS School for Business and Society, National Institute of Public Health and the Environment, the Netherlands

**koster@essb.eur.nl*

†info@rivm.nl

Abstract

Innovation projects are prone to "escalation of commitment" (the tendency to continue projects even if it is clear that they will be unsuccessful). In this study, we introduce a construct measuring the escalation prevention potential (EPP) of innovation projects as perceived by individuals in the organization. EPP consists of three components: (1) goals, (2) process, and (3) ability, to shield projects from escalation to commitment. A survey was conducted among 1,062 clinicians working in hospitals implementing electronic medical records (EMRs). The empirical results show that the three theoretical components of EPP sum up to a single measure. Four organizational characteristics of organizations (organizational routines, leadership reflexivity, employee involvement, and support staff quality) explain a large share of the variation in EPP.

Keywords: Innovation, escalation prevention potential, escalation of commitment, electronic medical records.

1. Introduction

This study investigates escalation prevention potential (EPP) as the ability of an organization to stop or steer unsuccessful innovation projects. Theoretically, EPP is rooted in the literature about "escalation of commitment", which focuses on the tendency to continue projects even if they are unsuccessful (Staw, 1976; Sleesman *et al.*, 2012). Research shows that escalation is caused by several determinants at different levels of analyses (project, psychological, social, and structural) (Ross and Staw, 1993) and is explained by multiple theoretical mechanisms (e.g., subjective expected utility, self-justification, framing, goal substitution, self-presentation, and agency problems) (Sleesman *et al.*, 2012). Basically, this literature challenges rational models of project management (Cooper and Zmud, 1990), as it shows that many innovation projects do not reach their intended outcomes.

In this chapter, we propose that the more EPP organizations have, the better they are equipped to steer projects and to abandon them if they turn out to be unsuccessful. To date, most of the research focuses on what may be called the negative side of escalation of commitment, namely, the list of studies aimed at understanding why projects fail (Brockner, 1992; Keil and Robey, 1999; Ku, 2008; Montealagre and Keil, 2000; Pan *et al.*, 2009; Ross and Staw, 1993; Schulz-Hardt *et al.*, 2009; Simonson and Staw, 1992; Staw, 1976). Far less attention is paid to the other side of the process, namely, the factors that prevent escalation behavior. In other words, from previous studies we know a lot about *why* escalation takes place, but far less is known about *how* to stop it. Furthermore, studies that do focus on the question how escalation may be prevented (Keil and Robey, 1999; Montealagre and Keil, 2000; Pan *et al.*, 2009; Pan and Pan, 2011) have a limited scope as they focus on a *specific kind of action* to prevent escalation, only focusing on its *project and psychological determinants* and rely either on *experiments* or a *qualitative case* study (which may limit their generalizability). This study broadens the existing view on escalation prevention by looking at *general mechanisms* underlying EPP, by also including *social* and *structural determinants* (Sleesman *et al.*, 2012) and by developing a *survey* instrument to assess the level of EPP of an organization (which can also be applied across different kinds of organization).

We test our model of EPP in a specific kind of organization and focus on one particular kind of innovation. The study is conducted in healthcare organizations. As in other organizations, healthcare organizations implement new technologies to increase efficiency and customer satisfaction. We focus on the introduction of electronic medical records (EMRs), which serve as an example for innovations in general. EMRs are IT tools to store patient information and enable the exchange of information among healthcare professionals within hospitals, assist professionals in decision-making, and can improve patient safety. While EMRs explicitly aim at improving the work performance in healthcare organizations, it turns out that it does not do so automatically. In the Netherlands, where this study was conducted, doctors and nurses are not forced to use EMRs. This means that hospitals have a lot of freedom in applying EMRs, both in the sense of whether they use them and how they use them. As a result, EMR use varies among hospitals in the Netherlands. Studies on implementation of EMRs show that it is difficult to determine the objective added value of working with EMRs and that resistance of users or other barriers reduces the potential benefits of using an EMR in hospital care (Chaudoir *et al.*, 2013; Greenhalgh *et al.*, 2004). This implies that purely rational models of technological innovation, according to which innovations by definition have added value to all stakeholders in an organization and do not regard change process as a part of a larger social system that need continuous attention, do not suffice to understand successful innovation.

This study develops and tests a survey instrument providing an overall indicator of an organization's EPP. Having such an instrument allows comparing EPP between individuals and organizations. And, ultimately, it can be used as a diagnostic tool. To do so, we developed a measurement scale and investigate whether the proposed building blocks measure the EPP construct. The empirical part of this study relies on survey data that were gathered among 1,062 respondents (doctors and nurses) from a random sample of hospitals in the Netherlands.

2. Theory

2.1. *Escalation prevention potential*

The *EPP* construct refers to the mechanisms that organizations possess to steer or stop a project. This construct is based on the de-escalation activities and conditions suggested in earlier studies (see, for example, Pan and Pan, 2011). However, while in this previous work only a list of possible de-escalation activities was presented, we take the next step by conceptualizing them and analyzing them at a more abstract level. We propose that there are three general mechanisms shielding projects from escalating, which are termed (1) goals, (2) process, and (3) abilities. A basic assumption of the proposed model is that the level of EPP is higher if these mechanisms are in place. And, if they are aligned, they may be even more successful to prevent escalation. This assumption closely follows the idea that organizational policies are more effective if they are internally consistent, as it signals a clear message to members of the organization (Huselid, 1995; Koster, 2011). What is more, the management of an organization with a higher level of EPP allows for feedback on their performance, as innovation projects are more transparent to the whole organization. Hence, it is assumed that the more transparency they instill in these projects on all three aspects, the more EPP they have.

2.1.1. *Goals*

Innovation projects are characterized by outcome uncertainty (Eisenhardt, 1989). In response to outcome uncertainty, decision-makers (and others involved in the project) may try to find means to justify what they are doing and why they do it. Hence, outcome uncertainty paves the way for sunk cost issues, self-justification, and agency problems (Whyte, 1986; Shapiro, 2005). According to Nilakant and Rao (1994), there are several ways to reduce outcome uncertainty. Stating clear goals at the start of a project and formulating measurable success factors at the beginning of it lead to a reduction of outcome uncertainty as it defines the direction of the project and how it can be assessed whether it develops as preferred. Or the other way around, projects lacking clearly stated goals and success factors are more likely to escalate as participants may look for other means to justify their actions. If the purpose of the innovation project is unclear and no success factors are formulated, projects may go on without intervention because there is no reason for it (Satyashankar *et al.*, 2007).

2.1.2. *Process*

Escalation of commitment is a dynamic process through which projects become gradually entrapped (Ross and Staw, 1993). This is allowed to happen if there are no clear guidelines and if the progress of the project is not monitored. Breaking up the project in smaller parts makes it easier for participants to intervene in the process and adjust or stop a project that is heading in an undesirable direction (Pich *et al.*, 2002). This can be done by defining projects in terms of sub-projects and by having regular meetings in which the progress of the project is evaluated. Piecing projects into smaller parts reduces the influence of some of the escalation determinants (Sleesman *et al.*, 2012), such as sunk cost problems (as the amount of resources that are already used remains limited), self-justification (as there is more information about the actual success of the project), embarrassment (because decision can be justified by referring to external rules), and agency problems detected in an early stage of the project. Again, to put it the other way around, projects that lack predefined phases and that are not regularly evaluated are more likely to escalate.

2.1.3. *Ability*

Finally, the skills of the project members and the clarity of the tasks they perform matter for instilling EPP (Pant and Baroudi, 2008). Project management is demanding in the sense that it expects a lot of the information processing capabilities of project participants in order to make informed decisions about the project. Hence, projects benefit if people with the right qualifications participate in them. Furthermore, according to the "responsibility effect" (Schulz-Hardt *et al.*, 2009), projects can escalate because a small group of individuals are responsible for it. This is reinforced if the ones starting the project are also the ones responsible for the implementation and success of the project (Simonson and Staw, 1992). A clear distribution of tasks (planning, implementation, and performance) among a larger number of participants can reduce these tendencies (Katz and Allen, 1985). In combination with ensuring that participants possess the necessary knowledge and capabilities to manage and fulfill the project (Yang, 2014), clear tasks can contribute to the de-escalation capacity of an organization. The escalation prevention mechanism "ability" reduces the risk that a small group of people becomes too greatly involved and dependent upon the project, while a large share of the organizational members are not involved at all. For example, by also including skeptics in the team (Pan and Pan, 2011), the likelihood of self-justification decreases.

2.2. *Determinants of escalation prevention potential*

The core theoretical explanations of escalation of commitment (Brockner, 1992; Sleesman *et al.*, 2012) provide the basis for defining and measuring the perception of the EPP of organizations and offer suggestions regarding its determinants. The extent to which organizations are able to develop and maintain the three components of escalation prevention according to its members depends on other characteristics of the organization. It is assumed that the perception of an organization's EPP depends on the availability of means to reduce outcome uncertainty, a focus on improving decision-making, and actions that encourage a shared understanding that lead to a less stronger connection between persons and projects. In a recent overview, Boonstra *et al.* (2014) show that there are several context, content, and process factors contributing to its successful implementation. Following that study, we conclude that the process of EMR implementation should be treated as an innovation project that is led by implementers or change managers and that the quality of change management is important for the success of such a project. In addition to that, Greenhalgh *et al.* (2009) find that realistic evaluation of goals and preliminary goals during the implementation process can be a valuable source of information for those involved. Periodic and realistic evaluation can provide valuable lessons on how certain preconditions make anticipated outcomes more likely. This study focuses on four of these contextual factors and preconditions of innovation projects.

2.2.1. *Routines*

Organizations have different ways of dealing with changes and innovation processes. Organizational routines (patterns of behavior, action, or interactions) provide stability in the course of organizational change (Feldman, 2000). These routines can contribute to the performance of organizations in different ways, for example through the reduction of outcome uncertainty (Becker, 2004), by decreasing the need for gathering information, or by gathering more information to improve the decision-making capacity (March and Simon, 1958).

With regard to decreasing the need for information, organizational routines can refer to certain rules, like standard operating procedures (Cyert and March, 1963) and programs

(Simon, 1977), prescribing how organization members ought to behave in certain situations. A consequence of such standard procedures is that it is not necessary to consider every new project completely but that parts of it may be organized in a similar (and effective) way. This kind of stability is likely to decrease the uncertainty associated with new projects and, hence, minimize chances of excessive risk taking and agency problems, given that organizational routines and rules can function as effective coordination and control mechanisms (Becker, 2004), which in turn can be strong mechanisms in dealing with agency problems in organizations (Eisenhardt, 1989).

In addition to minimizing the need to search for new information, organizations can possess learning routines (March, 1991), providing stability to the organization and hence reduce outcome uncertainty. Organizational learning means that organizations adapt their routines gradually based on past performance. Hence, if organizations have more experience with implementing new technology, if they are willing to take negative feedback seriously, and are able to experiment with new rules to further improve performance, the introduction of each new technology project becomes easier as project members can rely on existing rules. Since learning routines are not held by individuals, but are part of the repertoire of aggregates like teams and even the whole organization (Becker, 2004), their presence is a strong counterbalance to self-justification mechanisms in organizations. Based on these arguments, the first hypothesis states the following relationship between organizational routines and an organization's EPP.

H1: *Organizational routines contribute to the perception of escalation prevention potential of organizations.*

2.3. *Authentic leadership*

Authentic leadership (Avolio and Gardner, 2005) refers to the extent to which managers allow themselves to have a critical look at their own functioning and performance. Hence, this kind of reflexivity means that managers are actively involved in gathering information from project participants, acknowledging their own failures and are open to suggestions.

A reflexive attitude of organizational leaders establishes additional mechanisms that contribute to the potential of an organization to prevent escalation. Most and for all, authentic leaders generate their own critics and skeptics, rather than constituting a close circle of yes-sayers who do not dare or wish to critically approach the management of their organization (Prusak, 1997). Authentic leadership, thus, counterbalances many of the escalation determinants. In the presence of authentic leadership, self-justification and self-presentation are difficult to sustain as they force organization leaders to come to terms with themselves rather than keeping up an image for the outside world (Sleesman *et al.*, 2008). By critically considering their own performance, the management of the organization ensures that they actively aim for de-escalation of their projects. Hence, the second hypothesis reads as follows.

H2: *Authentic leadership is positively related to the perception of escalation prevention potential of organizations.*

2.3.1. *Employee involvement*

Escalation of commitment is more likely if there is a strong divide between organizational members who are involved in the innovation project and those who are not. If only a small fraction of the organization is engaged in a project, while the rest of the people in the organization remain rather distant, self-justification, self-presentation, and agency problems will lead to escalation of commitment more easily compared to projects in which more organization members are involved and feel responsible for its success. In that regard, it can be expected that organizations in which projects are carried out and managed by a small group of participants leads to neglect among the majority of the organizations or even exit among those who dislike the project altogether (Farrell, 1983). While projects that are managed in such a way can be more efficient, they are less effective if they lead to escalation of commitment.

Creating a voice within an organization increases its de-escalation potential. Expanding the project and involving more organization members (for example, starting with those who are affected most by the innovation) has the potential to turn neglect into voice and loyalty through increased efficacy (Withey and Cooper, 1989). Obviously, in many instances, voice may be seen as a pain and part of the complaints about projects results from a resistance to change instead of constructive comments and critical reflection (Oreg, 2003). However, if employees are not consulted in the innovation process, there will still be resistance to change, but it is simply not heard (and can therefore be neglected by the leaders of the project). Employee involvement itself can even be a means of taking away a lot of the resistance among employees. Thus, it can lead to more loyalty to the project, at least compared to the situation in which employees do not have the feeling that their opinions matter. Management techniques like Total Quality Management, for example, heavily rely on employee involvement (Lawler, 1994).

As is the case with authentic leadership, employee involvement means that projects get criticized, providing a strong counterbalance to self-justification and self-presentation forces. Agency problems are reduced because those leading the project are less able to only work on their own behalf since they need to incorporate the needs and interests of other members of the organization as well. Finally, employee involvement contributes to the outcome of the project. Provided that the success of many projects depends on whether employees apply certain techniques, taking their opinions into account at an early stage ensures that projects are legitimized. Given these considerations, it is hypothesized that employee involvement is an important precondition of an organization's de-escalation potential.

H3: *Employee involvement is positively related to the perception of escalation prevention potential of organizations.*

2.3.2. *Support staff quality*

Information processing and quality of decision-making are means to prevent escalation of commitment. Support staff plays a crucial role in facilitating the users of new technologies (Blank and Valdmanis, 2013; Struik *et al.*, 2014). In organizations where the human resource department manages to attract, attain, and develop necessary personnel, where the information and communication technology manages to develop and sustain well-functioning computer and software systems and where administrative processes run smoothly thanks to the administrative department, the EPP is expected to be higher than in organizations lacking such support (Ahire, 1997). A major reason for this is that each of the three components of the EPP construct suffers if the support staff is functioning sub-optimally. The required information to monitor goals and success of the project will not be delivered in time or is of inferior quality. The process will be hard to manage if the organization's own administration is not up to date. And, having a knowledgeable workforce presumes a HR department that is able to find the right people for the project (Abraham *et al.*, 1999).

Not having the right information in time undermines effective decision-making, which in turn makes projects susceptible for escalation. The information to decide to move in a different direction or to dismantle the project may simply not be available. Therefore, the EPP of organizations is expected to be higher if the support departments are capable.

H4: *Support staff quality is positively related to the perception of escalation prevention potential of organizations.*

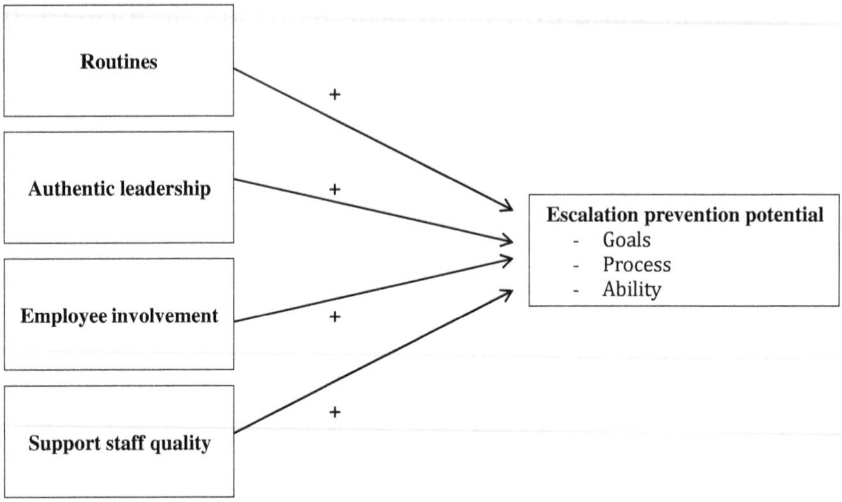

Figure 1. Content and determinants of EPP.

Figure 1 presents the conceptual model linking escalation prevention to its four hypothesized determinants.

3. Methods

3.1. *Sample and data collection*

The data for this research were collected using a questionnaire. This questionnaire enables to gather information across a large number of respondents located at different hospitals. Hence, the questionnaire intends to cover the variation in EPP as much as possible. In this study, we focus on a specific issue regarding the use of EMRs. As noted in the introduction, researchers have shown that hospitals are slow in adopting EMRs. This may result from the preferences and attitudes of the persons who have to work with the EMRs on a daily basis. Therefore, instead of focusing the survey on administrators (who are the key initiators of EMRs in hospitals), the survey was held among doctors and nurses.

An online questionnaire was sent to 2,000 doctors and 3,623 nurses who participated in the existing panels. They were asked to fill in an online questionnaire via email. The questionnaire contained items measuring the constructs of the theoretical model, questions on personal information, and basic information about their work. The nurses received an email with an invitation to fill in the same online questionnaire as the doctors. Participants were selected if they worked in hospitals where the implementation of an EMR took place at the time of data collection. The respondents could access the questionnaire via the Internet, where it was published by an external research agency. When respondents completed the questionnaire, they received a small monetary reward (the doctors received cash and the nurses received a voucher that they could spend on items or gifts through the research agency). No reminders were sent.

3.2. *Measures*

3.2.1. *Escalation prevention potential*

The three escalation prevention measures were operationalized by a series of questions about how the organization deals with projects concerning the introduction of new technologies. For each of the three sub-mechanisms, questions were asked reflecting the mechanisms defined in the theory about the EPP of organizations. All questions were measured on a 5-point Likert scale (1 = completely disagree and 5 = completely agree). For the selection procedure of these items, the factor analysis is as follows:

- **Goals** are measured with the items asking whether new information technology projects in the organization have a clearly defined aim, whether success factors are formulated and if there are measurable goals.
- **Process.** Regarding the process of new IT projects, it is asked whether such projects consist of predefined stages and whether the project is regularly evaluated.
- **Ability.** The two items measuring how new IT projects are organized ask whether responsibilities are clearly defined and whether the project participants have sufficient knowledge.

3.2.2. *Determinants of escalation prevention potential*

The four determinants of escalation prevention that were hypothesized in the theoretical model are operationalized as follows. These variables are also measured on a 5-point Likert scale.

- **Routines.** Two items are used to measure whether the organization possesses certain routines if new technology is implemented. The items reflect opinions about the following statements. *Standardized procedures* are measured by asking respondents whether a standard procedure is used when new technologies are introduced. The variable *Learning routine* is measured by asking respondents whether the organization learns from its past mistakes.
- **Authentic leadership.** Respondents are asked to score the level of authenticity of their leaders with the following 8 items: improving communication, analyzing relevant information before making a decision, providing performance feedback to individuals, acknowledging its own mistakes, taking different points of view into consideration before arriving at a conclusion, knowing when to reassess points of view and encouraging voice and support employees.
- **Employee involvement.** A scale with four items is used to measure the extent to which an organizational member can influence decisions. This scale asks respondents about the way in which a technological device was introduced. The items ask about whether respondents had a say in the process, if they were consulted about their needs to improve performance, to what extent they could voice their opinions about the new device, and whether they could make suggestions for improvement during the process.
- **Support staff quality.** Respondents are asked to rate the quality of the HR department, the IT department, and the administrative department with a set of similar items as follows:

  HR department quality — The quality of the human resource department is indicated with a scale consisting of three items about training related to the new technological device, the extent to which the HR department listens to the needs of the respondents, and whether the department has sufficient resources to provide training.

ICT department quality — Three items are used to measure the quality of support staff responsible for the functioning of information and communication technology within the organization based on the experiences with the introduction of the new technological device. Questions are asked about the adequacy of responses, whether the department has sufficient knowledge and expertise, and the departments' knowledge about adjusting the device to the needs of the respondent.

Administrative department quality — The quality of this department is assessed with three items measuring the adequacy of responses, whether the department has sufficient knowledge and expertise, and their knowledge about adjusting the device to the needs of the respondent.

The dependent variable is constructed based on our theoretical ideas. A pilot was conducted by discussing the parameters, namely five nurses and two doctors. The resulting items are the first efforts to measure EPP quantitatively. The independent variables are based on existing measures, which means that they have been validated in earlier research. Table 1 summarizes the core concepts, along with the individual items, and the sources from which they are drawn.

3.2.3. *Control variables*

To take into account that responses can be affected by background variables of the respondents, a number of control variables are added to the analysis. The control variables are *gender* (0 = male and 1 = female), *age*, *position* (0 = doctor; 1 = nurse), and *level of implementation*. The level of implementation is based on the answers of respondents on how computerized the EMR in their hospital is (or whether it is partly administrated on paper). The score is higher for respondents

Table 1. Overview of concepts and measures.

Concept	Measures	Source
Escalation prevention potential		Own measures
New IT projects in this hospital....	... have a clearly defined aim	
	... have success factors	
	... have measurable goals	
	... consist of predefined stages	
	... are regularly evaluated	
	... have clearly defined responsibilities	
	... have project participants with sufficient knowledge	
Routines		
Standardized procedures	In this hospital standard procedures are used to implements innovations	Based on Feldman (2005)
Learning routines	In this hospital people learn from past mistakes	Based on March (1991)
Authentic leadership		Cummings *et al*. (2010)
The management of this hospital...	...discusses matters to improve communication within the hospital	
	... analyzes relevant information before making a decision	
	... provides performance feedback	
	... acknowledges its own mistakes	
	... considers different opinions before drawing a conclusion	
	... reassesses points of view from time to time	

	... encourages employee voice	
	... supports employees	
Employee involvement		Sassen (2009)
	In this hospital people are encouraged to offer suggestions to improve work processes	
	My colleagues are open to suggestions to improve work processes	
	It is not a problem if attempts to improve work processes fail	
	My supervisor listens if I voice my opinion	
HR department quality		Greenhalgh *et al.* (2004)
The HR department...	... offers IT training	
	... offers need-based training	
	... has sufficient resources	
ICT department quality		Kraatz, Lyons and Tomkinson (2010)
The IT department...	... responds adequately	
	... has sufficient knowledge to make the EMR work	
	... has sufficient knowledge to adjust the EMR to my job	
Administrative department quality		Miller and Sims (2004)
The administrative department...	... responds adequately	
	... has sufficient knowledge to make the EMR work	
	... has sufficient knowledge to adjust the EMR to my job	

working with a completely computerized EMR. If the complete EMR was reported to be in one system, the score on this variable is higher and if the EMR functioned in multiple systems, the score is lower. And when the data of the nurses were visible for physicians and vice versa, the score of implementation level is higher.

3.3. *Data analysis*

3.3.1. *Factor analysis and reliability analysis*

The first part of the analysis (Kim and Mueller, 1978) aims at investigating whether the proposed conceptualization of de-EPP is corroborated by the data. To find out whether the three components of the theoretical construct (goals, process, and ability) actually form a single dimension and add up to a measurement scale, the underlying items are analyzed using factor analysis. The exploratory factor analysis revealed that seven of the nine items load on a single factor. The two items that did not load on this factor are as follows: "When a technological change is implemented many people benefit from its success" and "Stopping the process is seen as a personal letdown". These outcomes lead to the conclusion that these items do not reflect EPP as was expected. Hence, these two items are dropped from the analyses. Besides that, a factor analysis is conducted with all constructs of the theoretical model (see the ensuing sections for the outcomes). Finally, we performed a reliability analysis per scale to check for the internal consistency of the items.

3.3.2. *Regression analysis*

The second research question is which factors are associated with an organization's EPP. An ordinary least squares (OLS) regression analysis (Fox, 1991) is performed with EPP as the dependent variable and the four proposed determinants (routines, authentic leadership, employee involvement, and support staff quality) as well as the control variables as the independent variables. As mentioned above, Dutch hospitals have considerable leeway in adopting EMRs. As a result, the level of implementation of EMRs varies between hospitals. Measurement between the hospitals is likely to yield sufficient variation in regression analyses of both dependent and independent variables to be able to find associations.

4. Results

4.1. *Response and sample characteristics*

A total of 474 doctors replied and 699 nurses returned the questionnaires (response rates of 24% and 19%, respectively). Of the doctors, 72% were male and 28% were female. Around 94% of the doctors were specialists, 4.5% were residents, and 1.5% were specialist-assistants not in training. Of the respondents, 24% reported to be working in an academic hospital, 71% in a general hospital, 1% or 3% in specialized or private, respectively. The mean age of the 474 doctors in our study was 49.2 years (SD = 10.10), which corresponds with the average age of the Dutch population of male physicians (48.4 years).[1] The mean age for female physicians was a little higher in our study, namely 44.1 (SD = 8.2) compared to 40.2 in the Dutch population of female physicians (see footnote 1). In this study, more male physicians responded to the survey compared to the overall physicians' population of 2012 (national sample: 50% male and 50% female physicians; our sample: 71% male and 29% female) (see footnote 1).

---

[1]CBS StatLine — Medically qualified, employment status, position in employment, by occupation. Retrieved from http://statline.cbs.nl/StatWeb/publication/?DM=SLNLandPA=81551NEDandD1=0,2,9,14,19-20andD2=1-2andD3=1-10andD4=4,65andD5=landHDR=TandSTB=G3,G1,G4,G2andVW=T. Information retrieved from http://www.zorgatlas.nl/zorg/ziekenhuiszorg/algemene-en-academische-ziekenhuizen/aanbod/.

Of the nurses, 20% were male and 80% were female (The national average: 15% male and 85% female, see footnote 1). The mean age of the total group of nurses was 43.8 years. The mean age of the male nurses was 48.9 years (SD = 10.5). The mean age of male nurses in the Netherlands was 48.6 in 2012 (see footnote 1). The mean age of female nurses was 42.6 years (SD = 11.5), compared to 44 years in the Netherlands in 2012. A total of 17% of the nurses reported to work in an academic hospital, 22% in a top clinical hospital, 50% in a general hospital, 3% in a specialized hospital, 7% in a mental hospital, and 1% in a private hospital. In the Netherlands, eight of 85 hospitals are academic (9.4%), and 90.6% are general or specialized (see footnote 1). This means that nurses and doctors from academic hospitals are overrepresented in the sample, which is due to the fact that academic hospitals in the Netherlands precede the other hospitals in the implementation of EMRs. Due to item non-response and respondents indicating to work on paper patient files, 1,062 respondents were included in the analyses (626 nurses and 436 doctors). To investigate whether the non-response influenced the outcomes, we performed the following analyses. A marker variable was constructed for early responders and late responders. The population was split into two groups, based on the median response date (e.g., half of the population responded before that date and half of the population responded after that date). Including this variable in the regression model did not change the results and the variable itself was not significantly related to EPP. Subsequently, we tested all variables included in the regression model by comparing the mean values of the early responders and the late responders. ANOVA analysis and *t*-test showed no statistically significant results. These analyses lead to the conclusion that the time of response did not affect the outcomes.

4.2. *Factor analysis and correlations between the scales*

Table 2 presents the results of the factor analyses and reports the Cronbach's alpha of each measurement scale. The factor

Table 2. Factor analysis of the measurement scales.

	1	2	3	4	5	6
Escalation prevention potential ($\alpha = 0.88$)						
Success factors defined	**0.74**	0.17	0.08	0.10	–0.01	0.17
Clearly defined aim	**0.70**	0.29	0.16	0.07	0.10	0.09
Predefined phases	**0.70**	0.14	0.10	0.05	0.02	0.12
Clear responsibilities	**0.66**	0.30	0.17	0.17	0.23	0.07
Sufficient knowledge	**0.55**	0.26	0.14	0.35	0.31	0.11
Measurable targets	**0.60**	0.34	0.08	0.21	0.32	0.09
Regular evaluations	**0.55**	0.35	0.17	0.22	0.32	0.06
Authentic leadership ($\alpha = 0.92$)						
Improves communication	0.25	**0.69**	0.14	0.11	0.16	0.11
Analyses relevant information	0.30	**0.70**	0.15	0.07	0.20	0.09
Provides performance feedback	0.22	**0.65**	0.09	0.18	–0.07	0.12
Acknowledging own mistakes	0.11	**0.78**	0.11	0.09	0.08	0.09
Considers different opinions	0.19	**0.82**	0.18	0.08	0.16	0.10
Reassesses points of view	0.20	**0.80**	0.14	0.09	0.18	0.07
Encourages voice	0.15	**0.75**	0.13	0.14	0.07	0.11
Supports employees	0.18	**0.77**	0.12	0.12	0.09	0.11
Employee involvement ($\alpha = 0.90$)						
Suggestions about process	0.08	0.20	**0.83**	0.10	–0.06	0.08
Consulted about improvements	0.11	0.22	**0.84**	0.10	0.02	0.11
Consulted about process	0.18	0.16	**0.85**	0.11	0.08	0.05
Able to voice opinion	0.16	0.12	**0.83**	0.12	0.13	0.04
HR department quality ($\alpha = 0.90$)						
Offers IT training	0.13	0.16	0.13	**0.86**	0.07	0.13
Offers need-based training	0.20	0.20	0.15	**0.85**	0.15	0.14
Has sufficient resources	0.20	0.20	0.14	**0.82**	0.17	0.10
IT department quality ($\alpha = 0.91$)						
Adequate response	0.16	0.16	0.03	0.16	**0.75**	0.34

(*Continued*)

Table 2. (*Continued*)

	1	2	3	4	5	6
Sufficient knowledge	0.18	0.18	0.05	0.16	**0.80**	0.37
Adjustment to need	0.20	0.22	0.09	0.11	**0.77**	0.38
Administrative department quality (α = 0.93)						
Adequate response	0.15	0.18	0.12	0.15	0.25	**0.81**
Sufficient knowledge	0.17	0.16	0.08	0.14	0.33	**0.84**
Adjustment to need	0.20	0.20	0.09	0.13	0.34	**0.82**
Eigen value	2.80	11.26	2.22	1.70	1.45	0.78
Explained variance	10.00	40.22	7.92	6.06	5.19	2.79
Cronbach's alpha	0.92	0.88	0.90	0.90	0.91	0.91

Notes: $N = 1{,}062$. Method: PCA; Rotation: Varimax. Coefficients of 0.55 and higher in bold.

analysis shows that the theoretical constructs in the research model (evaluation prevention potential, authentic leadership, employee involvement, and support staff quality) refer to different measures. Looking at Table 2, all items that were included in the analyses belong to 1 particular dimension (the items measuring EPP belong together, the items measuring authentic leadership belong together, and so forth) and are not (or only weakly) related to the other dimensions. This outcome shows the strength of the measures that were validated in earlier research (such as authentic leadership and employee involvement) and that EPP forms a measurement construct that differs from these existing measures. Furthermore, Table 2 shows that these measures form reliable scales. Cronbach's alpha ranges from 0.88 for EPP to 0.93 for the scale measuring the quality of the administrative department.

Table 3 presents the descriptive statistics and the correlation coefficients of the variables. Constructs 1–8 represent the variables presented in the theoretical model. On average, the level

Table 3. Descriptive statistics.

	M	SD	1.	2.	3.	4.	5.	6.	7.	8.	9.	10.	11.
1. Escalation prevention potential	3.32	0.69											
2. Standardized procedures	3.29	0.85	0.45**										
3. Learning routines	3.28	0.94	0.57**	0.49**									
4. Authentic leadership	3.09	0.75	0.64**	0.35**	0.62**								
5. Employee involvement	2.71	1.03	0.41**	0.28**	0.34**	0.41**							
6. HR department quality	3.20	0.94	0.51**	0.34**	0.36**	0.42**	0.35**						
7. ICT department quality	3.42	0.97	0.52**	0.37**	0.44**	0.43**	0.22**	0.41**					
8. Administrative department quality	3.35	0.84	0.48**	0.35**	0.42**	0.41**	0.27**	0.39**	0.70**				
9. Job (1 = nurse)	60%	—	0.18**	0.08*	0.12**	0.11**	–0.20**	0.03**	0.27**	0.19**			
10. Gender (1 = female)	59%	—	0.11**	0.05	0.11**	0.10**	–0.13**	0.03**	0.19**	0.15**	0.51**		
11. Age	45.4	11.07	–0.08*	0.01	–0.10**	–0.08*	0.04	–0.01	–0.13**	–0.12**	–0.17**	–0.27**	
12. Level of implementation	1.74	0.80	0.13**	0.16**	0.10**	0.10**	0.02	0.10**	0.21**	0.22**	0.16**	0.07	0.02

Notes: $N = 1062$. $^{*}p < 0.01$; $^{**}p < 0.001$.

of EPP is somewhat above the theoretical mean ($m = 3.32$) and varies across hospitals (SD = 0.69). Furthermore, it is noteworthy that all means are above 3 except employee involvement. Also for these variables it holds that they vary across hospitals.

The correlation coefficients show that the dependent variable (EPP) is related to the other constructs ($r = 0.48$ or higher). Besides that, some of the independent variables are strongly related. Of the correlations between the independent variables, two may be problematically high: the quality of IT staff was 0.70 and the quality of administrative staff was 0.62 between routines and authentic leadership. To account for this, we examined whether multicollinearity is problematic using the variation inflation factor (Fox, 1991) and assessed alternative model specifications. The results of the analyses are reported in the next section.

4.3. *Analyses of the determinants of escalation prevention potential*

The factor analysis and the reliability analysis show that the three components of an organization's EPP indeed sum up to a single dimension. Next, it is investigated how the capacity to prevent escalation of commitment relates to the four determinants, while accounting for other background variables. The results are reported in Table 4.

To start with the control variables, Table 4 shows that age and tenure are not significantly related to perceptions of the EPP ($b = 0.00$). The effect of gender is positive, but not significant. The control variable "job" shows that nurses report a higher EPP to their organization than doctors do. However, it should be noted that this variable explains only 1% of the variation in EPP. The control variable level of implementation is negative but not significant.

Turning to the four factors that are hypothesized to be associated with the EPP of an organization, the following results stand out. First, the four organizational characteristics

Table 4. Regression results of EPP.

Variable	**b**	**SE**	**β**
Routines			
Standardized procedures	0.08**	0.02	0.11
Learning routines	0.09**	0.02	0.13
Authentic leadership	0.28**	0.03	0.30
Employee involvement	0.09**	0.02	0.13
Support staff quality			
HR department	0.14**	0.02	0.18
IT department	0.10**	0.02	0.14
Administrative department	0.04	0.02	0.05
Control variables			
Gender (1 = female)	–0.05	0.03	–0.03
Age	0.00	0.00	–0.01
Job (1 = nurse)	0.17**	0.04	0.12
Level of implementation	–0.01	0.02	–0.01
Constant	0.70**	0.10	
Adjusted R^2		0.57	
F		128.45**	

Notes: $N = 1062$. Dependent variable: EPP measured on a 5-point scale. Unstandardized regression coefficients and standard errors reported. Adjusted R^2 without the control variables is 0.56. $^{**}p < 0.001$.

explain 57% of the variation in an organization's EPP. All four hypotheses are supported by the regression analysis: apart from the quality of the administrative department, each of these factors is significantly associated with the EPP of the organization.

The variance inflation factor (VIF) of each variable is computed to test for multicollinearity. These results show that all VIFs are lower than 2.5, meaning that there is no reason to believe that outcomes are the result of multicollinearity between the variables. To be sure that the strong correlations did not affect the outcomes, we also conducted separate analyses for each of the variables. These additional analyses lead to the same outcomes. Finally, looking at the standardized coefficients in Table 4, authentic leadership is the main predictor of EPP ($\beta = 0.30$).

Based on these results, it is concluded that Hypotheses 1–3 are fully supported by the data and Hypothesis 4 is supported for quality of the HR and ICT department, but not for the administrative department. With regard to the latter department, Hypothesis 4 is rejected.

5. Discussion and Conclusion

5.1. *Discussion*

While the study provides insights about what EPP is and how organizations can facilitate this, it also has several restrictions that should be taken into account. Focusing on a specific innovation (the implementation of EMRs) enables comparison across healthcare organizations, but the downside is that the outcomes are restricted to specific kind of organizations. Besides that, the focus is more on developing the construct of EPP and its determinants and less on its outcomes. As a result, we do not know whether and how EPP contributes to de-escalation in organizations. Another point worth mentioning is that EPP is investigated using a questionnaire, which has strengths and also some weaknesses. One of the main weaknesses is that the answers represent the perceptions of doctors and nurses, besides the actual level of EPP. Finally, some issues could not be investigated in this study due to limited time and length of the questionnaire. Following these restrictions, a number of questions should be addressed in future studies.

First, a major question concerns the validity of EPP across other types of organizations and innovation projects. Scholars are encouraged to apply the instrument developed in this chapter in other kinds of organizations and projects. The second question is how EPP relates to actual prevention of escalation and other outcomes, like quality of the innovation and organizational performance. While some work has been done in that direction (Lambooij and Koster, 2016), additional work is needed. Third, the question is how the perceptions of EPP relate to actual EPP. Comparing objective and subjective measures would further deepen our understanding of the concept. Then, finally, there are different routes for future studies. For example, what is not touched upon here, but would require further investigation, are issues of privacy and security in IT systems like EMRs (Cremonini *et al.*, 2005; Korte and Koster, 2016). And, with regard to the factors influencing EPP, it is worthwhile to focus on solutions such as the business rules approach (Cisternino *et al.*, 2009) and how competency management influences the knowledge process within project teams (Ceravolo *et al.*, 2008). Finally, an issue that was not investigated here relates to the size of the project team. In theory, two opposing mechanisms can be at work here. While large project teams may be harder to steer and stop than small ones, it is likely that larger teams have fewer difficulties to fulfill the aspects of EPP. Smaller project teams may be more flexible, but for them it may be more difficult to have all EPP components in place. To figure out how EPP relates to the size of the project team, additional work is needed. If these points are addressed, we will know more about the use of EPP and its performance effects.

5.2. *Theoretical implications*

This study contributes to existing theories of escalation and de-escalation in five ways. First, while a large share of the literature focuses on determinants of escalation, this study examines what organizations can do to manage their EPP rather than investigating the dynamics of escalation. Second, it offers a theory-guided measure of the EPP that consists of three components and, thus, shows that it is possible to integrate these different activities and conceptualize them under the heading of a more general notion of de-escalation potential of organizations. Third, this study shows that EPP consists of different activities. While prior studies that list several of these activities do not distinguish between activities contributing to actual and the determinants enhancing the EPP (e.g., Pan and Pan, 2011), this study shows that it is worthwhile to make such a distinction. Fourth, this study included social and structural factors to investigate their relationship with the EPP of organizations. The empirical results emphasize the value of including these social contextual factors in understanding escalation and de-escalation. Fifth, this study contributes to leadership studies. Leadership research is largely concerned with the question on how certain leadership styles affect the behavior of employees. The question how an authentic leadership style can contribute to the functioning of projects is largely ignored in the literature.

Another contribution that this study offers concerns the measurement of EPP. While it was tested in a specific setting (hospitals) and focuses on a specific kind of project (IT project and more specifically the use of EMRs), the measures are formulated in general terms, meaning that it should be possible to apply them to other kinds of projects and in other kinds of organizations. The simplest way of doing that is changing the introductory text: "New IT projects in this hospital..." and formulating this in such a way that it matches the research question. Researchers are encouraged to use these measures and apply them in different organizations and investigate different kinds of projects. Doing that would say more about the value of this measure.

5.3. *Practical implications*

The outcomes of this study have practical implications for managing innovation projects. Viewing escalation studies may make someone pessimistic about the possibility to prevent escalation. Somewhere in the background of escalation research, it looks as if the main message is that projects are bound to grow beyond the control of decision-makers. What this study shows is that such forces may be managed by organizations if they follow a number of principles.

The first three principles relate to how projects are organized. Clearly defining and stating the goals of the project, dividing the project into different parts, and guaranteeing the responsibilities and capabilities of the project participants are of major concern here. Projects that do not apply these principles face the risk of failing due to escalation dynamics. Paying attention to goals, processes, and abilities simultaneously enhances the escalation-preventing potential of organizations.

Whether organizations manage to get these three components in place depends on other factors. Both the stability of the organization and the ability to learn contribute to its EPP. These conditions may therefore be necessary for managing projects and the results of this study have consequences on how organizations can deal with projects. First, it emphasizes the importance of gradually developing the ways in which projects are handled by the organization. Evaluating past projects and using these experiences in new projects guarantees a step-by-step improvement of projects. Second, there is also a strong need for ongoing criticism and even skepticism, from both the management of the organization and the employees of the organization, during the course of the projects to keep it on track. Hence, organizations should encourage and even reward self-criticism and even encourage whistle-blowing as they increase its EPP. Support staff plays an essential role here, given its ability to gather the information required for feedback.

For organizations, the challenge is how to ensure that the three components of EPP are in place. Some advice can be distilled from this research. The first thing that organizations can do is to take the measure of EPP and use it as a diagnostic tool. With every new project they are advised to ask questions like: Do our projects have clear aims? Are the responsibilities of the participant formulated clearly enough? If they can answer the questions positively, their EPP is in place. If they do not pass this EPP test, they should try to fix it. And, ultimately, if they realize that it is not possible to have a high level of EPP, they may question whether they should start a new project at all.

The beta weights in the model indicate that authentic leadership is relatively important in the EPP in organisations. Managers who implement measures that increase the EPP of their organizations have made themselves vulnerable to a certain extent since the goals of their project are clearly defined and monitored. The existence of these goals and evaluations of processes enable employees to control the performance of their management. However, it may be the best way to introduce transparency in the organization, to activate and involve all employees in an organization in realizing its organizational goals. By working according to the principles of EPP, management moves toward a model of rational management, because it acknowledges the dangers related to escalation of commitment, for instance, group thinking, readjusting goals during the project, or denying responsibilities when the project has failed. Management that has equipped their organization with more EPP acknowledges that they are part of the social system in their organization. By explicating the goals and sub-goals, a potential gap between current processes and needed processes becomes more apparent, and consequent necessary skills and resources (i.e., becomes) clearer. Then management can evaluate which ability is present in the organisation and which abilities need to be acquired to realize the goals. They are likely to be better connected to their organization and are therefore better able to successfully manage their organization. By acknowledging the social dynamics that also exist in management, they are able to enforce the rationality in their decisions during (implementation) projects. By this, they potentially de-escalate commitment and prevent excessive failure of implementation processes.

5.4. *Conclusion*

In this study, we investigate the management of new technologies. The literature on escalation of commitment provided the theoretical lens to identify important characteristics of innovation projects. Based on this literature, this study develops the concept of EPP, provides a measurement instrument, and investigates how it relates to other factors. To test these theoretical ideas, a survey was held among doctors and nurses using EMRs. The empirical results of the study are in line with the theoretical expectations. There is a single dimension of EPP and this dimension is strongly related to the four factors. The only exception is that the quality of the administrative department is not related to EPP.

References

Abraham, M., Crawford, J. and Fisher, T. (1999). Key factors predicting effectiveness of cultural change and improved productivity in implementing total quality management, *International Journal of Quality and Reliability Management*, 16(2), 112–132.

Ahire, S. J. (1997). Management science — total quality management interfaces: An integrative framework, *Interfaces*, 27(6), 91–105.

Avolio, B. J. and Gardner, W. L. (2005). Authentic leadership development: Getting to the root of positive forms of leadership, *The Leadership Quarterly*, 16(3), 315–338.

Becker, M. C. (2004). Organizational routines: A review of the literature, *Industrial and Corporate Change*, 13, 643–677.

Blank, J. L. T. and Valdmanis, V. G. (2015). Technology diffusion in hospitals: A log odds random effects regression model, *The International Journal of Health Planning and Management*, 30(3), 246–259.

Boonstra, A., Versluis, A. and Vos, J. F. (2014). Implementing electronic health records in hospitals: A systematic literature review, *BMC Health Services Research*, 14(1), 370.

Brockner, J. (1992). The escalation of commitment to a failing course of action: Toward theoretical progress, *Academy of Management Review*, 17, 39–61.

Ceravolo, P., Corallo, A. and Elia, G. (2008). Semantic web-based profiled knowledge discovery in community of practice, *International Journal of Business Process Integration and Management*, 3(4), 256–270.

Chaudoir, S. R., Dugan, A. G. and Barr, C. H. I. (2013). Measuring factors affecting implementation of health innovations: A systematic review of structural, organizational, provider, patient, and innovation level measures, *Implementation Science*, 8(1), 22.

Cisternino, V., Corallo, A., Elia, G. and Fugazza, C. (2009). Business rules for semantics-aware business modelling: Overview and open issues, *International Journal of Web Engineering and Technology*, 5(1), 104–131.

Cooper, R. B. and Zmud, R. W. (1990). Information technology implementation research: A technological diffusion approach, *Management Science*, 36, 123–139.

Cremonini, M., Damiani, E., di Vimercati, S. D. C., Corallo, A. and Elia, G. (2005). Security, privacy, and trust in mobile systems and applications, in Pagani (ed.), *Mobile and Wireless Systems Beyond 3G: Managing New Business Opportunities*, IGI Global, pp. 312–341.

Cummings, G. G., MacGregor, T., Davey, M., Lee, H., Wong, C. A., Lo, E., Muise, M. and Stafford, E. (2010). Leadership styles and outcome patterns for the nursing workforce and work environment: A systematic review, *International Journal of Nursing Studies*, 47, 363–385.

Cyert, R. M. and March, J. G. (1963). *A Behavioral Theory of the Firm*, Prentice Hall, Englewood Cliffs, NJ.

Eisenhardt, K. M. (1989). Agency theory: An assessment and review, *Academy of Management Review*, 14, 57–74.

Farrell, D. (1983). Exit, voice, loyalty, and neglect as responses to job dissatisfaction: A multidimensional scaling study, *Academy of Management Journal*, 26, 596–607.

Feldman, M. S. (2000). Organizational routines as a source of continuous change, *Organization Science*, 11, 611–629.

Fox, J. (1991). *Regression Diagnostics: An Introduction*, Sage, Newbury Park, CA.

Greenhalgh, T., Potts, H. W., Wong, G., Bark, P. and Swinglehurst, D. (2009). Tensions and paradoxes in electronic patient record research: A systematic literature review using the meta-narrative method, *Milbank Quarterly*, 87(4), 729–788.

Huselid, Huselid, M. A. (1995). The impact of human resource management practices on turnover, productivity, and corporate financial performance, *Academy of Management Journal*, 38(3), 635–672.

Katz, R. and Allen, T. J. (1985). Project performance and the locus of influence in the R&D matrix, *Academy of Management Journal*, 28(1), 67–87.

Keil, M. and Robey, D. (1999). Turning around troubled software projects: An exploratory study of the de-escalation of commitment to failing courses of action, *Journal of Management Information Systems*, 15, 63–87.

Kim, J. O. and Mueller, C. W. (1978). *Factor Analysis*, Sage, London.

Korte, M. and Koster, F. (2016). *Gebruik van een online platform. Een overzicht van de internationale literatuur.* (Using an online platform. An overview of the international literature), ICOON Paper 5, ICOON, Tilburg.

Koster, F. (2011). Able, willing, and knowing: The effects of HR practices on commitment and effort in 26 European countries, *International Journal of Human Resource Management*, 22(14), 2835–2851.

Ku, G. (2008). Learning to de-escalate: The effects of regret in escalation of commitment, *Organizational Behavior and Human Decision Processes*, 105, 221–232.

Lambooij, M. S. and Koster, F. (2016). How organizational escalation prevention potential affects success of implementation of innovations: Electronic medical records in hospitals, *Implementation Science*, 11, 75.

Lawler, E. E. (1994). Total Quality Management and employee involvement: Are they compatible? *Academy of Management Executive*, 8, 68–76.

March, J. G. (1991). Exploration and exploitation in organizational learning, *Organization Science*, 2, 71–87.

March, J. G. and Simon, H. A. (1958). *Organizations*, Wiley, New York.

Montealagre, R. and Keil, M. (2000). De-escalating information technology projects: Lessons from the Denver international airport, *MIS Quarterly*, 24, 417–447.

Nilakant, V. and Rao, H. (1994). Agency theory and uncertainty in organizations: An evaluation, *Organization Studies*, 15, 649–672.

Oreg, S. (2003). Resistance to change: Developing an individual difference measure, *Journal of Applied Psychology* 88, 680–693.

Pan, G. and Pan, S. L. (2011). Transition to IS project de-escalation: An exploration into management executives' influence behaviors, *IEEE Transactions on Engineering Management*, 58, 109–123.

Pan, G., Pan, S. L. and Newman, M. (2009). Managing information technology project escalation and deescalation: An approach-avoidance perspective, *IEEE Transactions on Engineering Management*, 56, 76–94.

Pant, I. and Baroudi, B. (2008). Project management education: The human skills imperative, *International Journal of Project Management*, 26(2), 124–128.

Pich, M. T., Loch, C. H. and De Meyer, A. (2002). On uncertainty, ambiguity, and complexity in project management, *Management Science*, 48(8), 1008–1023.

Prusak, L. (1997). *Knowledge in Organizations*, Butterworth-Heinemann, Boston.

Ross, J. and Staw, B. M. (1993). Organizational escalation and exit: Lessons from the Shoreham nuclear power plant, *Academy of Management Journal*, 36, 701–732.

Satyashankar, P., Rinkoo, A. V. and Somu, G. (2007). Management by objectives as a motivational, appraisal and effective management tool: Experience of a tertiary care teaching hospital, *Journal of Health Management*, 9(3), 459–465.

Schulz-Hardt, S., Thurow-Kröning, B. and Frey, D. (2009). Preference-based escalation: A new interpretation for the responsibility effect in escalating commitment and entrapment, *Organizational Behavior and Human Decision Making Processes*, 108, 175–186.

Shapiro, S. P. (2005). Agency theory, *Annual Review of Sociology*, 31, 263–284.

Simon, H. A. (1977). *The New Science of Management Decision*, Prentice Hall, Englewood Cliffs, NJ.

Simonson, I. and Staw, B. M. (1992). De-escalation strategies: A comparison of techniques for reducing commitment to losing courses of action, *Journal of Applied Psychology*, 77, 419–426.

Sleesman, D. J., Conlon, D. E., McNamara, G. and Miles, J. E. (2012). Cleaning up the big muddy: A meta-analytic review of the determinants of escalation of commitment, *Academy of Management Journal*, 55, 541–562.

Staw, B. M. (1976). Knee-deep in the big muddy: A study of escalating commitment to a chosen course of action, *Organizational Behavior and Human Performance*, 16, 27–44.

Struik, M. H., Koster, F., Schuit, A. J., Nugteren, R., Veldwijk, J. and Lambooij, M. S. (2014). The preferences of users of electronic medical records in hospitals: Quantifying the relative importance of barriers and facilitators of an innovation, *Implementation Science*, 9(1), 69.

Whyte, G. (1986). Escalating commitment to a course of action: A reinterpretation, *Academy of Management Review*, 11, 311–321.

Withey, M. J. and Cooper, W. H. (1989). Predicting exit, voice, loyalty, and neglect, *Administrative Science Quarterly*, 34, 521–539.

Yang, C. W. (2015). Implementing hospital innovation in Taiwan: The perspectives of institutional theory and social capital, *The International Journal of Health Planning and Management*, 30(4), 403–425.

Chapter 15

Influence of Personal Communication Networks on the Adoption of a Medical Device

Christian Barrot[*,§], Jan Kuhlmann[†,¶] and Andrea Popa[‡,‖]

[*]*Department of Management & Economics, Kühne Logistics University, Hamburg, Germany*

[†]*Institute of Innovation Research, Christian-Albrecht-University at Kiel, Germany*

[‡]*Institute for Social Medicine and Epidemiology, University Medical Center Schleswig-Holstein, Lübeck, Germany*

[§]*christian.barrot@the-klu.org*

[¶]*kuhlmann.jan@gmail.com*

[‖]*andrea.popa@uksh.de*

Abstract

Adoption processes are often heavily influenced by interpersonal communication. Marketing managers are increasingly trying to use these relationships to foster the market penetration of their products. In an empirical study of the US market for an innovative medical device, we survey the social network of (mostly chief) anesthetists from 151 hospitals. We confirm the influences from personal communication on individual adoption decisions through hazard regressions. We then use a multi-agent modeling framework trying to identify what seeding strategies would have been optimal to achieve a fast market penetration, i.e., which and how many anesthetists should be selected to initiate personal communication processes.

Keywords: Adoption, seeding, social networks, agent-based modeling, medical innovation.

1. Introduction

Adoption processes are often heavily influenced by interpersonal communication, both on a personal as well as on a professional level. Thus, any comprehensive analysis of such processes must incorporate various layers of social networks through which information can reach the targeted individual and thereby affect product awareness as well as adoption decisions. Furthermore, influences of corporate communication — such as advertising or detailing — must also be considered in a marketing context. A general assumption is that potential adopters, especially of complex and high-risk innovations, actively seek advice from trusted expert sources, who thus act as key influential or opinion leaders. The identification of such key influentials and the optimal sequence of sales calls is a major challenge for marketing managers. By doing so, managers hope to optimize their marketing spending through the activation of social contagion processes.

To address this problem, our study combines empirical data with multi-agent simulation: the first step consists of a field test in which the network relations surveyed were (mostly chief) anesthesiologists from 151 hospitals in the US who were adopters of an innovative medical device, i.e., a new-generation anesthesia workstation. Using a hazard modeling framework, we identify the influences from personal communication on individual adoption decisions. We then use this social network of adopters as the basis for multi-agent modeling framework in order to identify the optimal sequence of adoption, which would have achieved the fastest market penetration. In other words, we seek to identify which node of the anesthesiologists network sales force personnel should have been addressed (*seeded*) first to initiate personal communication processes with the maximum impact on diffusion.

The aims of this study were as follows: (1) to outline a model of personal communication influence on adoption behavior, (2) to collect and analyze an empirical personal communication network affecting an actual adoption process, and (3) to model different seeding strategies in order to optimize the speed of market penetration. We show that once an underlying structure of a social network has been identified, agent-based modeling (ABM) can be applied to simulate the impact of social contagion on the real-life market diffusion of an innovative product.

2. Literature Review

2.1. *Diffusion theory*

According to Rogers (2003), diffusion is a process in which, over time, information regarding an innovation is communicated over specific channels between members of a social system. Individuals begin adopting a product once it has been introduced into a market; this ideally continues until market saturation occurs, i.e., all potentially interested individuals have actually adopted the innovation. This process is similar to a viral contagion process in a population, which also typically follows an S-shaped pattern (Mahajan *et al.*, 1990).

Diffusion research seeks to model this contagion process as individual adoptions aggregated over an entire population in order to generate predictions regarding market success, diffusion velocity, and an innovation's market penetration (e.g., the Bass Model, Bass (1969)). Along with the viral contagion process (Mahajan *et al.*, 1990), a number of other approaches to modeling innovation diffusion exist. For example, Garber *et al.* (2004) use a *Small-World* network system approach in order to generate early predictions of innovation success, which allows for a flexible description of an underlying network connection structure. The seminal paper dealing with the diffusion of medical innovations by Coleman *et al.* (1966) documents the influence of network effects on the adoption of an innovative antibiotic in four U.S. communities in the Midwest; however, subsequent studies question the validity of the work, as it fails to account for advertising and other marketing measures (Burt, 1987; Van den Bulte and Lilien, 2001).

Gatignon and Robertson (1985) consider marketing activities as one of the main influential factors of diffusion; since the majority of marketing-mix activities are captured in the product-specific factors, i.e., price influences the relative advantage, product covers compatibility and complexity, and place reflects testability and observability, the final marketing activity, promotion or communication, must still be addressed. Interpersonal communication, on the contrary, is the direct exchange of information between two individuals. Since the initial work by Dichter (1966) and Arndt (1967), such Word-of-Mouth (WOM) has found particular attention in a marketing context (for an overview, see Hartmann *et al.*, 2008). The advent of the Internet and its opportunities for company-initiated WOM, often referred to as "viral marketing" has since led to a further extension of this research field (Hinz *et al.*, 2011; van der Lans *et al.*, 2010). One main advantage of WOM is the ability to engage in dialogue, fostering the ability to exchange information even more. Furthermore, the fact that interpersonal communication takes place among individual members of a trusted personal network increases the value of the opinions being communicated. This is particularly relevant in high-risk environments such as healthcare professions, where recommendations for drugs, therapies, or medical appliances necessitate a high level of trust. Thus, researchers frequently choose communication between physicians as setting for analysis (Iyengar *et al.*, 2011; Manchanda *et al.*, 2008; Nair *et al.*, 2010). Following the research stream initiated by Katz and Lazarsfeld (1955), we assume that the adoption process is more greatly influenced by interpersonal rather than by mass media communication.

As previously mentioned, Coleman *et al.* (1966) attempt to analyze the effects of numerous marketing-mix variables on the diffusion of an innovative drug using a descriptive empirical analysis, and criticism has been voiced regarding the study's ability to correctly verify the existence of factor impact on the network. However, the persistence of the study's uniqueness in nature is due to the difficulty of observing and collecting such network data. Because of this, the data set has been frequently reanalyzed using different methods yielding different results. To rectify this weakness, we emphasized the collection of new data catered to our research question.

2.2. *Agent-based modeling*

Once we have analyzed the underlying network structure of our sample, the key contribution of this study is to apply ABM in order to identify the path of maximum diffusion of information regarding the innovation, i.e., which anesthesiologists, had they been initially contacted, would have triggered the optimal diffusion of the innovation.

Previous empirical studies document the increasing reliance of consumers on advice from others in personal or professional networks during their purchase decision process (Hill *et al.*, 2006; Iyengar *et al.*, 2011). The increasing importance of consumer relationships in the purchasing process has led to the rise of "viral marketing" — the deliberate dispersion of initial, marketing-relevant information to consumers meant to capitalize upon WOM behavior (van der Lans *et al.*, 2010). An extension of this marketing approach is the implementation of seeding strategies: the targeting of specific members of social networks to capitalize on social contagion and ensure more rapid diffusion (Iyengar *et al.*, 2011). Seeding strategies distinguish between three types of individuals in networks: *hubs*, or individuals with a high number of connections to others, *fringes* who are poorly connected, and *bridges* that serve to connect two otherwise independent parts of the network (Hinz *et al.*, 2011). Although a number of studies, including those by Watts and Dodds (2007) and Van den Bulte and Lilien (2001), question the importance of social contagion on the rapidity of diffusion, Hinz *et al.* (2011) compare four seeding strategies in an large-scale empirical study and find that the best seeding strategies can be up to eight times more successful than others. The highest success of seeding strategies can be achieved when marketers target hubs (using high-degree seeding) or bridges (high-betweenness seeding). The results of Hinz *et al.* (2011) support the assertion by Becker (1970) that hubs are more likely to result in higher rates of diffusion due to increased activity of the hubs rather than increased persuasiveness, also in line with other studies (Iyengar *et al.*, 2011; Scott, 2000).

Because the diffusion process on the macro-level depends on the underlying network structures, we chose to apply ABM to model different adoption sequences that would be triggered by various seeding strategies. The applicability of ABM is given because of the complexity of the individual interactions between individual system members, and the reliance of the diffusion process development on the interactions of these individual members (Siebers *et al.*, 2007). Furthermore, since we are able to collect comprehensive information regarding the structure and levels of influence between individual anesthesiologists, ABM can be utilized to simulate alternative strategies and thus identify the paths which would have generated a higher rate of diffusion — an application with potentially great value to marketing managers (Garber *et al.*, 2004; Goldenberg *et al.*, 2001, 2002). In contrast to analytical and heuristic approaches to model our diffusion process, ABM offers flexibility and autonomy in the modeling of the action of individual agents based on their environment; since relatively simple relationships and ties can be programmed as behavioral rules, ABM is an effective method to model the development of a system over time (Siebers *et al.*, 2007).

3. Identification and Replication of the Underlying Social Network

The first step of our study is to empirically identify and analyze a personal communication network and to determine its influences on an actual adoption process. This will later serve as the basis for our simulation.

3.1. *Data description*

Medical specialists must always be up-to-date with the newest technological advances in order to offer the highest quality of care, which implies that the communication within this group is especially high when compared to other professions, due to the continuing education requirements fulfilled via seminars, conferences, and trade shows (Rogers, 2003). Searching for a highly innovative, B2B market within the field of medicine led us to the market for technical medical devices. According to Espicom (2011), the sales of medical devices are estimated at about US$106 billion in the US alone in 2011, making it the largest market for such devices.

The fact that the creation of innovative medical devices heavily relies on the knowledge of specialized doctors contributes to the uniqueness of the underlying communication network: because of the early involvement of doctors in the innovation process, doctors, for one, are innovators themselves since it is with their knowledge that innovative medical devices are developed in the first place; second, the early involvement implies that at least some of the doctors are highly informed about the innovation at the point of the innovations' introduction into the market, implying very early interpersonal contact, thus reducing potential adopters' uncertainty about the innovation. Fulfilling all of these demands, we chose to analyze the market for an innovative anesthesia workstation developed by one of the international leaders in the field, who cooperated with us for this study. Product-relevant advertising is limited to general presentations of the company's whole product palette at trade shows, presentations of the considered anesthesia workstation at anesthesiologist conferences, and the running of advertisements in professional anesthesiology journals. Finally, although the advantages of innovative anesthesia workstations are quite obvious, their reliability and durability are first revealed after being in use for an extended period of time. The fact that a patients' life can depend on the perfect functionality of the device raises the stakes attached to anesthesia workstations when compared to other medical devices and heightens the need of product awareness, i.e., the communication of information.

3.2. *Data collection*

The scope of collecting network data was to identify the communication structures among US anesthesiologists. By tracking who communicates with whom, and how frequently, a picture of information flow between the anesthesiologists can be derived and used to identify what influence which anesthesiologist had on the adoption timing of a respective colleague. The network structure was surveyed in the form of an ego-centered network, in line with the standard scientific practice when it is not feasible to collect information on the network as a whole (Burt, 1982; Wasserman and Faust, 1994).

The anesthesia workstation used in our study was introduced to the US market in 2001, providing us with diffusion data over a period of more than three years. We collected the data for our analysis both through secondary data from the sales information system of our collaborating partner (i.e., hospital order, dates, contact person information at each of the hospitals, the size of the hospital given by the number of operating rooms, advertising expenditures) and through primary data collection done via a written survey.

The questionnaire was designed to be short and simple and consisted of three parts. In addition to questions about the respondents' network contacts, an additional 52 items were included. The first part of the survey included personal and occupational questions and requested details about the respondents' work-related network, i.e., people with whom he or she discusses anesthesiology or related topics. Specifically, the network connections were surveyed in that the respondent was asked to name up to six persons in their network. To expand the reach of the survey, we then asked the respondent to name any known network connections between any of the contacts listed by using a matrix fill-in form. This enabled us to gather, in addition to direct connections of a specific ego, the connections existing between the alteri as well. Because of the importance of this item, we developed this section of the questionnaire with the help of US industry experts and anesthesiologists. Part two of the survey requested details about the respective hospital where the respondent was employed, and part three covered specifics about the first-time purchase of the anesthesia workstation being considered. Because the very nature of a network relies on individual persons, we can disregard any dependencies or biases that may arise from surveying the key informant (Kumar *et al.*, 1993; Marsden, 1990).

The written survey of our analysis was conducted from February to May of 2005. The survey was replicated in an online survey tool enabling respondents to return the mailed survey via post or complete it online; this was done in order to boost response rates. We offered respondents the possibility to donate US$50 to one of the anesthesiologist organizations listed on the response form, either in their name or anonymously. The questionnaires were addressed to the manufacturer's contact person at the hospital as provided in the company's sales database; we included an item asking for the questionnaire to be forwarded in case this person was not responsible for the final purchase decision. After the survey was sent, personal phone calls were made at appropriate time intervals until either a definitive decline to participate was expressed or the completed questionnaire was returned. Although the survey was conducted anonymously, respondents were required to provide the name of the hospital they worked for and their position in order to correctly place them in the network. The target market of the anesthesia workstation consisted of 141 hospitals. In our survey, we were able to gather network information directly from 48 hospitals and indirectly (through the respective ego-networks) for an additional 98 hospitals, out of which 15 were not part of the initially defined target market. For five hospitals, we could not gather any network information, as they neither responded to our survey nor were named as a contact by another hospital. As a result, a total of 151 hospitals were ultimately considered in our network. As with all survey-based network research, missing data on relevant connections could pose a severe threat to the validity of the network structure (Borgatti *et al.*, 2006). However, after extensive exploratory analysis and feedback from salespeople and selected participants, we are confident to have captured a valid representation of the communication network. In addition, previous research has shown that results from network analysis hold even if a certain number of links are missing (see, for example, Robins *et al.*, 2004).

The combination of primary and secondary data sources utilized allows us to avoid common source biases (Podsakoff *et al.*, 2003). We further reduce the risk of Common Method Bias in the data collection context by offering two ways of responding to the written survey: online and via post, and foregoing personal interviews. Furthermore, we utilize established response methods to reduce the complexity and ambiguity of the items included in the survey; endogenous and exogenous variables are alternately asked in order to avoid a context bias. A run of Harman's Single-Factor Test resulted in a 10-factor solution, thus displaying no sign of a Common Method Bias in our data collection.

Similar studies verifying the reliability of network data confirm ego and alter responses with rates between 70% and 90% (Jansen, 2006). Contact frequencies are validated with rates between 80% and 90%. The ego-centered method of collecting network data on specific relationships is considered to be valid and reliable (Marsden, 1990) so that, despite limits in further verifying the network results, the collected network data can be considered to be valid and reliable.

3.3. *Selection of variables*

The focus of our first step of analysis is to determine how the individual adoption decisions are influenced by either *corporate communication* (such as advertising in various forms) or *personal communication* (with colleagues on a professional or friendship level). As we employ a Hazard Model, we are able to consider both time-variant and time-invariant covariates in our analysis of both forms of communication.

At the heart of this study is the influence of interpersonal and network communication that we have elicited through our survey. We include such influences in two ways: the variable *network fix* is operationalized as the total penetration within the complete network of a focal hospital at the time of adoption. This variable reflects a threshold concept: depending on their individual innovativeness and risk function, hospitals would wait for a certain number of others to adopt first to ensure that the product is safe and economically viable. This reflects a time-invariant variable as *network fix* is only measured once, at the time of adoption. The personal communication covariate, *network variable*, is operationalized as time-varying. For every month and focal hospital, we aggregate the communication activity with those other contacts that have adopted within the previous six weeks. We assume that the intensity of relevant WOM is highest around the time of the actual purchasing decision. Furthermore, we extend the circle of adoption to include adoptions beyond those of first-degree contacts: An individuals' ability to influence others' adoption processes does not stop at his or her direct contacts but can reach others through intermediaries (Granovetter, 1974; Wellman, 1988). Since the flow of information rarely survives two intermediaries (Scott, 2000; Granovetter, 1974), we consider an anesthesiologists' influence of others' adoption processes up to three degrees of separation. For this variable, we use ties weighted by communication intensity (i.e., conversations per month).

In a similar way, we include corporate communication in our model. The covariate *advertising fix* measures all advertising expenditures of the firm until the month of adoption in USD. We use a carry-over function to discount earlier spending. The time-varying covariate *advertising variable* captures all monthly advertising expenditures of the firm in USD.

The remaining covariates are selected using an exploratory factor analysis to identify the main components of the sample variance. This multi-step analysis ultimately leads to the four additional covariates we include in our analysis: *source of initial information* (categorical variable with −1 = salesperson, 1 = WOM, and 0 = advertising as reference category), *conference participation* (dummy variable, 1 = participation at *American Society of Anesthesiologists Conference*), and *opinion follower* (aggregation of four items asked using a 1–7 Likert scale, high values are tied to opinion following). Finally, we consider *hospital size* (metric, measured through number of operating theaters) to serve as a proxy for a host of other characteristics including budget size and average length of the buying process, which is why it is necessary to be included. The selected set of variables was tested for multicollinearity with all of the standard diagnostics within the acceptable ranges.

3.4. *Analysis of factor influence on the adoption process*

The first part of our study seeks to identify which factors influence the timing of an individual's decision to adopt. We chose a special variant of Hazard-Rate Models for our analysis, the Accelerated Failure Time (AFT) model. This method allows for the inclusion of both time-varying and time-invariant covariates in a parametric framework.

We incorporate time-varying covariates into our model by integrating sub-episodes into our time component, i.e., the adoption process of an individual is divided into *k* non-overlapping episodes according to the time-varying covariates. The episodes of discrete covariates change with the values of the covariate; continuous covariates' episodes are divided into the smallest possible interval, estimated using a step function (Petersen, 1991). In order to estimate these episodes for each individual in our network, two new variables are introduced using LIMDEP: one is a censoring indicator, which tells whether each case is censored or a change of circumstance; the second variable indicates the number of episodes per individual, which may vary. This generated data are treated as a single observation. This episode estimation requires an adaptation of the general hazard model likelihood function:

$$\ln L = \sum_{i=1}^{t} \left(C_i \ln\left[h(t_i \mid X_i) \right] + \ln\left[S(t_i \mid X_i) \right] \right), \tag{1}$$

to a likelihood function incorporating episode splitting:

$$\ln L_i = C_i \ln\left[\alpha\lambda_k \left(\lambda_k t_k \right)^{\alpha-1} \right] - \left[\left(\left(\lambda_j t_j \right)^{\alpha} - \left(\lambda_{j-1} t_{j-1} \right)^{\alpha} \right) + \cdots + \left(\left(\lambda_k t_k \right)^{\alpha} - \left(\lambda_{k-1} t_{k-1} \right)^{\alpha} \right) \right], \tag{2}$$

where L_i is the likelihood function of individual *i*, T_k is the episode *k*, and X_k and X_j represent the manifestation of the covariates in the sub-episodes *k* or *j*.

The goodness of the model fit is tested using McFadden's Pseudo R^2 (McFadden, 1974), resulting in a seemingly poor model fit of $R^2 = 0.07$. However, running a likelihood ratio test assessing the validity of the considered covariates provided a test statistic of LR = 47.5788, meaning that despite the poor R^2, the covariates are significant in explaining the model, with $\rho < 0.005$. The results of the analysis are displayed Table 1. Note that negative signs for a coefficient correspond to shorter time to adoption (thus an acceleration of adoption), while a positive sign corresponds to a delaying effect on adoption. As can be seen, all variables with the exception of the *Advertising variable* are significant at the 10% level. Furthermore, all covariates display the anticipated influence, with the exception of conference participation.

The positive influence of an individual being an *Opinion follower* can be explained as such: the more an individual trusts the opinion and judgment of others, the longer he or she will take in adopting an innovation in order to be able to gather more information about the product. In our case, the fact that an anesthesiologist is an opinion follower lengthens his or her adoption process by ca. 16%. *Hospital size* displays the expected influence, being that the larger the hospital, the quicker

Table 1. Influences on adoption decisions (hazard model).

Covariate	**Beta**	**Wald**	**Expected sign**
Opinion follower	0.1244	0.0109	+
Conference participation	0.2158	0.0887	–
Hospital size	–0.0283	0.0000	–
Initial contact	0.2465	0.0039	+
Advertising fix	–0.1968	0.0021	–
Advertising variable	–0.0105	0.7962	–
Network fix	0.0631	0.0000	+
Network variable	–0.3626	0.0000	–
Constant	7.6193	0.0000	
α	2.6345	0.0000	

the adoption process. Greater purchasing power and better information flow between the hospital and manufacturer can accelerate the purchasing process by up to 27%.

Contrary to expectations, *Conference Participation* has a delaying effect on the adoption process of an anesthesiologist. A possible explanation for this is that a potential adopter postpones their adoption decision in order to attend a conference (only held annually) to gather more information about innovative products. This behavior would lead to a deceleration of the adoption process by up to 24% by postponing purchasing decisions until future points in time. The *Source of Initial Information* has a positive effect on the adoption process; the interpretation of this variable is twofold due to its coding: since contact with a sales representative is coded with −1, the variable is interpreted to mean that those individuals first contacted by a sales representative had a 28% shorter adoption process than those not initially contacted by a sales rep, or those whose initial source of information was advertising, coded with 0. Conversely, a personal initial contact was coded with +1 so that if the source of initial innovation information for an anesthesiologist was of personal nature, the anesthesiologist demonstrated a 28% longer adoption process than if he or she had first received information via advertising. Such an anesthesiologist would generally not partake in conferences or read professional journals, meaning that he or she would belong to a lag group of adopters.

The insignificance of the covariate *Advertising variable* is, at first, puzzling since *Advertising fix* is significant in its influence, which supports the idea that advertising accelerates the adoption process of innovations. The main reason might be more econometric: the variance of this covariate is rather low as the company applied rather steady marketing budgets. However, the expected effect of corporate communication is substantially captured through the *Advertising fix* covariate, indicating that a change in advertising pressure over the course of an innovations' diffusion process can accelerate the adoption process by 16%.

As expected, both network covariates are significant in their influence and play a more important role in an individuals' decision to adopt than advertising measures do. Concretely, the threshold effect captured by the covariate *Network fix* has the expected delaying impact on an individuals' adoption process; i.e., an individuals' communication threshold can lengthen the adoption process by 73%. Every decision of a potential adopter to collect a further opinion regarding the innovation extends the length of the adoption process by 6.5%. On the contrary, *Network variable*, capturing monthly contacts, accelerates the adoption process by 40%. This means that each additional monthly contact an individual has can shorten the time to adoption by 30%. Both variables act independent of each other.

In summary, our Hazard regression model reveals a significant and substantial accelerating effect of personal communication prior to adoption as well as a significant accelerating effect of advertising. In the second step of our study, we now apply ABM to determine how these influences hold when accounting for the underlying network structure and investigate whether there is potential to use seeding strategies to stimulate contagion processes and, thus, foster and accelerate diffusion.

4. Application of Agent-based Modeling

Even though a significant effect of personal influences on adoption decisions and timing has been found, the ability to foster this effect through marketing activities and the aggregate effects resulting from an optimized procedure remain unclear.

Firms can stimulate social contagion processes by specifically targeting influential or central actors in a network of (potential) customers. Such seeding strategies are common in both the consumer field as well as in a business context — in a way, strategies like *lead customer* programs are adapted forms of seeding in an industrial context. Alternatively, such a seeding strategy would be used to allocate the initial detailing efforts.

Two aspects are relevant for this type of approach: (1) Managers need to know who to specifically address and (2) managers need to know what the aggregate outcomes are in terms of adoption or sales curves from such strategies. Both aspects are particularly well addressed with the application of social network analysis and, especially, ABM. On the basis of such simulations, managers can make informed decision about whether or not a strategy focused on social contagion is reasonable and, if so, who to target for the initial seeding.

In previous research, ABM simulations are mostly based on generic networks that have only been defined by some network properties such as degree distributions, total number of ties, and average degree centrality. In this study, we use the empirically observed network presented in the preceding sections as our basis — exactly as it was elicited in the field. This can be easily implemented in widely used spreadsheet software programs such as Microsoft Excel: Think of a simple table structure — each column represents a time period and each row a network actor (i.e., a hospital). For each row t, a specific cell (hospital) c_{it} is then linked with each other cell cj_{t-1} for which a personal relationship in the field has been observed. This linkage follows an approach proposed by Garber *et al.* (2004) and Goldenberg *et al.* (2001).

Goldenberg *et al.* (2001) use the basic Bass diffusion model as their starting point. In the Bass model (Bass, 1969), the individual adoption probability is influenced by P, the so-called external innovation coefficient, and Q, the imitation coefficient. P incorporates all effects that stem from outside an individual's social network, i.e., influences that are independent of the behavior of others, such as advertising. On the contrary, Q incorporates all effects stemming from within the social network of an individual, i.e., influences that are dependent on the behavior of others, such as WOM communication and peer pressure or network effects, collectively referred to as *social contagion* (van den Bulte and Lilien, 2001).

Goldenberg *et al.* (2001, 2002) transfer the aggregate-level Bass model to an individual-level model, i.e., the influences of Q are disaggregated into the coefficient q^i that captures the effect of *one* direct relationship to another individual in the target market (see Goldenberg *et al.*, 2002, for details on this transformation).

The time-dependent (noncumulative) individual probability of adoption, given that the individual has not yet adopted, is based on the following binomial formula (Goldenberg *et al.*, 2002):

$$\text{prob}(t) = 1 - (1-p)\,(1-q^i)^{r(t-1)}, \tag{3}$$

where prob(t) represents the individual transition probability for an adoption in time t. For the external influences, the coefficient p is equivalent to the p value found in the Bass model, since all individuals are assumed to be exposed to external influences to a similar extent as postulated by Bass (1969). Internal influences are captured at the individual level through q_i and are directly linked to $r(t)$, the number of related individuals who have adopted the innovation up until period $(t-1)$. Thus, the individual adoption probability increases with an increasing number of adopters within the ego-network. Contrary to most other ABM studies, $r(t-1)$ is empirically observed in our study.

Each individual has the initial state $S = 0$ (non-adoption; the transition rule to the (irreversible) event state $S = 1$ (adoption) is given by

$$S(t) = \begin{cases} 1, & S(t-1) = 1 \\ 1, & U \geq prob(t), \\ 0, & U < prob(t) \end{cases} \tag{4}$$

where U represents a random number drawn from a uniform distribution in the range (0,1) and, thus, incorporates unobserved heterogeneity in the model (see Goldenberg *et al.*, 2001) for more details). By definition, the starting value $S(0)$ is 0 unless exogenous seeding is undertaken by the firm.

Since we aim to identify the applicability of different seeding strategies and their respective outcomes when compared to a base scenario, we first have to define different sets of parameter values as both p and q_i are unobserved in our data. Fortunately, diffusion literature offers very specific guidelines on what ranges potential internal and external influence vary. In their seminal meta-analysis of empirical diffusion research, Sultan *et al.* (1990) report an average value of $P_A = 0.03$ for the coefficient of innovation and $Q_A = 0.38$ for the coefficient of imitation. Following the approaches of Goldenberg *et al.* (2001, 2002) and Garber *et al.* (2004), we convert these values to our individual-level framework. This is unproblematic for the innovation coefficient, as both P and p have the same order of magnitude representing the impact of external sources on adoption probability (Goldenberg *et al.*, 2002). Thus, we use $p = 0.03$ as our base scenario and add a very low ($p = 0.01$) and very high ($p = 0.10$) scenario to test for extreme values. The conversion is more complicated for the imitation coefficient, as Q reflects the overall internal influence of the ego-network of an individual, while q^i only does so for a specific dyadic relationship to one other individual. Thus, the coefficient value needs to be converted: since Q is, conceptually, an aggregation of all individual-level influences q^i, Goldenberg *et al.* (2002) suggest that q^i is smaller than Q by a magnitude of the total market potential M:

$$Q = 1 - (1 - q^i)^M.\text{[1]} \tag{5}$$

For the average Q_A value reported by Sultan *et al.* (1990), applying this conversion to our case (with a market potential $M = 151$) leads to

[1]Note that the original Goldenberg *et al.* (2002) paper contains a typo in the conversion equation of Q to q — the closing parenthesis is placed incorrectly.

$$Q_A = 0.38 = 1-\left(1-q^{I}\right)^{151}$$
$$=> q^{I} = 0.0032. \tag{5a}$$

Again, we use this value as a base case and add a very low ($q^I = 0.001$) and very high ($q^I = 0.020$) scenario to test for possible extreme values. The lower boundary corresponds on the aggregated level to Q_A /3 and the upper boundary to Q_A *3.

Both the q^I and the p coefficient values are held constant over time for ease of interpretation. While a temporal adjustment of both values could easily be implemented, most diffusion models refrain from doing so since Bass *et al.* (1994) show that such variations would not lead to substantially improved estimation results in their *Generalized Bass Model* formulation.

In order to analyze the impact of different seeding strategies, we systematically vary the number of initial seeds. In our specific industrial context, "seeding" may be realized through a lead customer program, such as the installation of the new medical devices in a central hospital or through the specific deployment of experts holding, for example, exclusive presentations of the device at central hospitals. Because both strategies are associated with significant costs, the number of such seeds needs to be limited. Consequently, we incorporate a variation of seeds ranging from 0 in the base case to 1, 3, 5, and 10 hospitals being purposefully addressed. Note that the latter value corresponds to a threshold of 5–10% of the total market that is often reported as the upper bound for seeding strategies (see, for example, Hinz *et al.*, 2011).

To identify the best seeding points for the respective group sizes, we use the KeyPlayer software (Borgatti, 2003) add-on for the social network analysis software UCINET (Borgatti *et al.*, 2002). UCINET allows for a simple data exchange with other spreadsheet-based software such as Microsoft Excel. Based on the undirected, unweighted representation of our observed network, we ran the KeyPlayer algorithm (Borgatti *et al.*, 2006) for each of the required seeding sample sizes. The selection of optimal seeds is primarily based on centrality-based measures (for details, see the documentation by Borgatti, 2003) and is therefore in line with the recent empirical findings regarding defining characteristics of optimal seeds by Hinz *et al.* (2011).

Overall, our simulations span $3 \times 3 \times 5 = 45$ scenarios. For each of these scenarios, we ran 100 repetitions (4,500 in total) of the diffusion process in order to reach stable averages. Again, this process can efficiently be implemented in Excel.

5. Discussion of the Results

For each of the 45 scenarios, we ran simulations of diffusion processes lasting for 24 periods, which is in accordance with the experience of the manufacturer that a new medical device spreads across the major part of the market within the first 2 years.

In the first step, we assess how sensitive the simulation model is with regard to the input values of the coefficients of innovation p and imitation q^{I}. For this purpose, we compare various levels of the respective coefficient values while holding all else constant. Exemplary results are visualized in Figure 1 for external influences and in Figure 2 for external influences. A comparison of both charts reveals a somewhat surprising result.

Considering external influences, we observe a very substantial effect on the diffusion process for the three different scenarios: In the base scenario with both coefficient values set according the mean values reported by Sultan *et al.* (1990), the diffusion process would have reached 84 (out of 151) hospitals by the end of period 24. This coverage drops drastically if we set the external coefficient value to the "low external influence" scenario, i.e., we now observe only 36 adoptions (less than 24% of the simulated market). For the "high external influence scenario", the simulation runs result in a nearly complete market penetration, i.e., 141 out 151 hospitals within the first two years.

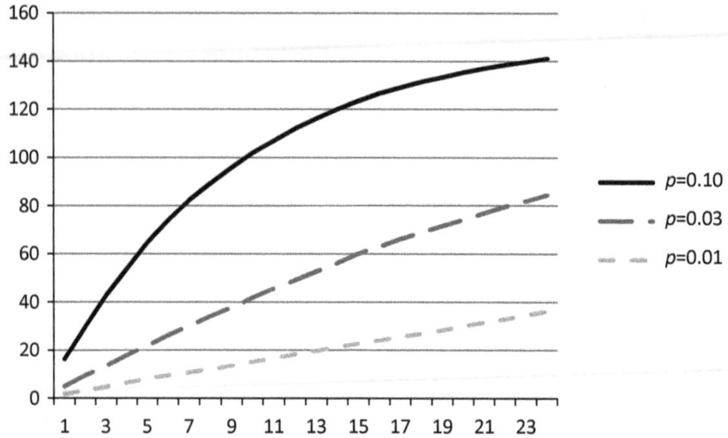

Figure 1. Effect of external influences on diffusion.
Note: Seeds held constant at 0; internal influence held constant at $q' = 0.0032$.

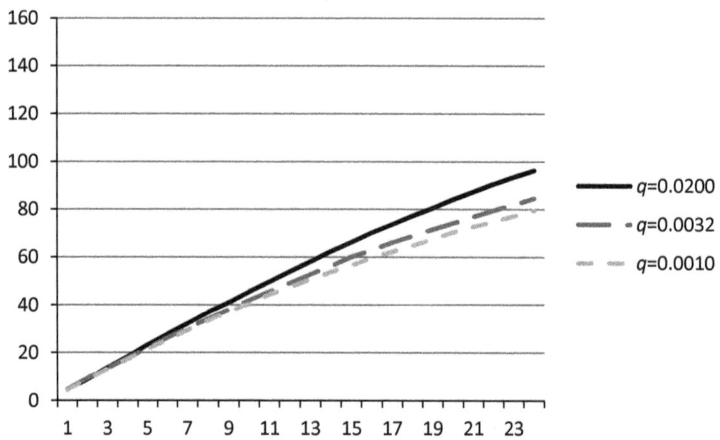

Figure 2. Effect of internal influences on diffusion.
Note: Seeds held constant at 0; external influence held constant at $p = 0.03$.

The results for the variations of the internal influences lead to a totally different result: The spread between the "high internal influence scenario" and the "low internal influence scenario" is surprisingly small: Total market penetration reaches

79, 84, and 96 for the low, base, and high scenarios, respectively. Thus, even if the input value for the internal influences is increased by a factor 20, the simulated market penetration rate would only increase by about 10 percentage points.

In the next step, we now incorporate different seeding strategies in the model. For this purpose, the identified central hubs are used as "seeds" by setting their starting values to 1, simulating an adoption prior or at launch, for example, through a lead customer program. Figure 3 reports the results of the five different seeding levels for the base case ($p = 0.03$ and $q^I = 0.0032$) as an example of the simulation.

The key result of this analysis is clearly displayed in Figure 3: Seeding is ineffective in this market. While the base scenario without seeding leads to 84 adoptions, even an initial seeding of 10 hospitals (ca. 7% of the total market) fails to increase this value higher than 91 adopting hospitals within the first two years. We observe neither an acceleration of the diffusion process nor any significant increase in adoption, results which hold across all scenarios in our simulation. In fact, the increase in

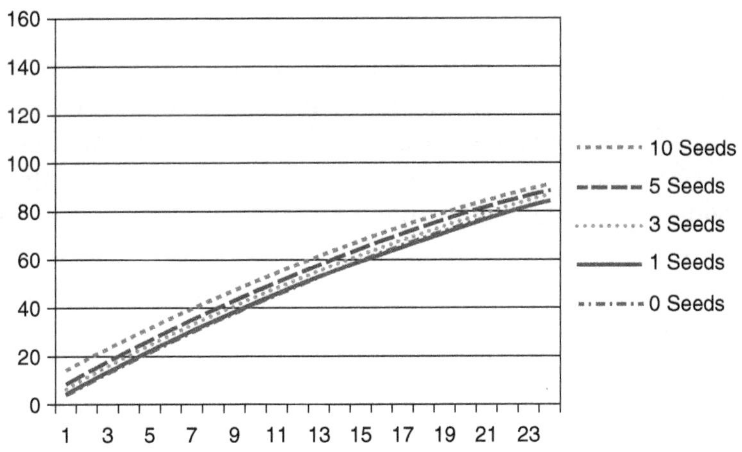

Figure 3. Effect of seeding levels on diffusion.
Note: Internal influence held constant at $q^I = 0.0032$; external influence held constant at $p = 0.03$.

terms of adoption is sometimes even smaller than the number of initial seeds — for example, by seeding to 5 hospitals the company would end up with 4 more adoptions after two years.

Thus, any hope the manufacturer placed in stimulating WOM or garnering viral marketing effects are destined to fail. At the same time, the market seems to be very responsive to variations in the external influences — a fact that could be addressed using traditional marketing instruments such as advertising.

But what are the reasons for this surprising result which seemingly contradicts our earlier findings that an individual-level (hazard) regression analysis shows significant effects of personal influence, social networks, and the like? The answer seems to lay in the observed network structure of this market for medical devices: While customers do form communication networks and certain relationships between different actors show a very strong interaction, the overall analysis of the customer base reveals a decisively different picture. First, the customer base does not consist of a single, connected network, but is fragmented into many, often very small clusters. The main component of the network contains 63 customers (41.7%), and all other customers are split between 29 other additional clusters, none of which contains more than seven nodes (five hospitals are unconnected). Similar results are revealed for the density of the network: The most central node (part of the main component, as all other well-connected hospitals) has 11 ties to other hospitals; only 14 hospitals have five or more ties, while 106 have two or less connections. The average degree centrality of 2.1 reveals a very sparsely connected network. Thus, while a viral process might be stimulated within the main component, any broader campaign is doomed to fail due to the fragmentation and low density of the network. This leaves the manufacturer with the unexpected recommendation to focus on strategies that increase the external influences that impact the complete market, overcoming the fragmented sub-networks — in this case, improvements in the diffusion process could be achieved with simply increasing traditional marketing budgets (such as advertising, symposiums, or detailing) rather than any "new" social marketing instrument.

6. Conclusions

This study has several implications for both researchers as well as marketing managers planning to employ ABM methods to real-life marketing problems.

Methodologically, we show that it is possible to use observed, real-life social networks rather than synthetic network data to analyze and optimize specific marketing problems even when using relatively simple, widely used spreadsheet software such as Microsoft Excel. This is imperative because a meaningful diffusion of this powerful simulation and analysis tool for managerial decision-making is heavily reliant on the ease with which ABM approaches can be adapted to managerial practice.

Substantially, we show that simple existence of social contagion processes detected through regression-based analysis not incorporating the actual network structure are prone to error: even if customers widely profess to be influenced by others and econometric analysis leads to significant results for social influences, the underlying network structure is the crucial element for diffusion or contagion processes. Whenever a network is too sparse or unconnected clusters too small, any intended viral or WOM marketing campaign will fail.

Our study faces certain limitations that need to be addressed in further works. We only include a single B2B market in a specific, yet economically highly relevant field. Thus, we cannot generalize our substantial findings — however, the failure of instruments aiming at viral processes in highly fragmented markets is obvious. Furthermore, the existence of similar network structures in other B2B markets seems rather likely according to feedback we have received from marketing managers targeting other industries. As in all network studies, missing values could lead to potential distortions. Given the very thorough data collection process, though, we are confident that the wide majority of ties have been captured, at least for this sample, and that the overall network structure is a valid representation of the communication network. And, finally, we do not incorporate any measures on the strength in this initial model. Since this information was gathered for our focal network, this aspect could be incorporated in further evolutions of the model. Such evolutions could also test alternative distributions with regards to modeling the unobserved heterogeneity of individual adoption thresholds.

ABM approaches are well suited to test the applicability of WOM-based marketing strategies, particularly when they use empirically observed networks as a starting point. Such simulations allow for a fast analysis of the applicability of such strategies, and, if indeed applicable, to what extent corporate seeding strategies can foster the resulting spreading process. And even if the analysis shows — such as in this study — no improvement through specific seeding strategies, these results are of significant value to the marketer: They can clearly indicate that the intended viral marketing strategies will not be successful and therefore, contrary to management's expectations, traditional marketing instruments should be upheld to penetrate the market. Even at a time when social networks, such as Facebook, prevail and seemingly "next big thing" strategies such as viral or social marketing are *en vogue* in many marketing departments, such approaches are not appropriate for every market. In particular, industrial goods markets such as the innovative medical devices market considered in our study may still best be addressed by a mixture of "old school" instruments — even if it needs newly developed methods such as ABM to come to this conclusion.

Acknowledgments

This research was supported by the *Deutsche Forschungsgemeinschaft* (*DFG*) through sponsorship of the postgraduate research program "Business Aspects of Loosely Coupled Systems and Electronic Business" at the Christian-Albrechts-University at Kiel. The authors also want to thank their industry partner that wishes to remain anonymous for their extensive support during the course of this study.

References

Arndt, J. (1967). Role of product-related conversations in the diffusion of a new product. *Journal of Marketing Research*, 4(3), 291–295.

Bass, F. M. (1969). A new product growth model for consumer durables. *Management Science*, 15(5), 215–227.

Bass, F. M., Krishnan, T. V. and Jain, D. C. (1994). Why the Bass model fits without decision variables. *Marketing Science*, 13(3), 203–223.

Becker, M. H. (1970). Sociometric location and innovativeness: Reformulation and extension of the diffusion model. *American Sociological Review*, 35(2), 267–282.

Borgatti, S. P. (2003). *KeyPlayer*. Analytic Technologies, Boston.

Borgatti, S. P., Carley, K. M. and Krackhardt, D. (2006). On the robustness of centrality measures under conditions of imperfect data. *Social Networks*, 28(2), 124–136.

Borgatti, S. P., Everett, M. G. and Freeman, L. C. (2002). *Ucinet for Windows: Software for Social Network Analysis*, Analytic Technologies, Harvard.

Burt, R. S. (1987). Social contagion and innovation: Cohesion versus structural equivalence. *American Journal of Sociology*, 92(May), 1287–1335.

Coleman, J. S., Katz, E. and Menzel, H. (1966). *Medical Innovation: A Diffusion Study*, Bobbs-Merrill, NY.

Dichter, E. (1966). How word-of-mouth advertising works, *Harvard Business Review*, 44(6), 147–166.

Espicom. (2011). *USA Medical Device Market Intelligence Report*, Espicom Business Intelligence, Princeton.

Garber, T., Goldenberg, J., Libai, B. and Muller, E. (2004). From density to destiny: Using spatial dimension of sales data for early prediction of new product success, *Marketing Science*, 23(3), 419–428.

Gatignon, H. and Robertson, T. S. (1985). A propositional inventory for new diffusion research, *Journal of Consumer Research*, 11(4), 849.

Goldenberg, J., Libai, B. and Muller, E. (2001). Talk of the network: A complex systems look at the underlying process of word-of-mouth, *Marketing Letters*, 12(3), 211–223.

Goldenberg, J., Libai, B. and Muller, E. (2002). Riding the saddle: How Cross-market communications can create a major slump in sales *Journal of Marketing*, 66(2), 1–16.

Granovetter, M. S. (1974). *Getting a Job: A Study of Contacts and Careers*, Harvard University Press, Cambridge.

Hartmann, W., Manchanda, P., Nair, H., Bothner, M., Dodds, P., Godes, D., Hosanagar, K. and Tucker, C. (2008). Modeling social interactions: Identification, empirical methods and policy implications, *Marketing Letters*, 19(3), 287–304.

Hill, S., Provost, F. and Volinsky, C. (2006). Network-based marketing: Identifying likely adopters via consumer networks, *Statistical Science*, 21(2), 256–276.

Hinz, O., Skiera, B., Barrot, C. and Becker, J. U. (2011). Seeding strategies for viral marketing: An empirical comparison. *Journal of Marketing*, 75(6), 55–71.

Iyengar, R., Van den Bulte, C. and Valente, T. W. (2011). Opinion leadership and social contagion in new product diffusion, *Marketing Science*, 30(2), 195–212.

Jansen, D. (2006). *Einführung in die Netzwerkanalyse*, 3rd edn., Leske und Budrich, Opladen.

Katz, E. and Lazarsfeld, P. F. (1955). *Personal Influence — The Part Played by People in the Flow of Mass Communications*, The Free Press, NY.

Kumar, N., Stern, L. W. and Anderson, J. C. (1993). Conducting interorganizational research using key informants, *Academy of Management Journal*, 36(6), 1633–1651.

Mahajan, V., Muller, E. and Bass, F. M. (1990). New product diffusion models in marketing: A review and directions for research, *Journal of Marketing*, 54(1), 1–26.

Manchanda, P., Ying, X. and Youn, N. (2008). The role of targeted communication and contagion in product adoption, *Marketing Science*, 27(6), 961–976.

Marsden, P. V. (1990). Network data and measurement, *Annual Review of Sociology*, 16(1), 435–463.

McFadden, D. L. (1974). Conditional logit analysis of qualitative choice behavior, in Zarembka, P. (ed.), *Frontiers in Econometrics*, Academic Press, NY, pp. 105–142.

Nair, H. S., Manchanda, P. and Bhatia, T. (2010). Asymmetric social interactions in physician prescription behavior: The role of opinion leaders, *Journal of Marketing Research (JMR)*, 47(5), 883–895.

Petersen, T. (1991). The statistical analysis of event histories, *Sociological Methods & Research*, 19(3), 270–323.

Podsakoff, P. M., MacKenzie, S. B., Lee, J.-Y. and Podsakoff, N. P. (2003). Common method biases in behavioral research: A critical review of the literature and recommended remedies, *Journal of Applied Psychology*, 88(5), 879–903.

Robins, G., Pattison, P. and Woolcock, J. (2004). Missing data in networks: Exponential random graph (p*) models for networks with non-respondents, *Social Networks*, 26(3), 257–283.

Rogers, E. M. (2003). *Diffusion of Innovations*, 5th edn., Free Press, NY.

Scott, J. P. (2000). *Social Network Analysis: A Handbook*, 2nd edn., Sage, London.

Siebers, P.-O., Aickelin, U., Celia, H. and Clegg, C. W. (2007). Using intelligent agents to understand management practices and retail productivity, in *Proceedings of the 39th Conference on Winter Simulation: 40 Years! The Best is Yet to Come*, IEEE Press, Washington DC, pp. 2212–2220.

Sultan, F., Farley, J. U. and Lehmann, D. R. (1990). A meta-analysis of applications of diffusion models, *Journal of Marketing Research*, 27(February), 70–77.

Van den Bulte, C. and Lilien, G. L. (2001). Medical innovation revisited: Social Contagion versus marketing effort, *American Journal of Sociology*, 106(5), 1409–1435.

van der Lans, R., Bruggen, G. v., Eliashberg, J. and Wierenga, B. (2010). A viral branching model for predicting the spread of electronic word of mouth, *Marketing Science*, 29(2), 348–365.

Watts, Duncan J. and Dodds, Peter S. (2007). Influentials, networks, and public opinion formation, *Journal of Consumer Research*, 34(4), 441–458.

Wellman, B. (1988). Structural analysis: From method and metaphor to theory and substance, in Wellman, B. and Berkowitz, S. D. (eds.), *Social Structures: A Network Approach*, Emerald, Cambridge, pp. 19–61.

Lightning Source UK Ltd.
Milton Keynes UK
UKHW021018311219
356158UK00001B/22/P

9 789811 204685